Interpretation and Uses
of Medical Statistics

Interpretation and Uses of Medical Statistics

Leslie E. Daly
MSc, PhD (Hon) MFPHM
Lecturer in Community Medicine
and Epidemiology,
University College, Dublin

Geoffrey J. Bourke
MA, MD, FRCPI, FFPHM, FFPHMI
Professor of Community Medicine
and Epidemiology,
University College, Dublin;
Consultant in Epidemiology and
Preventive Medicine,
St. Vincent's Hospital,
Elm Park, Dublin

James McGilvray
MA, MLitt
Professor of Economics,
University of Strathclyde

FOURTH EDITION

b

**Blackwell
Science**

© 1969, 1975, 1985, 1991 by
Blackwell Science Ltd
Editorial Offices:
Osney Mead, Oxford OX2 0EL
25 John Street, London WC1N 2BL
23 Ainslie Place, Edinburgh EH3 6AJ
238 Main Street, Cambridge
  Massachusetts 02142, USA
54 University Street, Carlton
  Victoria 3053, Australia

Other Editorial Offices:
Arnette Blackwell SA
  1, rue de Lille, 75007 Paris,
  France

Blackwell Wissenschafts-Verlag GmbH
  Kurfürstendamm 57
  10707 Berlin, Germany

  Feldgasse 13, A-1238 Wien
  Austria

First published 1969
Second edition 1975
Reprinted 1978
Third edition 1985
Fourth edition 1991
Reprinted 1992, 1995, 1996

Set by Setrite Typesetters, Hong Kong
Printed and bound in Great Britain by Hartnolls
Limited, Bodmin, Cornwall

DISTRIBUTORS

Marston Book Services Ltd
PO Box 87
Oxford OX2 0DT
(*Orders:* Tel: 01865 791155
        Fax: 01865 791927
        Telex: 837515)

North America
  Blackwell Science, Inc.
  238 Main Street,
  Cambridge, MA 02142
  (*Orders:* Tel: 800 215-1000
          617 876-7000
          Fax: 617 492-5263)

Australia
  Blackwell Science Pty Ltd
  54 University Street
  Carlton, Victoria 3053
  (*Orders:* Tel: 03 347-0300
          Fax: 03 349-3016)

British Library
Cataloguing in Publication Data

Daly, L. E.
  Interpretation and uses of medical statistics
  I. Title   II. Bourke, G. J.   III. McGilvray, J.
  610.212

ISBN 0-632-02911-0

Contents

Appendix B: Statistical Tables, 328

Appendix C: Statistical Analysis, 398

Appendix D: Sample-Size Calculations, 425

Bibliography and References, 428

Preface

The first edition of this book appeared in 1969, and was designed to introduce the basic concepts of statistics and their medical application to readers who had no formal training in statistical theory or methods. The book emphasized interpretation rather than techniques of calculation, and sought to make readers familiar with the expressions and methods commonly employed in the analysis and presentation of data in medical research. Its success demonstrated the need for such a book, and a second edition, incorporating a number of revisions and extensions, was published in 1975.

The third edition published in 1985, while retaining its basic aim of interpretation, entailed a comprehensive revision of the scope and content of the book. Taking account of the developments in the range and sophistication of statistical techniques in medical research, and the need for a greater understanding of statistics by medical undergraduates and graduates, the book included details for calculation of the common statistical tests, and chapters on research design and methodology.

This new edition greatly expands on the material covered previously. The broad structure of the book remains the same but there are a number of new sections and chapters, and some material has changed position. In line with current thinking on the analysis and presentation of medical research much more emphasis is now placed on confidence intervals. New sections have been incorporated on the analysis of counts, rates and comparative risk measures and on data transformations, and exact confidence interval tables for the binomial and Poisson distributions have been included. The sections on life table analysis have also been expanded and include computations for the logrank test and associated measures.

An entire chapter is now devoted to an explanation of the analysis of variance, a technique that many have difficulty with. A new chapter (incorporating some material from the previous edition) considers the whole area of multivariate analysis and the control of confounding, with detailed discussion relating to the interpretation of such analyses. Computational details are given for the Mantel−Haenzel methods for the analysis of a series of 2 × 2 tables. The chapters on vital statistics and computing have also undergone major revisions.

The choice of material for this new edition was determined on the basis of statistical techniques currently being used in the analysis of medical research. The book now covers over 95% of the statistical methods used in papers from a general medical journal according to a survey of a few years ago (Emerson & Colditz, 1983). Derivations of formulae are avoided in general but instead their logic is explained. Although alternative methods are available for some of the more advanced techniques discussed, we decided that confusion is avoided if only one is presented. The approach chosen by us however should prove acceptable in most situations.

With the availability of computers to a large percentage of research workers, the necessity for statistical computation has decreased over the past number of years. On the other hand many studies profit from a 'hand analysis'. Computational details of tests are only given in this book if they are feasible with a pocket calculator. This will enable those without computer access to perform their own analyses. On the other hand, for those using more advanced methods on a computer, the book's concentration on the interpretation of results from procedures such as multiple regression should also prove useful. One problem with a computer analysis is that confidence interval estimations are generally not directly available, nor are the commonly used comparative measures of risk or the Mantel–Haenzel summary measures. The descriptions in this book will allow such calculations to be performed as an adjunct to a computer output.

Despite this expansion in content we hope that the book will continue to appeal to those who, less interested in the actual statistical calculations, seek a basic understanding of statistical concepts and their role in medicine. This book contains much more than a 'cookbook' of statistical techniques, and much less than the detailed and often difficult texts that cover advanced methods. We have tried to steer a middle course by introducing concepts slowly and carefully, by avoiding any proofs or unnecessary formulae, and yet going far enough to cover most of the important topics in what we hope is an understandable manner.

Parts of the book may be skipped over by those who want only a basic introduction to statistics or who wish to understand what they read in the journals, while enough detail is given to enable it to be used as a practical guide to data analysis. It should be suitable as a text book for a range of courses taken by medical and para-medical students at both undergraduate and postgraduate levels.

To assist the reader, a brief guide to the structure of the book is included in the following pages. Appendix C also provides an overview of the statistical methods covered in the text together with a detailed step by step description of the computational approaches. This appendix should be a useful guide to those seeking an appropriate analytical method.

We hope that this new edition of *Interpretation and Uses of Medical Statistics* will fulfil our hopes for it, and prove suitable for undergraduate students, for those who just want to find out more about medical statistics and for researchers who wish to analyse their own data.

L. D., G. J. B., J. M.

Structure of the Book

Chapter 1 introduces the reader to the different types of data, to tables, bar charts, histograms and polygons. The section on drawing histograms is somewhat technical and can be omitted without loss of continuity. The second chapter introduces the mean, median and mode together with percentile indices and the standard deviation.

Chapter 3 introduces the notion of probability and chance at a basic level and describes sampling techniques commonly employed. The normal distribution is introduced. Chapter 4 introduces the reader to estimation using confidence intervals. Methods for estimating a single mean, proportion, count and rate are described. The Student's t distribution is introduced. This chapter is a cornerstone on which much of the book is built.

Chapter 5 introduces the idea of hypothesis tests and significance levels using a simple non-mathematical approach. In Chapter 6 the general principles of significance or hypothesis tests are explained, and the concept of power is introduced. Applications in the one-sample case are described. Again the concepts in this chapter are a key to understanding the body of this work.

Chapter 7 gives a detailed description of confidence interval estimation and hypothesis tests for the comparison of two groups. Paired and independent data are considered and the material covers all the procedures commonly encountered in the medical literature. Chapter 8 considers the comparison of more than two groups and introduces the reader to the analysis of variance. Computations for a one-way analysis of variance (ANOVA) and the test for a trend in proportions are detailed, while other methods are discussed more generally. Chapter 9 covers the topic of simple regression and correlation, with computational details.

Chapter 10 of the book is concerned with research methodology and the statistical methods used in analysing epidemiological type research. Cross-sectional, prospective and retrospective (case-control) studies are described, and confidence intervals and hypothesis tests for the analysis of relative risks, odds ratios and the clinical life table are detailed. Chapter 11 devotes itself entirely to the randomized controlled trial in the evaluation of medical interventions.

Chapter 12 is perhaps the most difficult in the book. It considers the statistical control of confounding and multivariate analysis. Analysis of variance and covariance, multiple regression and logistic regression are discussed in detail from the point of view of interpreting results but details of calculations are not given. Calculations are given however for the Mantel−Haenzel analysis of a series of 2 × 2 tables.

Chapter 13 defines and discusses the most commonly used measures of mortality, fertility and morbidity, usually referred to as 'vital statistics', and explains the construction and interpretation of population life tables. Chapter 14 provides a brief review of the use of computers in medical research. The concluding Chapter 15 examines the sources of bias present in many studies and comments on relevant points. Some brief guidelines are presented for critical reading of the medical literature and the setting up of a research project.

Four appendices are included for the benefit of those who wish to perform their own analyses. Appendix A details short-cut computational methods for some of the measures discussed in the text. Appendix B contains a set of statistical tables and Appendix C outlines, in step-by-step form, the computational procedures for the statistical tests described in the book: Appendix D presents some simple sample size formulae that can be used to determine the number of subjects required for a particular study.

Descriptive Statistics: Data Presentation

1.1 Introduction

A first step in the description and analysis of statistical data is usually to present the data in the form of a table, graph or diagram. This is a convenient way of summarizing the statistics, and also serves to demonstrate to the reader the principal characteristics of the data. In effect, it presents the reader with a compact view of what would otherwise be a jumbled mass of figures. The exact form in which the data are presented will naturally depend upon the subject matter as well as upon the methods and aims of the statistical analysis. Most readers will already be familiar with the use of tables and diagrams for these purposes. It is not intended here to give a detailed account of the numerous ways in which data can be presented, but some general features of tables and diagrams will be explained.

It is important to distinguish between descriptive and inferential statistics. Descriptive statistics embody the techniques used to organize, summarize and describe data in a scientific manner. This chapter and the following one introduce the topic. The other area of statistical analysis involves generalizing from a sample of observations to a larger group and is referred to as inferential statistics. The remainder of the book is chiefly concerned with this topic.

1.2 Types of data

Suppose that one wanted to study certain characteristics in a group of medical students such as age, sex, city of birth, socio-economic group and number of brothers/sisters. Each of these characteristics may vary from person to person and is referred to as a *variable* and the values taken by these variables (e.g. 18 years of age; male; born in Dublin, etc.) are referred to as *data*. Data and the variables that give rise to them can be divided into two broad categories — qualitative and quantitative.

Qualitative data are not numerical and the values taken by a qualitative variable are usually names. For example, the variable 'sex' has the values male and female, and the variable 'city of birth' values such as London or Dublin. Socio-economic group is also, essentially, a qualitative variable although often people may talk of socio-economic group I or II. The numerical unit is not a unit of measurement however, but merely a tag or label. Qualitative variables are also called *nominal*, *categorical* or *attribute* variables. In the special case where a variable assumes two values only (e.g. alive/dead) it is called a *binary* or *dichotomous variable*. Some qualitative variables also have an intrinsic order (e.g. socio-economic group I is, in some sense, higher than or above socio-economic group II) and are referred to as *ordinal* variables.

The variables 'age' and 'number of brothers/sisters' are examples of quantitative variables. They assume numerical values which are a result of measurement. In essence, qualitative data refer to qualities and quantitative data to quantities.

A *discrete* (quantitative) variable is one whose values vary by finite specific steps. The variable 'number of brothers/sisters' takes integral values only; numbers such as 2·6 or 4·5 cannot occur. A *continuous* variable, on the other hand, can take any value. Given any two values, however close together, an intermediate value can always be found. Examples of continuous variables are 'birth weight', 'age', 'time' and 'body temperature', while examples of discrete variables are 'number of children per family', 'number of hospital admissions' or 'number of tablets in bottles of different sizes'. In practice, variables which are continuous are measured in discrete units and data may be collected accurate to the nearest kilogram (for weight) or centimetre (for height) for example. The distinction between continuous and discrete variables is important however.

1.3 Tables and bar charts

Obviously, it is necessary to have some way of presenting data other than by means of a long list of the values for each variable looked at, in each individual studied. The basic rule for displaying qualitative data is to count the number of observations in each category of the variable and present the numbers and percentages in a table. The object of a table is to organize data in a compact and readily comprehensible form. A fault which is fairly common is to attempt to show too much in a table or diagram. In general, a table should be self-explanatory without the need for over-elaborate explanations including 'keys' or notes. Examples have often been seen in which it is more difficult to interpret a table or diagram than to read the accompanying text, and this defeats the whole purpose of the presentation.

In Table 1.1 the results of a study of smoking in 2724 persons are presented. The smoking variable has three categories, non-, ex- and current smokers, and the number of persons falling into each category was counted. The table also presents the results separately for each sex. Such a table shows the relationship or association between two qualitative variables, here smoking status and sex. The figures which appear in the body of the table are referred to as the *frequencies* and

Table 1.1. Smoking status of the Irish population, based on a study of 2724 persons. O'Connor & Daly (1983) with permission

	Male		Female		Total	
	No.	%	No.	%	No.	%
Current smokers	669	(49·5%)	499	(36·4%)	1168	(42·9%)
Ex-smokers	328	(24·2%)	215	(15·7%)	543	(19·9%)
Non-smokers	356	(26·3%)	657	(47·9%)	1013	(37·2%)
	1353	(100·0%)	1371	(100·0%)	2724	(100·0%)

record the total number of observations in each group or class; the sum of the frequencies in each column makes up the *total frequency* or the total number of observations.

It will be seen that the percentage frequencies are also shown. *Percentage* or *relative* frequencies are quite often used in tables and are advantageous for comparative purposes. In the example, the percentage distributions facilitate a comparison of smoking habits between males and females. Such a table with two qualitative variables is called a *contingency table*.

Qualitative data can also be presented in a diagrammatic form such as a *bar chart* (Fig. 1.1). The categories of the variable are shown on the horizontal axis (abscissa) and the frequency, or if required the relative frequency, is measured on the vertical axis (ordinate). (Sometimes, the variable is shown on the vertical axis and the frequencies on the horizontal with the bars going across the page.) Bars are constructed to show the frequency, or relative frequency, for each class of the attribute. Usually the bars are equal in width, although this is not always the case, as will be explained later. Figure 1.1 is a simple bar chart illustrating the data relating to females in Table 1.1. The height of the bar shows the frequency of each group and gives a useful 'picture' of the distribution. When bar charts are being constructed it is important that the scale should start at zero, otherwise the heights of the bars are not proportional to the frequencies, which is the essential thing. They could then be very misleading as a source of information.

Another method for displaying qualitative data is by means of a *pie chart* or *pie diagram*. Essentially, a circle is drawn whose total area represents the total frequency. The circle is then divided into segments (like the slices of a pie) with the area of each proportional to the observed frequency in each category of the variable under examination. While the pie diagram has its uses, in most cases the pictorial representation of a qualitative variable given by the bar chart is preferred. Moreover, the bar chart is easier to construct and with slight adaptations extends to the display of quantitative data as discussed in the following section.

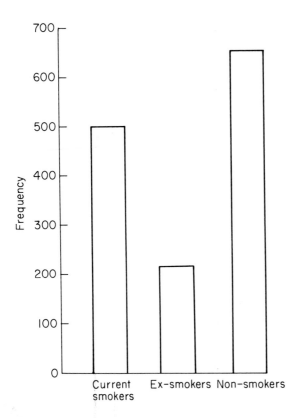

Fig. 1.1. Bar chart of data (females only) in Table 1.1. Distribution of 1371 females by smoking status.

1.4 Frequency distributions, histograms and polygons

It was explained in the previous section that the basic rule for displaying qualitative data was to count the number of observations or units in each category of the variable and to display these frequencies in a table or bar chart. The same rule can also be used for quantitative data but categories may have to be created by grouping the values of the variable.

Tables 1.2 and 1.3 show what are called the *frequency distributions* for two quantitative variables. Family size in Table 1.2 is a discrete variable and birth weight in Table 1.3 is a continuous variable. Since family size is a discrete variable and there are not too many different values, no grouping is required for the tabular presentation in Table 1.2 apart from the last category which includes all families sized seven and over. The birth weight data however, being continuous, had to be grouped for tabular presentation. Fourteen classes were created: the first is from $1 \cdot 76 - 2 \cdot 00 \, \text{kg}$, the second is $2 \cdot 01 - 2 \cdot 25 \, \text{kg}$ and so on as shown in Table 1.3. The limits for these classes ($1 \cdot 76$, $2 \cdot 00$, $2 \cdot 01$, $2 \cdot 25$, etc.) are referred to as the *tabulated class limits* and must take account of the accuracy to which the data were recorded. The birth weight data in this study were recorded to the

Table 1.2. Distribution of family size in 20 coronary heart disease patients who had at least one sibling

Family size	Frequency (numbers)
2	2
3	2
4	2
5	3
6	4
7 and over	7
Total	20

Table 1.3. Birth weight distribution of 1260 female infants at 40 weeks gestation. Original data from Hayes *et al.* (1983) with permission

Birth weight (kg)	No. of births
1·76 − 2·00	4
2·01 − 2·25	3
2·26 − 2·50	12
2·51 − 2·75	34
2·76 − 3·00	115
3·01 − 3·25	175
3·26 − 3·50	281
3·51 − 3·75	261
3·76 − 4·00	212
4·01 − 4·25	94
4·26 − 4·50	47
4·51 − 4·75	14
4·76 − 5·00	6
5·01 − 5·25	2
Total births	1260

nearest 0·01 kg. Thus, a value of 1·764 kg would have been recorded as 1·76 kg and a value of 2·008 kg would have been recorded as 2·01 kg. Values like 2·255 kg would have been recorded as 2·26 or 2·25 kg according to the judgement of the person taking the measurements. (The sensitivity of the weighing scales would, in practice, probably not allow for a reading of exactly 2·255 anyway.) The upper tabulated limit of one class, 2·00 kg say, is just 0·01 kg (the recorded accuracy of the data) below the lower tabulated limit, 2·01 kg, of the next class. All recorded values must fit into one of the tabulated classes.

The *true class limits* on the other hand are the limits that correspond to the actual birth weights included in each class. Thus, all weights from 1·755 to 2·005 kg (ignoring weights of exactly these values) are included in the class 1·76 to 2·00 kg; weights between 2·005 and 2·255 kg are included in the class 2·01 to 2·25 kg, etc. The tabulated limits depend on the accuracy to which the data are recorded, while the true limits are those that would have been employed if it was possible to measure with exact precision. The true class limits are the more important for later applications, although it must be remembered that these depend on the tabulated limits chosen, which in turn depend on the degree of accuracy in the recorded data (see Table 1.4).

The *class interval* is the difference between the true upper class limit and the true lower class limit. Thus, the class 1·76 kg to 2·00 kg has true upper and lower limits of 2·005 and 1·755 and a class interval of 2·005 − 1·755 = 0·25 kg. In the birth weight example all the class intervals are equal.

Another important concept is the *class midpoint*, the use of which will be referred to later. This is the value of the variable midway between the true lower class limit and the true upper class limit. It can be calculated by adding together these upper and lower limits, then dividing by 2. The midpoint for the first class in Table 1.3 is, thus, (1·755 + 2·005)/2 = 1·88 kg. The midpoint for the second class is 2·13, for the third 2·38, and so on (see Table 1.4).

Usually, measurements are rounded up or down, to give a particular degree of accuracy, and the true class limits are determined as described above, midway between the upper and lower tabulated limits of two adjacent classes. In medical applications however, age is often measured as 'age last birthday'. In this case,

Table 1.4. Tabulated limits, true class limits, class intervals and class midpoints for the birth weight data (kg)

Tabulated limits	True class limits	Class interval	Class midpoint
1·76 − 2·00	1·755 − 2·005	0·25	1·88
2·01 − 2·25	2·005 − 2·255	0·25	2·13
2·26 − 2·50	2·255 − 2·505	0·25	2·38
2·51 − 2·75	2·505 − 2·755	0·25	2·63
2·76 − 3·00	2·755 − 3·005	0·25	2·88
3·01 − 3·25	3·005 − 3·255	0·25	3·13
3·26 − 3·50	3·255 − 3·505	0·25	3·38
3·51 − 3·75	3·505 − 3·755	0·25	3·63
3·76 − 4·00	3·755 − 4·005	0·25	3·88
4·01 − 4·25	4·005 − 4·255	0·25	4·13
4·26 − 4·50	4·255 − 4·505	0·25	4·38
4·51 − 4·75	4·505 − 4·755	0·25	4·63
4·76 − 5·00	4·755 − 5·005	0·25	4·88
5·01 − 5·25	5·005 − 5·255	0·25	5·13

tabulated limits of $20 - 24$ years, $25 - 29$ years, etc. correspond to true limits of $20 - 25$, $25 - 30$, etc. and class midpoints of $22\cdot5$ and $27\cdot5$ years respectively. The difference between the method for dealing with age compared to that used for most other variables often causes confusion, but it is still most important to understand how the accuracy to which data are recorded affects calculation of the true class limits and midpoints.

The notion of class intervals cannot be applied in quite the same way to discrete frequency distributions. Thus, in Table 1.2 the values 2, 3 and 4 cannot be interpreted as $1\cdot5 - 2\cdot5$, $2\cdot5 - 3\cdot5$, $3\cdot5 - 4\cdot5\dots$ The variable takes only the integral values $2\cdot0$, $3\cdot0$ and $4\cdot0$, and there are no class intervals as such.

Quantitative data can be represented diagrammatically by means of a *histogram*. A histogram is a 'bar chart' for quantitative data. Figure 1.2 shows the histogram for the birth weight data. For equal class intervals ($0\cdot25$ kg in the example) the heights of the bars correspond to the frequency in each class but, in general (see below), it is the area of the bars that is more important. With equal class intervals, the area is of course proportional to the height. The total area of all the bars is proportional to the total frequency.

The main differences between a histogram and a bar chart are that in the latter there are usually spaces between the bars (see Fig. 1.1) and the order in which the bars are drawn is irrelevant, except for the case of an ordered qualitative variable.

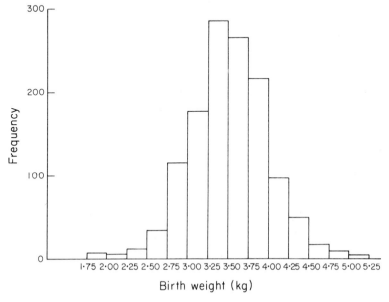

Fig. 1.2. Histogram of data in Table 1.3. Birth weight distribution of 1260 female infants at 40 weeks gestation.

The histogram gives a good picture of the shape of the distribution, showing it to rise to a peak between 3·25 and 3·50 kg and to decline thereafter. An alternative method of presenting a frequency distribution is by means of a *frequency polygon* which in Fig. 1.3 has been superimposed on the histogram of Fig. 1.2. The frequency polygon is constructed by joining the midpoints of the top of each bar by straight lines and by joining the top of the first bar to the horizontal axis at the midpoint of the empty class before it, with a similar construction for the last bar. The area under the frequency polygon is then equal to the area of the bars in the histogram. Earlier it was mentioned that the area of the bars of the histogram was proportional to the total frequency. It follows that the area enclosed by the frequency polygon is also proportional to the total frequency. Figure 1.4 shows the frequency polygon for the birth weight data with the histogram removed.

Quantitative data are sometimes presented in the form of a *composite bar chart*. In Fig. 1.5 two frequency distributions have been superimposed on the same diagram. By means of this, a visual comparison can be made between the total number of patients at each age and the mortality at 6 months in relation to age, among patients with infective endocarditis.

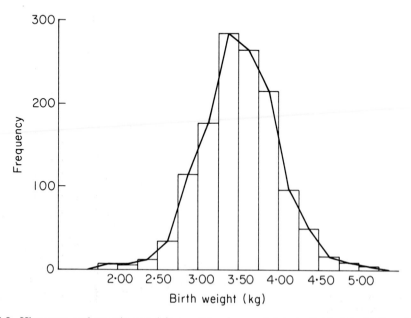

Fig. 1.3. Histogram and superimposed frequency polygon of data in Table 1.3. Birth weight distribution of 1260 female infants at 40 weeks gestation.

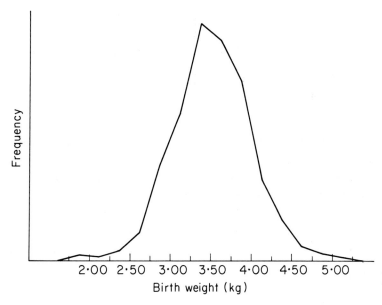

Fig. I.4. Frequency polygon. Birth weight distribution of 1260 female infants at 40 weeks gestation.

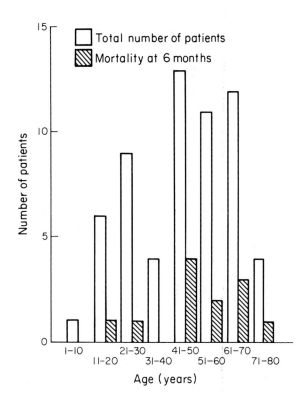

Fig. I.5. Mortality in relation to age in 60 patients with infective endocarditis. Lowes *et al.* (1980) with permission.

1.5 Drawing histograms

This section considers some of the points that must be observed when constructing frequency histograms in practice, and can be omitted at a first reading.

When preparing quantitative data for presentation, the chosen class intervals should not overlap each other and should cover the full range of the data. Depending on the total number of persons or units studied, the data should be divided into somewhere between five and twenty intervals. If too many intervals are employed the resulting histogram may have too many peaks and valleys instead of rising to a maximum and falling off as in Fig. 1.2. This is most often due to small frequencies in each class and when it occurs a larger class interval should be employed. If too few intervals or classes are used, too much information may be lost. Creating appropriate classes is often a trial and error procedure. Sometimes the number of persons or units in a study may be too small for a histogram to be drawn.

The edges of the bars in the histogram should, ideally, be drawn on the true class limits, but for presentation purposes, to give 'nice' units on the horizontal axis, the bars are sometimes shifted over slightly. This should only be done, however, if the class intervals are much larger than the accuracy to which the data were recorded. In the birth weight example the accuracy, 0·01 kg, is 4·0% of the class interval of 0·25 kg and the bars are drawn at 1·75, 2·00 ... instead of at the true class limits of 1·755, 2·005 ... These differences could not be detected by the naked eye, but in other situations the true class limits may have to be employed.

In this example too, equal class intervals of 0·25 kg were used throughout and such a practice is to be strongly encouraged. If class intervals are unequal, problems can arise in drawing the histogram correctly. Note too, that open-ended intervals such as ≥ (greater than or equal to) 4·76 kg will also lead to problems and should be avoided if possible.

Suppose, for example, that the two classes 3·76 − 4·00 and 4·01 − 4·25 were combined. From Table 1.3, the frequencies in these classes were 212 and 94 persons, so there are 306 persons in the new combined class of 3·76 − 4·25. If the histogram was drawn with the height of the bar over this class as 306, Fig. 1.6 would be obtained. Something seems very wrong here and it is due to the fact, already noted, that the *area* of each bar should be proportional to the frequency, not its height. Since the class interval for this class at 0·5 kg is twice that for the other classes, the bar should only be drawn to a height of 306 divided by 2, which equals 153. If this is done, the areas of each bar will be proportional to the frequencies in their corresponding classes and Fig. 1.7 is obtained. This is similarly shaped to the histogram obtained with equal class intervals, which shows that unequal class intervals do not distort the picture of the data. It is much easier, however, to draw histograms with equal class intervals.

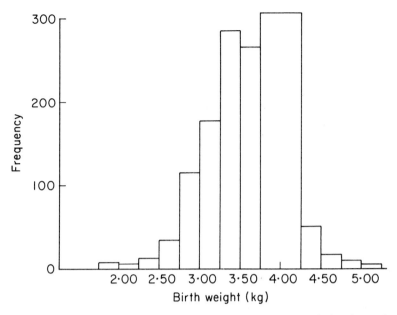

Fig. 1.6. Incorrectly drawn histogram due to non-allowance for unequal class intervals.

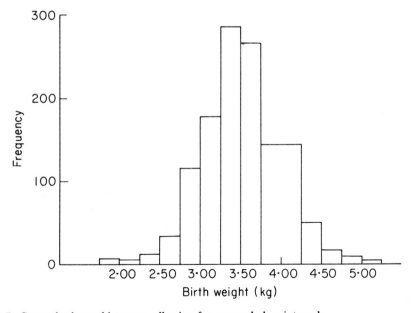

Fig. 1.7. Correctly drawn histogram allowing for unequal class intervals.

If one has a histogram — or its corresponding polygon — created from data broken into many different sized class intervals, it can be difficult to interpret the scale on the vertical axis. In fact, it is difficult to interpret the scale for any polygon without first knowing the class interval on which the original histogram was based. As has been said, it is area that is important and for this reason the frequency scale is often omitted from frequency polygons.

1.6 Frequency curves

The main importance of a frequency polygon is that it gives a picture of the shape of a variable's distribution. As is seen in later chapters, the shape of such a distribution can materially affect the type of statistical analysis that can be employed.

As opposed to a frequency polygon (made up of segments of straight lines), reference is often made to a variable's *frequency curve*. This is the frequency polygon that would be obtained if a very large number of units were studied. Suppose that 20 000 female births had been studied, instead of the 1260 in the example, and that a histogram with class intervals of 0·05 kg instead of 0·25 kg were constructed. The histogram of this distribution would, in all likelihood, be similar in shape to the earlier one and although there would be many more bars, each bar would be much narrower in width, in fact, one-fifth as wide. In the same way as before, a frequency polygon could be drawn. However, because the midpoints of each class are much closer together, the frequency polygon would approximate much more closely to a smooth curve. In appearance it might resemble Fig. 1.8.

By studying larger and larger groups, and by continually reducing the class interval, the frequency polygon will approximate more and more closely to a smooth curve. Thus, when frequency curves are mentioned it is usually the distribution of a variable based on a very large (infinite) number of observations which is being considered. In describing the shapes of distributions, frequency curves rather than polygons are often referred to.

There are three important concepts in describing the shape of a frequency distribution. The first question to ask is whether the distribution has one 'hump' or two 'humps'. Figure 1.9a shows a 'two-humped' frequency curve for a variable. The technical term for this is a *bimodal* distribution and although such distributions do occur the *unimodal* ('one-humped') distribution is much more common. In a unimodal distribution the frequency of observations rises to a maximum and then decreases again.

Unimodal distributions can be subdivided into *symmetrical* and *skewed* distributions. Symmetrical distributions can be divided into two halves by the perpendicular drawn from the peak of the distribution and each half is a mirror image of the other half. (Fig. 1.9b.)

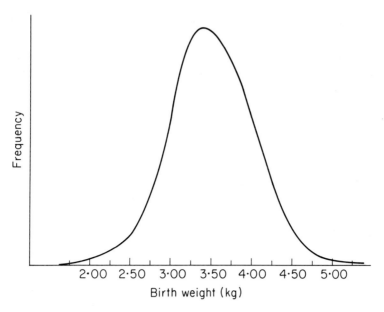

Fig. 1.8. Frequency curve for female birth weight at 40 weeks gestation.

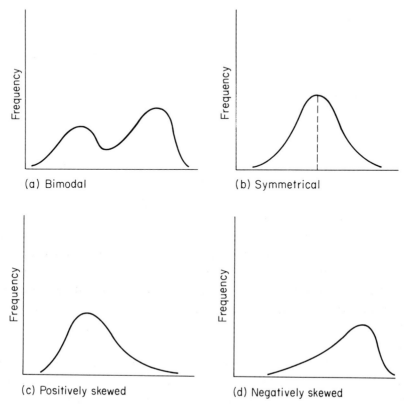

Fig. 1.9. Examples of frequency distributions.

Figures 1.9c and the 1.9d are skewed distributions. (This is a concept that really only applies to unimodal distributions.) Such asymmetrical distributions are said to be positively or negatively skewed depending upon the direction of the 'tail' of the curve. Figure 1.9c is a *positively skewed* distribution with a long tail at the upper end. Figure 1.9d is *negatively skewed*; there is a long tail at the lower end of the distribution. Since the curves shown on p. 13 are smooth continuous curves, the variable which is plotted along the horizontal scale must also be assumed to be continuous. Curves of frequency distributions may assume any particular shape, of which the four illustrated are common examples. When a distribution is positively skewed most of the observations are over to the left around the 'hump'. Some observations, however, are spread out to the right (positive direction) with no corresponding values to the left (negative direction). Often one can anticipate whether skewness is likely to be present or not, even before examining the data. One such case is the variable 'length of patient hospital stay'. Most patients will have a stay of about 5 or 6 days; there will be some lower values than this (but none lower than one day!) and perhaps a fair few higher values for those in hospital for considerable lengths of time. This essentially means that if the histogram of lengths of stay is drawn it will have a definite positive skew.

1.7 Data transformations to reduce skewness

As will be seen later it is often preferable to work with data that are symmetrical with a nice bell-shaped distribution. Data do not always behave as required, however, and often one is faced with a distribution that is quite skew. Although special techniques are available to analyse such data directly, there are advantages to performing what is called a *transformation* of the data to reduce the degree of skewness. Essentially a transformation of the data is a change of scale. Thus, instead of working with a variable like length of stay in a hospital (which as said above usually has a markedly positive skew), one might instead take the square root of each observation and perform all analysis on the transformed variable. The square root transformation will tend to reduce positive skewness and so the square root of hospital stay may be an easier scale to work with from the statistical point of view even though logically it leaves a lot to be desired. Figure 1.10 shows diagrammatically how the square root transformation tends to make the length of stay of seven patients more symmetrical than in the original scale. It is the lengths of stay of 14 and 16 days that essentially skew this distribution, and the diagram shows how the square root transformation brings these high values in the tail further back towards the left than lower value observations. The transformation thus reduces a positive skew.

There are a number of different transformations that can be applied to data to reduce the degree of skewness, and Fig. 1.11 illustrates their use. In most cases it

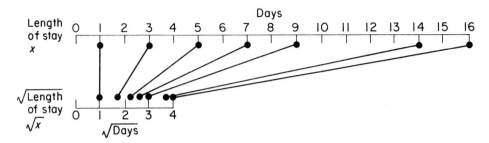

Fig. 1.10. The square root transformation applied to seven lengths of stay.

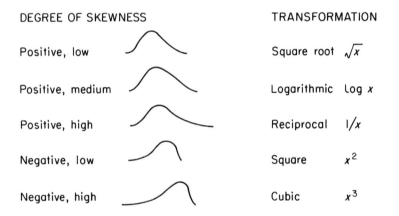

Fig. 1.11. Common transformations to reduce skewness. (x is the original observation.)

is a matter of trial and error by drawing the histograms of the transformed distributions to see which transformation works best. A very common transformation to reduce positive skewness is to take the logarithm of each value. (The log of a number is whatever power to which 10 must be raised to obtain it. The log of 100 is 2 because $10^2 = 100$. The log of any positive number can be obtained from tables or by using a pocket calculator.) If any of the observations has a value of zero or less then the log is undefined, and in this case a positive number should be added to each original value in the distribution so that all values are greater than zero. The log of these new values can then be taken.

In addition to the reduction of skewness these transformations can be used for other purposes which will be considered later (see Sections 7.4 and 9.6).

1.8 Cumulated frequency polygons

A further way of presenting quantitative data is by means of the *cumulated* (or *cumulative*) *frequency polygon* or *ogive*. In Table 1.5 the birth weight data have been rearranged by a process of successive cumulation of the frequencies in Table 1.3. Thus, four infants weigh less than or equal to 2·0 kg, seven (4 + 3) weigh less than or equal to 2·25 kg, 19 (7 + 12) weigh less than or equal to 2·5 kg, 53 (19 + 34) weigh less than or equal to 2·75 kg, and so on. These are the cumulated frequencies. The cumulated frequencies in Table 1.5 are given for values less than the upper tabulated limit for each class. This is done for convenience of presentation and the values in the first column should be more correctly given as the true upper class limits which are 0·005 kg above the tabulated limits (see discussion in last section). In Fig. 1.12 the cumulated frequencies have been plotted in the form of a cumulated frequency polygon or ogive. When the points have been plotted, successive points are joined by straight lines. In principle, the ogive can be used to estimate the number of female babies weighing less than or equal to a certain number of kilograms, by interpolation. Suppose one wanted to estimate the number of babies weighing less than or equal to 4·1 kg. By drawing a vertical line from the relevant point on the horizontal scale, noting where it meets the polygon and moving horizontally across to the vertical scale, it can be estimated that about 1133 infants weigh less than or equal to 4·1 kg (see Fig. 1.12). Obviously, it would be possible to give a mathematical formula for estimating this number but the graphical method is sufficient for most practical applications. If the original (ungrouped) measurements were available this calculation could, of course, be performed by direct counting.

Table 1.5. Cumulated frequencies for the birth weight data of Table 1.3. (The weights given should theoretically be increased by 0·005 kg — see text.)

Birth weight less than or equal to (kg)	Cumulated frequency
2·00	4
2·25	7
2·50	19
2·75	53
3·00	168
3·25	343
3·50	624
3·75	885
4·00	1097
4·25	1191
4·50	1238
4·75	1252
5·00	1258
5·25	1260

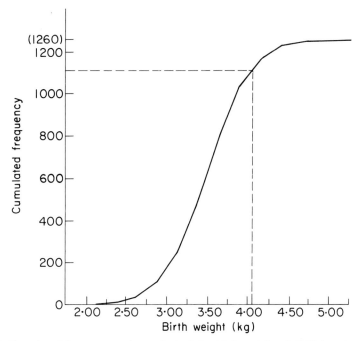

Fig. 1.12. Cumulated frequency polygon (ogive) for birth weight of 1260 female infants at 40 weeks gestation.

1.9 Graphs and scattergrams

Graphs and scattergrams are often a very effective means of presenting data and can be a considerable help to the reader. Graphs and scattergrams essentially display the relationship or association between two quantitative variables. A fault which is fairly common is to attempt to show too much material in a graph. In general, it should be self-explanatory, avoid excessive information and detail, and be self-contained in the sense that it should present the essential points without the reader having to search the text for explanations. The lines of the graph should be capable of being easily followed to observe a change in the value of the ordinate (vertical scale) for a given change in the value of the abscissa (horizontal scale). The choice of scales is of vital importance since the same material can be made to look very different by this choice. When observing graphs, the scales should be examined to determine if a *relative* or *absolute* scale has been used. This is another example of a transformation of scale. Relative scales and logarithmic scales are synonymous, and require to be interpreted with caution, otherwise they can create spurious impressions. Why use a logarithmic rather than an arithmetic scale? To understand this, the following property of a logarithmic scale may be noted: equal vertical distances on a logarithmic scale measure equal *proportionate distances*, whereas equal vertical distances on an arithmetic or absolute scale

Table 1.6. Subjects in a screening programme recorded over 4 years

Year	No. of subjects in screening programme
1980	5 000
1981	10 000
1982	20 000
1983	40 000

measure equal *absolute differences*. The use of a logarithmic scale implies that what is of interest is the relationship between one characteristic and proportionate changes in another. As a further illustration of this point consider the example in Table 1.6.

The absolute change in the number of subjects in the screening programme increases rapidly from year to year. The proportionate change from year to year is, however, constant at 100%. If two graphs of these data are drawn, one using an arithmetic scale and the other a logarithmic scale, and the two graphs super-imposed, a marked difference in the appearance of the graphs will be seen (Fig. 1.13). Note that the log scale in Fig. 1.13 records the natural numbers corresponding to the log values on the scale, rather than the log values themselves. Comparison of the two scales in the figure also shows how the use of a log scale enables a much greater range of values to be recorded on a given size of graph. In general, logarithmic scales are used when there is interest in proportionate changes, or the *rate* of change in a variable, rather than in the absolute amount of change. There is nothing esoteric or complex about logarithmic charts, but they must be carefully interpreted. The important point to bear in mind is that a logarithmic scale measures proportionate or percentage changes in a variable.

Figure 1.14 represents another important type of diagram called a *scattergram*. Like the graph, it displays a relationship between two variables (a bivariate relationship). Typically however, graphs display how one variable may change

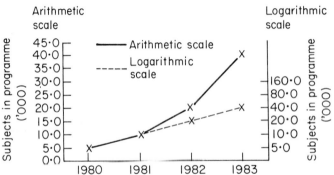

Fig. 1.13. Arithmetic and logarithmic scales.

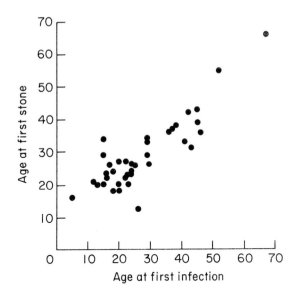

Fig. 1.14. Relationship between age at first stone and age at first infection in 38 women with two or more stone-associated urinary tract infections. Abbreviated from Parks *et al.* (1982) with permission.

over time with a line joining the corresponding points, while a scattergram is designed more to show the association, or lack of association, between two general quantitative variables. For each subject, or whatever the unit of observation might be readings are taken for each variable and a point is then plotted in relation to the two readings.

Figure 1.14 shows a scattergram relating 'age at first urinary tract infection' and 'age at development of first renal stone' among a sample of women with two or more stone-associated urinary tract infections. For example, one extreme point can be seen in the upper right-hand corner of the diagram. This point corresponds to an age, at first urinary tract infection in a female, of 68 years and an age at first renal stone which is approximately the same. On the other hand, another isolated point will be seen corresponding to an age at first urinary tract infection of about 25 years, in a female whose age at first renal stone was approximately 12 years. The spread of points on the scattergram shows an upward trend to the right. This indicates that there is an association or relationship between the two variables considered and that the older the women are at first infection, the higher the age at first kidney stone.

In Chapter 9 various techniques for measuring associations of this kind are explained.

1.10 Summary

This chapter has concentrated on the presentation of data relating to descriptive statistics. Distinctions have been made between qualitative and quantitative data and some methods for the diagrammatic presentation of these data have been outlined. The importance of the histogram, frequency polygon and cumulated frequency polygon has been stressed.

It was shown how a contingency table could display the association between two qualitative variables, and how graphs and scattergrams could perform the same task for two quantitative variables.

2
Descriptive Statistics: Summarizing Data

2.1 Introduction

In the previous chapter it was seen how a collection of quantitative data may be presented in the form of a frequency distribution, such as a histogram, which gives a useful picture of the 'shape' of the distribution. In this chapter the process of presentation and description is carried one stage further.

A variety of descriptive measures may be used to describe the same collection of data. Most readers are probably familiar with the idea of an 'average', which is used to describe the general level of magnitude of a particular variable. For example, it is common to refer to the average number of days spent in hospital by a given group of patients. There are a number of different ways in which the 'average' may be defined and measured and such measures are called *measures of central value* or *central location*. A measure of central value, as its name suggests, 'locates' the middle or centre of a collection of values; sometimes, however, as will be seen, extreme values may also be of interest. A measure of central value may be used to divide observations into two equal groups, so that it may be said, for example, half of a number of patients spent less than 7 days in hospital, and the remaining half spend 7 days or more in hospital. Other measures of location may be used to divide observations into two unequal groups.

Another type of measure frequently used in conjunction with a measure of central value is a *measure of dispersion*. The purpose of this measure will be explained more fully later in this and in subsequent chapters; suffice it to say here that it is an extremely important measure which is used to describe the dispersion or variability of values in a distribution around their central value.

2.2 Measures of central value

The most common measure of central value is the *arithmetic mean*; generally, this is what is meant by the 'average' of a collection of values. The arithmetic mean of a number of observations is calculated by adding up the values of all the observations and dividing this total by the number of observations. The purpose of the arithmetic mean is to summarize a collection of data by means of a representative value — an average value.

Table 2.1 shows the ages of 15 patients. The sum of all the ages is $4 + 5 + 5 \ldots$ which equals 139. Since there are 15 observations, the arithmetic mean is obtained by dividing 139 by 15, obtaining 9·3 years. If x represents the value of any variable measured on an individual, the mean is calculated by adding up all the xs and dividing by the number of persons studied which is denoted n. A special symbol Σ (sigma — the capital Greek 's') is used as a shorthand for 'add up all the' so that the arithmetic mean ($\bar{x}$; pronounced 'x-bar') of a variable is expressed as:

$$\bar{x} = \frac{\Sigma x}{n} . \tag{2.1}$$

In the example above, $\Sigma x = 139$, $n = 15$ and therefore $\bar{x} = 9·3$ years. Σ is also called the summation sign. When ambiguity can be avoided the term 'mean' is often employed for the arithmetic mean.

It is particularly easy to calculate the arithmetic mean from data such as those in Table 2.1. The actual age of each patient is known and it is a simple matter to add up all the individual ages and divide by 15. It has been pointed out however, that quantitative data are often presented in a frequency distribution, and the exact value the variable takes for each person is not then known, but only the class into which each person falls. Table 2.2 repeats the frequency distribution of birth weight presented in the last chapter. An estimate of the arithmetic mean birth weight can still be made by making a few assumptions.

Assume that the infants in each class all have a birth weight corresponding to the class midpoint. Thus, the four infants in the class $1·76 - 2·00$ kg are assumed

Table 2.1. Ages of 15 patients. Abbreviated from Lagos *et al.* (1980) with permission

Patient	Age (years)
1	4
2	5
3	5
4	6
5	6
6	6
7	6
8	7
9	8
10	10
11	12
12	12
13	16
14	18
15	18

Table 2.2. Birth weight distribution of 1260 female infants at 40 weeks gestation

Birth weight (kg)	Class midpoint (kg)	No. of births
1·76 − 2·00	1·88	4
2·01 − 2·25	2·13	3
2·26 − 2·50	2·38	12
2·51 − 2·75	2·63	34
2·76 − 3·00	2·88	115
3·01 − 3·25	3·13	175
3·26 − 3·50	3·38	281
3·51 − 3·75	3·63	261
3·76 − 4·00	3·88	212
4·01 − 4·25	4·13	94
4·26 − 4·50	4·38	47
4·51 − 4·75	4·63	14
4·76 − 5·00	4·88	6
5·01 − 5·25	5·13	2
Total births		1260

to have a birth weight of 1·88 kg, and the three infants in the next class are assumed to weigh 2·13 kg, and so on. Thus, the midpoint of each class is taken as being representative of all the values within that class. In doing this, it is not suggested that the four infants in the class 1·76 − 2·00 kg have an exact weight of 1·88 kg; it is suggested only that the *average* weight of these four infants will be about 1·88 kg, and since this is midway along the range of possible weights in this class it seems to be a reasonable assumption to make.

Using this approach, the mean birth weight of the 1260 infants is estimated by adding up the four assumed weights of 1·88 kg, the three weights of 2·13 kg, the 12 weights of 2·38 kg and so on, up to the final two weights of 5·13 kg. The sum of these weights is 4429·05 kg. Dividing by the total number studied, $n = 1260$, the mean birth weight of these infants is obtained as 3·52 kg. Of course, since the actual birth weight of each infant is not given this is only an estimate, but unless there is something peculiar about the distribution this estimated mean should be very close to the true mean which would have been obtained if all the actual weights were known.

The interpretation and use of the arithmetic mean requires little comment, since the concept of the 'average' is widely used and understood. The mean provides a useful summary measure for a particular collection of data, as in the example above, and it is also useful for purposes of comparison. If, for instance, it is wished to compare the ages of two groups of patients, the most convenient form of comparison is in terms of the mean ages in the two groups. Comparisons of this kind are very important in statistical analysis, and they are discussed at greater length in a subsequent chapter.

Although the arithmetic mean is the most common measure of central value, there are several other measures which are widely used. One of these is the *median*. The median is the value of that observation which, when the observations are arranged in ascending (or descending) order of magnitude, divides them into two equal sized groups. Consider the age data shown in Table 2.1. The 15 observations are already arranged in ascending order of magnitude, so the middle observation or median is the eighth one, which has the value of 7 years. This can be obtained either by counting up from the bottom until the eighth highest observation is reached, or counting down from the top until the eighth lowest observation is reached. Had the data not been in ascending order of magnitude it would have been necessary to order them.

The median can also be calculated for data where there is an even number of observations by taking the arithmetic mean of the two middle observations. The median would exceed in value not more than half the observations and be exceeded in value by not more than half the observations.*

A more complex method must be employed to calculate the median if only a frequency distribution of the variable is available. Although a mathematical formula can be derived, the easiest approach is to construct the cumulated frequency polygon for the observations. Figure 2.1 gives this for the birth weight data. (This was already presented in Fig. 1.12.) The vertical scale can be given as a percentage of all the observations (i.e. 1260 corresponds to 100%) or, as previously, in terms of the number of observations. The median is the birth weight below which half or 50% of the values lie. Given the construction of the frequency polygon this is obtained by drawing a horizontal line from the 50% point (or at 1260/2 = 630 observations)[†] to the polygon. The value where the vertical line dropped from this point meets the bottom axis gives the median of the distribution. From Fig. 2.1, the median birth weight can be estimated as 3·51 kg. Thus, half the infants have birth weights below 3·51 kg and half have birth weights above this figure. The assumption underlying this approach for estimation of the median is that observations are distributed evenly within each class. In terms of a frequency curve or polygon, a vertical line from the median divides the area under the curve in half. Fifty per cent of the area lies below the median, representing 50% of the total frequency (see Fig. 2.2).

To summarize then, the median is calculated by arranging the observations in

---

* If there are n observations, the median is the value of the $[(n + 1)/2]$th observation. If n is odd, $(n + 1)/2$ will be an integer. If n is even, $(n + 1)/2$ will involve the fraction 1/2.

[†] Note that with this approach the point on the axis corresponding to $n/2$ will define the median rather than $(n + 1)/2$ used with ungrouped data.

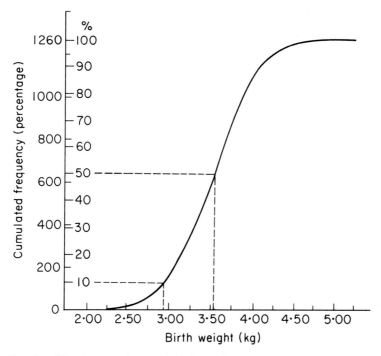

Fig. 2.1. Cumulated frequency polygon for birth weight data.

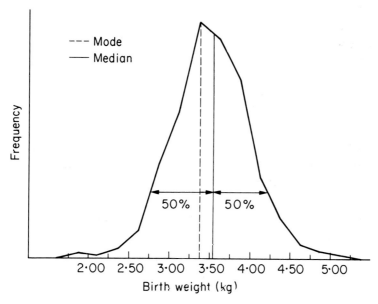

Fig. 2.2. Frequency polygon for birth weight data showing the position of the median and mode.

ascending (or descending) order of magnitude and the middle value of the series is selected as being a representative value for the variable. Thus, the median is an alternative to the arithmetic mean as a measure of the average for a given group of observations.

Although the median is quite simple to calculate and commonly used as a measure of central value, the arithmetic mean is generally preferred. The reasons for this are dealt with later, but at this stage it should be noted that, in general, the arithmetic mean and the median will be different in value. In the example of the ages of 15 patients (Table 2.1), the arithmetic mean is 9·3 years and the median is 7·0 years. In the birth weight example, the mean is 3·52 kg while the median is 3·51 kg. Whether the median is less than, greater than, or in rare cases equal to the mean depends upon the general shape and characteristics of the particular distribution concerned, a point which is discussed later in this chapter. However, for many types of distribution the mean and the median will be fairly close in value.

A third measure of central value is the *mode*. The mode may be defined as the most commonly occurring value, or as the value of the variable which occurs with the greatest frequency. Among the 15 patients in Table 2.1, four were aged 6 years. This can also be considered a representative value for these data since it occurs in 4/15 or 26·7% of the observations and is the most commonly occurring value. Six years is the modal value for this distribution.

The mode can also be calculated for data arranged in a frequency distribution. It may be remembered that in the previous chapter it was explained how a frequency distribution may be illustrated by means of a histogram or a frequency polygon. It was explained also, that as the number of observations is increased and the class intervals are reduced, the frequency polygon approximates more and more closely to a smooth unbroken curve. The point at which this curve reaches a peak represents the maximum frequency, and the value which corresponds to this maximum frequency is the mode.

In a histogram, the group into which most observations fall is the *modal group*, or more generally, the *modal class*. In the birth weight histogram the modal class is seen to be 3·26 − 3·50 kg which has a total of 281 observations (see Fig. 1.2). The value at which a frequency polygon reaches its maximum gives a single estimate of the mode, though a more precise estimate of exactly where the mode is within the modal class can be derived algebraically. In the birth weight data, the mode occurs at 3·38 kg — the midpoint of the modal class (see Fig. 2.2). In the sense that the mode is the most frequently occurring value, it may be said to be a representative or average value, and may also be used as a measure of central value like the mean or the median. The mode is usually different in value from both the mean and the median.

As a measure of central value the mode is less commonly used than either the arithmetic mean or the median. Moreover, some distributions do not have a modal value, while other distributions may have more than one such value. A 'one-humped' distribution with one mode is called unimodal while a 'two-humped' distribution is generally referred to as bimodal even if one of the 'humps' is higher than the other.

There is one further measure of central value which is sometimes used. This is the *geometric mean*. As explained, the arithmetic mean is calculated by adding up all the values in the distribution and dividing the resulting total by the number of observations. The geometric mean is calculated by adding up all the logarithm values of the variable, dividing the total by the number of observations and taking the antilogarithm of the answer. This is equivalent to taking the nth root of the product of all the observations where n is the number of observations. Thus, the geometric mean of 2, 3 and 5 is the cube root of 30 or 3·107.

This may be thought a rather peculiar method of calculating an average. However, the geometric mean is sometimes a more appropriate measure to use than the arithmetic mean, for instance in averaging ratios or for distributions which are markedly skewed. Since the geometric mean is the average of the logarithm values of a series of observations, it is also appropriate to use it in cases where data are transformed logarithmically. The geometric mean is always less than the arithmetic mean in value.

One should be careful in statistical calculations not to blindly employ techniques in situations where they may not be appropriate. One example of this is the use of the ordinary arithmetic mean when a *weighted mean* should be used. Table 2.3 shows the average length of stay observed in three wards of a hospital. It would be incorrect to calculate the overall average length of stay for all three wards by taking the mean of the three lengths of stay (9·0 + 12·0 + 20·0)/3 = 13·7 days.

The overall average length of stay should, in some manner, take account of the number of patients in each ward for which an individual length of stay was calculated. To calculate an overall representative value, each component length of stay in the average must be 'weighted' by the number of patients in the ward. The weighted average length of stay is then

Table 2.3. Average length of stay of patients in different hospital wards

Ward	No. of patients	Average length of stay (days)
A	30	9·0
B	20	12·0
C	5	20·0

$$\frac{(30 \times 9 \cdot 0) + (20 \times 12 \cdot 0) + (5 \times 20 \cdot 0)}{30 + 20 + 5} = 11 \cdot 1 \text{ days}$$

where one divides by the sum of the weights (patients). In notational form a weighted mean can be expressed by

$$\bar{x} = \frac{\Sigma wx}{\Sigma w} \tag{2.2}$$

where w represents the weights for each observation. Generally, it is incorrect to take an unweighted average of a series of means, and the approach outlined above should be used.

Four different measures of central value have now been described — the arithmetic and geometric means, the median and the mode. At this stage it may occur to the reader that the concept of an 'average' or 'central value' is not at all precise, and this is in fact the case. Each of the measures described may be claimed to be an 'average' in some sense, and yet they will generally be different in value when used to describe the same data. Yet this is less confusing than it may seem, because the same ambiguities occur when the word 'average' is used in normal conversation, even though one may be quite clear what is meant when the term is used. If, for instance, it is said that the 'average' number of children per family in Ireland is two, this does not mean that it is the precise arithmetic mean, which may be 1·8 or 2·3. What is probably meant is that two is the most commonly occurring family size — that more families have two children than have one, three or four for example. In this case, the mode is being used as the 'average' value. In contrast, if it is said that the average age of the Irish male population is 32·4 years, probably the arithmetic mean age is being referred to. Or again, if it was decided to say something about the average income of medical practitioners, the median might be preferred — this will indicate that half the doctors earn the median income or less and half earn the median income or more. In general, no hard and fast rules can be laid down about which measure to use — any one of the measures may be the most suitable in a particular instance. The mean, median and mode may be close together in value, or they may differ considerably in value; this depends upon the shape of the distribution.

In symmetrical distributions, the mean, median and mode all coincide; in asymmetrical or skewed distributions the values of these measures will generally differ. The arithmetic mean is sensitive to extreme values while the median and mode are not. For example, the mean of the following series of observations

$$4 \quad 5 \quad 5 \quad 5 \quad 5 \quad 5 \quad 75$$

is 14·9 which seems a poor representative value. The extreme value of 75 increases the mean, which uses all the observations in its calculation. The median, on the other hand, is not affected by the value of 75 and is seen to be 5. The median seems more appropriate as a central measure in this situation, although if it is necessary to take account of extreme values the mean could be used. In most practical situations, the mode is not a useful representative value. In the example above, the mode has the same value as the median (5) but many sets of data may have more than one mode (e.g. 1, 2, 2, 4, 4, 9 has modes of 2 and 4) or no mode (e.g. 1, 2, 4, 5, 9). Data with more than one mode are called *multimodal* or, as has been said, in the case of the two modes only, *bimodal*.

The example above with the extreme value of 75 is, in some sense, a very skewed distribution. If now, the mean, median and mode are examined in terms of their positions in a skewed frequency curve, what is happening can be seen more clearly. Figure 2.3 shows a positively skewed frequency distribution with some values far away from its 'centre' in the right-hand tail. The position of the mode at the peak of the distribution is easily found. Obviously, there is now a larger area to the right of the mode than to the left, so that the median, which divides the total area into halves, must be greater than the mode. Finally, the arithmetic mean is larger than either of the other measures because it is influenced by the extreme values in the upper tail of the distribution. (In a negatively skewed distribution the order of magnitude will, of course, be reversed to mean, median, mode — in alphabetical order!)

Looking at Fig. 2.3 it can be seen that in highly skewed distributions the median or mode may well be a more appropriate measure of central value than the arithmetic mean, and it has already been pointed out that the geometric mean is also a good measure for such distributions. The arithmetic mean, however, remains the most commonly used measure of central value, partly because it is very amenable to further mathematical manipulations. Whatever measure is used however, its purpose is the same — to describe or summarize a collection of data by means of an average or representative value.

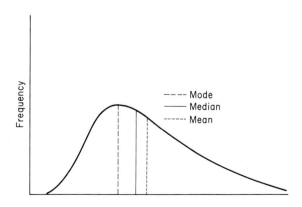

Fig. 2.3. A positively skewed distribution.

2.3 Other measures of location — quantiles

All the measures discussed so far are measures of central value; that is, they are designed to 'locate' the centre or middle of a distribution. However, it may also be of interest to locate other points in the distribution. Consider the polygon for the birth weight data shown in Fig. 2.4. The vertical lines divide up its total area in certain proportions and the values (of birth weight) at which the lines are drawn are given special names — *percentiles*. Ten per cent of the area of the polygon lies below 2·91 kg and 2·91 kg is called the 10th percentile of the distribution. (It is seen later how to actually estimate these percentiles.) Since area is proportional to frequency, this can be interpreted to mean that in the example 10% of female infants at 40 weeks gestation weigh less than (or equal to) 2·91 kg and 90% have birth weights above this figure.*

It has already been pointed out that the median divides a distribution in two halves so that 50% of infants weigh less than the median — 3·51 kg. For this reason, the median is also called the *50th percentile*. It is drawn in as the middle line in Fig. 2.4. Other percentiles are similarly interpreted. The 90th percentile of the birth weight distribution is, for instance, 4·10 kg. Ninety per cent of infants

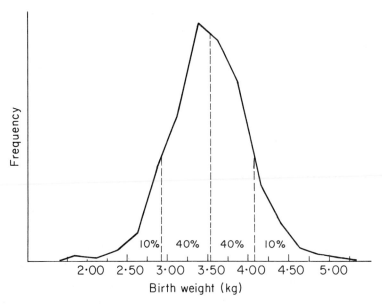

Fig. 2.4. 10th, 50th and 90th percentiles of birth weight distribution.

---

* The question of whether an individual with the exact value given by a particular percentile should be included in the upper or lower group is, for all practical purposes, immaterial in continuous distributions.

weigh less than 4·10 kg and 10% weigh more. The 90th percentile is sometimes called the 'upper 10th percentile'. Like the 50th percentile (the median), the 25th and 75th percentiles are sometimes given special names − the *lower quartile* and *upper quartile* respectively.

The percentiles divide the distribution into 100ths but sometimes it is more convenient to refer to a different set of divisions. Thus, quartiles divide the distribution into quarters, quintiles divide the distribution into fifths and deciles divide it into 10ths. For example, the third quintile is the same as the 60th percentile and the ninth decile is the 90th percentile. Note that some people refer to percentiles as plain 'centiles' and that the general term for all such divisions is *quantiles*.

Percentile values are calculated in a manner similar to that used for the calculation of the median described in the last section. The cumulated frequency polygon with the vertical scale marked in percentage terms should be used. To estimate the 10th percentile of the birth weight distribution, for instance, find the 10% point of Fig. 2.1, move horizontally across to the polygon, drop a vertical line from this intersection and read off the corresponding birth weight. It is, as already noted, approximately 2·91 kg. This graphical method is quite adequate for percentile calculations.

The measures included in the example and their interpretation should illustrate, without requiring formal definitions, the meaning and purpose of percentiles. They are used to divide a distribution into convenient groups. The median or 50th percentile locates the middle of a distribution. The other percentiles similarly locate other points or values in the distribution. All these measures are called measures of location. The median, like the mean and the mode, is a special (i.e. particularly important) measure of location and is called a measure of central value or central location. Whilst measures of central location are the most important, other measures of location assist in describing a distribution more fully. In certain circumstances, measures like the fifth and 95th percentiles may be of greater interest than the median. By using the median in conjunction with these other measures, a compact description of a distribution can be made.

The ability of percentile measures to summarize a frequency distribution is the basis of the *centile chart*. Figure 2.5 shows such a chart for the birth weight of female infants by gestational age. The chart displays the 5th, 10th, 50th, 90th and 95th percentiles of birth weight at each gestational age from 34 to 43 weeks. The chart is used to make a judgement if a newborn infant is heavier or lighter than would be expected. Suppose, for example, a female is born at 38 weeks weighing 2·9 kg. It can be seen from the chart that this weight is below the median (below 'average') but is well above the 10th percentile (about 2·68 kg) for this gestational age. Thus, the birth weight is not exceptionally unusual. On the other hand, a birth weight below the 5th percentile for a particular gestational age would

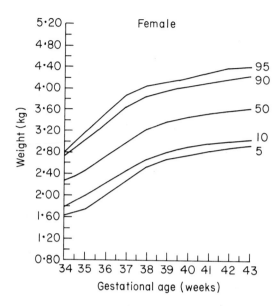

Fig. 2.5. Centile chart of birth weight for gestational age. Hayes *et al.* (1983) with permission.

suggest that an infant was much lighter than expected and would probably result in further investigation. Centile charts for height and weight by chronological age are also used to detect any growth retardation in children.

The centile chart in Fig. 2.5 was constructed by forming, for each gestational age (in completed weeks), the birth weight distribution of a large number of female infants. The percentiles of each separate distribution were then calculated and plotted on the chart.*

2.4 Measures of dispersion

When looking at a set of values or a frequency distribution it can be easily seen if the observations are widely dispersed from the measure of central value or are scattered fairly closely around it, but it may often be desirable to describe the dispersion in a single summary figure. One method of doing this is to calculate the *range* of the values, which is the difference between the highest and lowest values in the set. Although this measure may be of interest, it has the major disadvantage that it is based only on extreme values (i.e. highest and lowest) and ignores all the other values. For this reason, some further measure of dispersion is required,

---

* The birth weight distribution at 40 weeks is based on the data discussed in this text (Table 1.3). The percentile values on the chart may, however, differ slightly from those obtained from these data; this is because a statistical 'smoothing' technique was employed to 'even out' the plotted percentile lines.

which will include all the values in its calculation and which will, in addition, be amenable to further mathematical manipulation.

Table 2.4 shows two sets of data, each with the same mean of $\bar{x} = 13\cdot5$. The first set of data is far less spread out than the second, as can be seen by comparing the ranges. Concentrating on the second set of data, an intuitive approach to defining a measure of dispersion or spread might be to first see how far each individual observation is away from the (arithmetic) mean. The deviations of the four observations from the mean are

$$10\cdot0 - 13\cdot5, \quad 11\cdot0 - 13\cdot5, \quad 15\cdot0 - 13\cdot5, \quad 18\cdot0 - 13\cdot5$$

or $\qquad -3\cdot5, \qquad -2\cdot5, \qquad +1\cdot5, \qquad +4\cdot5.$

Now try taking an average of these deviations using the arithmetic mean. At this point an important property of the arithmetic mean will be noted. This is that the sum of deviations from the arithmetic mean is always zero. The minus deviations cancel out the plus deviations; a measure of variation cannot be calculated algebraically as the average of the deviations, since their sum is always zero. In calculating the dispersion of values around the arithmetic mean, however, it is immaterial whether the deviations are plus or minus; only the numerical magnitude of the deviation is of interest. Hence, to avoid getting zero when the deviations are added together, try squaring these deviations. The squared deviations are

$$(-3\cdot5)^2, \quad (-2\cdot5)^2, \quad (1\cdot5)^2, \quad (4\cdot5)^2$$

or $\qquad 12\cdot25, \qquad 6\cdot25, \qquad 2\cdot25, \qquad 20\cdot25.$

An average of these squared deviations would now appear to be a reasonable definition of variability. For reasons discussed in Section 4.6, the average value is determined by summing the squared deviations and dividing by one less than the total number of deviations. The resulting measure is called the *variance*. The sum of the squared deviation in the example is 41, so that the variance is $41/3 = 13\cdot66$.

Table 2.4. The variance and standard deviation

	12 13 14 15	10 11 15 18
Observations	12 13 14 15	10 11 15 18
Mean ($\bar{x}$)	13·5	13·5
Range	$15 - 12 = 3$	$18 - 10 = 8$
Squared deviations from the mean $(x - \bar{x})^2$	$(12\cdot0 - 13\cdot5)^2(13\cdot0 - 13\cdot5)^2$ $(14\cdot0 - 13\cdot5)^2(15\cdot0 - 13\cdot5)^2$	$(10\cdot0 - 13\cdot5)^2(11\cdot0 - 13\cdot5)^2$ $(15\cdot0 - 13\cdot5)^2(18\cdot0 - 13\cdot5)^2$
Sum of squared deviations $\Sigma(x - \bar{x})^2$	5·0	41·0
Variance $S^2 = \dfrac{\Sigma(x - \bar{x})^2}{n - 1}$	$5\cdot0/3 = 1\cdot66$	$41\cdot0/3 = 13\cdot66$
Standard deviation S	$\sqrt{1\cdot66} = 1\cdot29$	$\sqrt{13\cdot66} = 3\cdot69$

The divisor of $n - 1$ for the variance is called the *degrees of freedom* for the statistic which is a term that will be met with in a number of different contexts. The term essentially means the number of independent quantities, making up the statistic, that are free to vary. The variance in the example considered is calculated from the four original observations and their mean which of course is not independent of them. If, knowing nothing else, one was asked to guess at what the first observation might be, any value might be given. If one was asked to guess the second and third observations, again any values would suffice. However given these three guessed values, and the mean, the fourth value is predetermined. For instance if one chose the values 11, 12 and 15 the fourth value would have to be 16 since the mean must be 13.5. Thus, there are three degrees of freedom for this variance, and in general the degrees of freedom for a variance are one less than the sample size. The degrees of freedom for any statistic can usually be determined as the number of independent quantities used in the calculation of the statistic (e.g. the n individual observations), less the number of parameters in the statistic estimated from them (e.g. the sample mean).

To avoid working with 'squared' units, the square root of the variance can be taken and this is called the *standard deviation*. The square root of 13·66 is 3·69 which is the standard deviation of the four observations 10, 11, 15 and 18. The standard deviation can be defined in mathematical notation as

$$S = \sqrt{\frac{\Sigma(x - \bar{x})^2}{n - 1}} \qquad (2.3)$$

where S represents the standard deviation (S^2 is the variance), x is an individual observation, $\bar{x}$ is the arithmetic mean and n is the number of observations. The mean ($\bar{x}$) is subtracted from each observation or value (x), and the resulting deviation is squared. This is done for each of the values. Finally, the sum of the squares of the individual deviations from the mean is divided by the total number of observations less one ($n - 1$), and the square root of the result gives S. Appendix A details an equivalent computational method to determine the standard deviation, which is easier to use in practice. The standard deviation is sometimes called the *root mean square deviation*.

Table 2.4 shows the standard deviations and variances for the example just considered and for the four observations 12, 13, 14, 15, which have the same arithmetic mean, but are less spread out. Their standard deviation is 1·29 compared to the value of 3·69 obtained for the observations 10, 11, 15 and 18. The standard deviation then can be interpreted as a measure of the average dispersion of values around their central value. The arithmetic mean and the standard deviation are complementary measures. The arithmetic mean measures the general level of magnitude of the distribution, or its central value; the standard deviation shows how closely the individual values in the distribution are dispersed around the central value. The greater the spread of values in a particular distribution, the greater the value of the standard deviation.

Frequent references to the standard deviation and its properties are made in subsequent chapters of this book, and the reader should make a special effort to grasp the meaning of this measure. The variance and standard deviation may also be calculated for a grouped frequency distribution. As for the mean, the calculation is somewhat longer and is presented in Appendix A.

If one wanted to compare the variability of some measurement in two groups the standard deviation can be used. However, if the two groups have very different means, the direct comparison of their standard deviations could be misleading in cases when more variability in the group with the larger mean might inherently be expected. For instance, the standard deviation of doctors' salaries is likely to be greater than the total income of a grant-dependent medical student! Suppose that the annual mean income of a group of doctors is found to be £35 000 with a standard deviation of £4000, and that the mean income for medical students is £3500 with a standard deviation of £600. To compare the relative amount of variation, the *coefficient of variation* can be employed. This is simply the standard deviation expressed as a percentage of the mean.

$$\text{CV} = \frac{S}{\bar{x}} \times 100 \ . \tag{2.4}$$

This is independent of the unit of measurement and is expressed as a percentage. The coefficients of variation of doctors' and students' incomes are 11·4 and 17·1% respectively, showing that the income of a medical student is *relatively* more variable than that of a qualified practitioner, though it is of course less variable in absolute terms.

Other measures of dispersion are available. The *mean deviation* is calculated similarly to the standard deviation, by ignoring the minus signs in the individual deviations from the mean (rather than squaring them), adding the deviations together and taking the average. The *quartile deviation* (or *semi-interquartile range*) is calculated as half the difference between the upper and lower quartiles, and is the appropriate measure of dispersion to use if the median is used as the measure of central value.

In essence, measures of dispersion are designed to show how closely the values in a distribution are grouped around their central value. If there is a considerable variation or range of values in a distribution, a relatively high value for the measure of dispersion would be expected. At the other extreme, if all the values in a distribution were equal, then the measure of dispersion would be zero.

2.5 Summary

In the foregoing sections of this chapter, and in the previous chapter, methods which may be used to describe and summarize a collection of data have been discussed and illustrated. In the previous chapter it was explained how the data might be organized and presented. In this chapter it has been explained how the important characteristics of a distribution might be summarized by means of measures of location and measures of dispersion.

3

Probability, Populations and Samples

3.1 Introduction

Having read the first two chapters of this book, one should now understand how data collected in a particular study might be organized, summarized and presented. Descriptive statistics, however, form only one part of statistical analysis and the remainder of this book, for the most part, deals with what is called inferential statistics. In this chapter some of the groundwork is laid for the material that is to follow.

Essentially, statistical inference embodies a methodology which enables something about a large population to be discovered on the basis of observing a subgroup or sample from that population. This chapter starts with a brief foray into the notion of probability and then considers the properties required of a good sample. Sample survey techniques are considered and the normal distribution, one of the most important in statistics, is introduced. An understanding of the meaning of a variable's frequency distribution is needed for this chapter.

3.2 Definition of probability

Central to all statistical analysis is the mathematical theory of probability or chance. Interest in this area arose during the 17th century in the context of gambling, and since then the subject has been studied in depth and is a field of investigation in its own right. Although some purists might disagree, a fairly sound grasp of statistical concepts is possible without a deep understanding of probability theory. In line with the origins of the theory of probability, examples in this section tend to be from games of chance such as cards or dice.

Intuitively, everyone has an idea of what probability is. The probability of a coin landing heads is 1/2; the probability of getting a 3 on the roll of a die is 1/6; the probability of drawing an ace from a pack of cards is 4/52. The truth of such probability statements will depend on whether the coin or die is unbiased (not a two-headed coin or a loaded die) or whether all the aces are actually in the pack and that it is well shuffled.

What can be deduced about probability from the above examples? Firstly, a probability is measured on a numerical scale ranging from 0 to 1. An event with the probability of 0, for all practical purposes, cannot occur; an event with a probability of 1 is a certainty (e.g. death). Between these two extremes, a probability can take any value from 0 to 1 and can be expressed as a fraction (1/6) or a decimal (0·1667). Probabilities can also be expressed in terms of percentages; e.g., a probability of 16·67%. The second point about a probability of an event is that it can be calculated if it is known how many times the event can occur out of all possible outcomes, *provided that each outcome is equally likely*. Thus, there are six equally likely outcomes to the throw of a die; one of these is the appearance of a 3 on the upper face so that the probability of a 3 is 1/6. In a pack of cards, there are four aces in 52 cards. Of the 52 possible outcomes, all equally likely, four are favourable so that the probability of an ace is 4/52. The caveat that each outcome must be equally likely is important. For instance, to determine the probability of obtaining two heads after tossing a 10p coin and a 50p coin, it would be incorrect to conclude, because there are three possible outcomes (two heads, one head and zero heads) and only one is favourable, that the answer is 1/3. In fact, there are four *equally likely* outcomes for the 50p and 10p coin respectively; these are H/T, T/H, H/H and T/T, where H/T means a head on the 50p coin and a tail on the 10p coin. Of these four equally likely outcomes, only one is favourable so that the probability of two heads is 1/4.

The probabilities discussed above were all defined from outside the particular experiment (drawing of a card, tossing of a coin) and can, thus, be called *a priori* probabilities. Such probabilities have the property that if the experiment was repeated a large number of times, the proportion of times the event would be observed would approach the *a priori* probability. If a coin was tossed three times, three heads might be obtained, but if it was tossed a million times or more the proportion of heads should be very close to 0·5 or 50%.

This gives rise to the frequency definition of probability, which is an event's relative frequency in a very large number of trials or experiments performed under similar conditions. This suggests that a probability could be estimated on the basis of a large number of experiments. For instance, to determine the probability of a live-born child being a male, one could examine a large series of births and count how many males resulted (ignoring the problem of hermaphrodites!). In Ireland in 1989 there were 51 659 live births of which 26 613 were male. Thus, the best estimate of the probability of a male, on the assumption that the same underlying process in sex determination is appropriate, is 26 613/51 659 = 0·515 or 51·5%.

There is another type of probability which does not fit into the framework discussed above. A person may say, for instance, that the probability of their getting an honours in the first year medical examination is 0·6 or 60%. There is no way that such a probability may be interpreted as an event's long-term relative frequency as described above, and such a probability is referred to as a subjective probability. Such definitions are not considered in this book, although subjective probability can provide an alternative framework within which to view statistical inference.

3.3 Probability and frequency distributions

Having defined a probability in terms of an event's long-term relative frequency in repeated trials, it is now necessary to examine the relationship of probability to statistical calculations. A simple example will illustrate most of the concepts, and no mathematical rigour is attempted. Consider a bag of 10 coloured marbles, five red, three green and two blue (Fig. 3.1), from which one marble is drawn. The *a priori* probability that this marble will be red is 5/10 = 0·5, that it will be green is 3/10 = 0·3 and that it will be blue is 2/10 = 0·2. If now it was not known either how many marbles were in the bag or what colours they were, the proportions of each colour could be estimated by drawing one marble, noting its colour, replacing it and continuing in the same manner for a large number of trials. If a bar chart was drawn for the number of different times each colour was obtained, the results might be similar to those shown in Fig. 3.2 which is based on the results of 10 000 such draws: 4986 of the draws were of a red marble, 3016 were of a green marble and 1998 were of a blue marble. If each of these figures is divided by the total

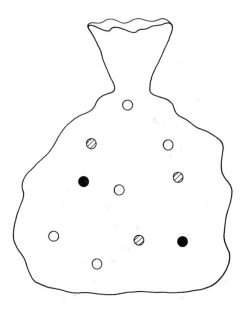

○   Red (5)

⊘   Green (3)

Fig. 3.1. A bag of coloured marbles.   ●   Blue (2)

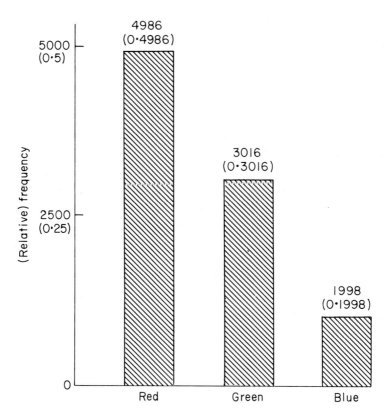

Fig. 3.2. A bar chart showing the colours obtained in 10 000 draws of a single marble (with replacement) from the bag in Fig. 3.1. Relative frequencies are given in parenthesis.

number of trials (10 000) relative frequencies for red, green and blue of 0·4986, 0·3016 and 0·1998 respectively are obtained. These relative frequencies are nearly identical to the actual *a priori* probabilities, as would be expected, given the original definition. When the number of observations on the bar chart is replaced by the relative frequency, a relative frequency diagram is obtained as also illustrated in Fig. 3.2. Note that the relative frequencies must sum to 1·0.

The experiment described then, gives rise to a relative frequency diagram showing the distribution of colours in the bag of marbles. From the opposite point of view however, given the relative frequency diagram in Fig. 3.2, the probability of obtaining a specific result in one draw of a marble from that particular bag could be known to a high degree of accuracy.

This example serves to illustrate the close connection between probability and frequency distributions. Instead of working with a bar chart, the frequency distribution of a quantitative variable such as birth weight at gestational age 40 weeks might be given, as in the last chapter. This may easily be transformed into a relative frequency distribution when, instead of the total area under the curve representing the 1260 births studied, it represents the total frequency of all observations, which is given a value of 1. Whereas in the bar chart example the relative frequencies of a particular colour were represented by the height of the bar, in a relative frequency distribution it is the area under the curve above a certain range of values that represents their relative frequency. (Remember — it was pointed out that it was the area of a bar that was important in frequency distributions of quantitative data, rather than its height.)

Figure 3.3 shows the relative frequency polygon for the birth weight data. Note that the vertical axis is not given a scale since it is relative areas under the curve that are of interest. As an illustration, the relative frequency of birth weights between 2·50 and 3·00 kg* is about 0·12 or 12%. Given this frequency distribution, it can be deduced that the probability of any one child in the study (female, 40 weeks gestation) having a birth weight within these limits is 0·12 or 12%.

Thus, the relative frequency distribution for a variable provides information on the probability of an individual being within any given range of values for that variable. It should be noted that with a continuous distribution such as weight, a probability cannot be ascribed to an exact weight of, say, 2·4 kg; such an exact

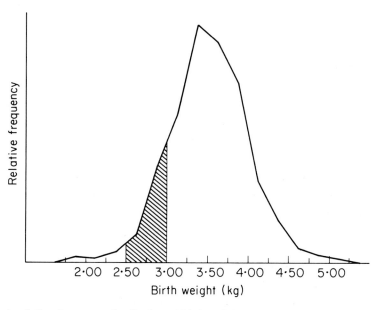

Fig. 3.3. A relative frequency distribution of birth weight at gestational age 40 weeks for females. The shaded area is 12% of the total area.

---

* Actually 2·505 to 3·005 kg. See discussion in Section 1.5.

weight would really signify a value of exactly 2·40 kg — the zeros continuing indefinitely — and the area over such a value is actually zero. However, the probability of an individual having a value, for instance between 2·395 and 2·405 kg, can be established, which is in the example as accurate as the original measures were in the first place.

3.4 Combining probabilities

Going back to the example of the bag of marbles, some simple rules of combining probabilities can be illustrated. Suppose that one wanted to determine the probability of obtaining, in one draw from the bag, either a red marble *or* a green marble. Of the 10 possible outcomes eight are favourable, therefore the probability of a red *or* green marble is 8/10 or 0·8. This result could, however, have also been obtained by adding together the separate probabilities of a red marble (0·5) and a green marble (0·3). This gives rise to the general addition rule of probability; the probability of the occurrence of *two mutually exclusive* events is obtained by adding together the probability of each event. If A and B are two such events,

$$P(A \text{ or } B) = P(A) + P(B), \tag{3.1}$$

where P(event) means the probability of an event. Mutually exclusive means that if one event occurs, the other event cannot occur, and the additive rule only holds under this condition. If a marble is red, it cannot be green at the same time. On the other hand, to determine the probability of an ace or a diamond in a pack of cards, the additive principle would not hold, since the existence of the ace of diamonds makes the two events not mutually exclusive.

Suppose now that a marble is drawn, returned to the bag and then a second marble drawn. What is the probability of obtaining a red marble first, and then a green one? In this situation, the multiplicative rule of probability holds and the probability of the joint occurrence of two *independent events* is given by the multiplication of the separate probabilities:

$$P(A \text{ and } B) = P(A) \times P(B). \tag{3.2}$$

Thus, the probability of a red and a green marble is $0·5 \times 0·3 = 0·15$. The requirement of independence means that the occurrence of the first event does not affect the probability of the second event, and this is required for the multiplicative rule. Since in the example the marbles were replaced, the result of the first draw could have no influence on the result of the subsequent draw. If the events are not independent, a different rule must be used. This is:

$$P(A \text{ and } B) = P(A) \times P(B \text{ given } A), \tag{3.3}$$

where $P(B$ given $A)$ means the probability of the event B given that the event A

has already occurred. An example of this more general rule follows. Suppose that the first marble was not replaced. What now is the probability of a red marble and a green marble? The probability of a red marble is 0·5, but if a red marble is drawn from the bag and not replaced, the probability of a green marble is not now 0·3. There are only nine marbles left after a red marble has been drawn: four red, three green, and two blue, and the probability of a green marble is, thus, 3/9 or 0·3333 if a red marble was drawn already. Thus, in this instance the probability of a red and a green marble in that order is 0·5 × 0·333 = 0·1666. Examples of the use of this rule in its application to the calculation of survival rates are seen in Chapter 10. $P(B$ given $A)$ is referred to as a *conditional probability* and the independence of two events A and B requires in probability terms that

$$P(B \text{ given } A) = P(B). \tag{3.4}$$

3.5 Populations and samples

When medical researchers collect a set of data, their interest usually goes beyond the actual persons or items studied. For instance, in the study of birth weights in the previous chapters, the purpose was to construct centile charts that would be applicable to future births. Because of this desire to generalize, describing the results of a particular study is only a first step in a statistical analysis. The second step involves what is known as statistical inference. In technical terms, a statistical inference is an attempt to reach a conclusion about a large number of items or events on the basis of observations made on only a portion of them. The opinion poll, which studies a small number of persons to estimate attitudes or opinions in a large population, is a good example of this. In the medical field, a doctor may prescribe a particular drug because prior experience leads him/her to believe that it may be of value to a particular patient. A surgeon too may use a particular operative technique because in previous operations it seemed to give good results. (As is seen in Chapter 11, however, such inferences may be erroneous, and the controlled clinical trial provides a sound scientific method to compare the efficacy of medical interventions.)

In statistical terminology, it is usual to speak of *populations* and *samples*. The term population is used to describe all the possible observations of a particular variable or all the units on which the observation could have been made. Reference may be made to a population of patients, a population of ages of Irishmen at death, or a population of readings on a thermometer. What is to be understood as the 'population' varies according to the context in which it is used. Thus, the population of patients in a particular hospital and the population of patients in the whole of Ireland are quite distinct populations. It is important to understand that the term 'population' has a precise meaning in any given context.

A population may be finite or infinite. The population of hospital patients in Ireland at or over any particular period of time is finite. On the other hand, the population of readings on a thermometer is infinite since, in principle, an infinite number of such readings can be taken. Many populations are so large that they may be regarded as infinite — for example, the number (population) of red blood cells in the human body.

In its broadest sense, a sample refers to any specific collection of observations drawn from a parent population. It is possible to have a sample of patients, a sample of temperature readings, and so on. The two properties required of any sample are that it be of reasonable size and that it be representative of the population from which it was taken. At one extreme, a sample may include all of the units in the parent population in which case it is referred to as a *census*. In many countries a census of the full population is taken at regular intervals. A census is, by definition, completely representative of the population. At the other extreme, a sample may consist of only one unit selected from the population. Although it is of theoretical interest, such a sample cannot in practice reveal very much about a parent population unless many assumptions are made. In this sense, a reasonably sized sample is somewhere between two units and all the population. Intuitively, however, it would be felt that sample sizes of two or three are also inadequate, and that the larger the sample, the more reliance can be placed on any inference made from it. Exactly what is an adequately sized sample depends on the precise nature of the study being carried out, and on many other factors which are considered at a later stage.

Why study samples at all? Why not always examine the full population, as in a census? There are two basic reasons which may be put forward. Firstly, it is usually too expensive and time-consuming to study an entire population and in fact it may not even be possible to define the population precisely. What for instance is the population of patients with coronary heart disease? The second reason, just as important, is that a sufficiently sized representative sample can give information concerning a population to whatever degree of accuracy is required. Thus, a census is, in many instances, a waste of resources and effort, although it is only with a census that the number of persons in a population can be determined precisely.

A large sample does not by itself, however, make for a representative sample. One of the best examples of this is taken from the early days of the opinion poll. In 1936, an American magazine, *The Literary Digest*, sampled telephone subscribers and its own readers to forecast the result of the forthcoming US presidential election. They received 2·4 million replies and predicted as a consequence that one of the candidates, Landon, would have a landslide victory over Roosevelt. Few people have ever heard of Landon, so what went wrong? A little thought might suggest that telephone subscribers and readers of a particular magazine could be of a different social class than the entire voting population, and that voting preferences may indeed depend on this factor. Such was the case, since few of the sampled groups were to have been found on the breadline or in the soup queues of those depression years. The voting preferences of the sample were not representative of the entire population, and so an erroneous inference was drawn. The large sample size could not alter the inherent *bias* of the sample. (A bias can be broadly defined as a factor which will tend to lead to an erroneous conclusion.)

How then, is it possible to ensure that a representative sample is selected? An intuitive approach might be to uniquely identify all the units in a (finite) population and 'put all the names in a hat', mix well, and draw out enough names to give a sample of whatever size is required. This is the principle used in the selection of winning tickets in a raffle or lottery, and it has many desirable properties. Every unit of the population has the same chance of being included in the sample, and biases such as in the opinion poll discussed above do not arise. Samples chosen in such a way are called *simple random samples* and form the theoretical basis for most statistical inference. Such samples are representative of the population insofar as no particular block of the population is more likely to be represented than any other. The definition of a simple random sample given above will suffice here, noting that the more general term 'random sampling' refers to the situation when each member of the population has a known (non-zero, but not necessarily the same) probability of selection. Random is thus a term that describes how the sample is chosen, rather than the sample itself.

When any data are to be studied, it must always be remembered that they are (usually) a sample from a far larger population of observations and that the purpose of the study is to make inferences about the population on the basis of the sample. Any time a frequency polygon for a variable is constructed, it is being used to estimate the underlying distribution of that variable. Although, in practice, it is never known precisely what this distribution looks like, one could imagine taking a measurement on everyone in the population and forming a population frequency curve. With such a large number of observations, and using very small class intervals, a curve rather than a polygon would be obtained. For the population of all female births at 40 weeks gestation, for example, a curve similar to that in Fig. 3.4 for birth weight might be obtained.

Now, considering only quantitative variables, the frequency distribution in the population will have a mean and standard deviation. These are given special symbols: μ (mu — the Greek letter 'm') refers to the population mean and σ (sigma — the lower case Greek letter 's') refers to a population standard deviation. Any such measures, when applied to a population, are called 'population parameters'. When, on the other hand, the mean and standard deviation refer to samples, they are often symbolized $\bar{x}$ and S respectively, and such measures in a sample are called 'sample statistics'. (A good way of remembering this is that

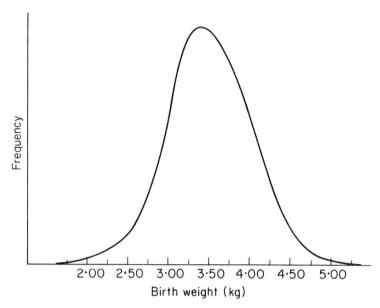

Fig. 3.4. The underlying frequency distribution of birth weight for females at 40 weeks gestation.

populations have parameters with a '*P*' and samples have statistics with an '*S*'.) With this terminology, it can be said that the purpose of sampling is to estimate population parameters on the basis of sample statistics.

3.6 Sample surveys

To draw a simple random sample from a given population, one needs to have some list of all the units in the population. Such lists are referred to as the sampling frame. Obviously, to put 'all the names in a hat' and draw a sample would be, in practice, a very tedious operation and fraught with potential biases, due to lack of mixing for example. An alternative and equivalent method is, however, available. This requires the use of a table of random numbers. One page from such a table is given in Appendix B (Table B.1). Essentially, a table of random numbers can be thought of as being produced by a little man sitting down in front of a hat containing the numbers 0 to 9 on 10 separate pieces of paper. He draws a number, notes it down, replaces it in the hat, mixes well and draws another number, repeating the process millions of times. Tables of random numbers are not, of course, produced by little men but are now generated by computers. They have the important property that every digit has a one in ten chance of being present at any particular position in the Table. Thus, such tables can be used to simulate the physical drawing of a sample from a hat. Suppose that a sample of size five is required from a population of 80 individuals. First, number the 80 units in the population from 01 to 80. Start at an arbitrary point (use a pin) in a table of random numbers and read down the nearest column. Since two digits are sufficient to identify any member of the population, read the first two digits of a column and continue reading down the column until five different two-digit numbers between 01 and 80 are obtained. Repeat numbers should be ignored, as should numbers outside this range. The numbers chosen in this way identify the particular members of the population who are in the sample. For example, start at the top of the sixth column in Table B.1. The first eight two-digit numbers are 72, 12, 90, 86, 15, 28, 28, 36; ignoring 90, 86 and the second 28 for the reasons stated, the remaining numbers identify the members of the sample.

A refinement of the simple random sample is the *stratified random sample*. The population is divided into groups, or strata, on the basis of certain character-istics, for example age and sex. A simple random sample is then selected from each stratum and the results for each stratum are combined to give the results for the total sample. The object of this type of sample design is to ensure that each stratum in the population is represented in the sample in certain fixed proportions which are determined in advance. For example, in determining the smoking habits of the national population, age and sex are obviously important factors, and it might be desirable to select a sample whose age and sex composition exactly reflects the age and sex composition of the whole population. With a simple random sample, it is unlikely that the age and sex composition of the sample would achieve this. However, by dividing the population into age/sex groups and selecting a random sample within each group it can be ensured that the proportions in each age/sex group in the sample will be identical with these proportions in the total population. Although the sample proportions may reflect exactly the proportions in the population, not all stratified random samples are selected in this way. Certain strata may be deliberately 'over-represented' in the sample, while others are 'under-represented'. The important point is that the sample proportions are predetermined. For this reason, stratified random samples are often preferred to simple random samples. If a stratified sample has been taken with some strata over- or under-represented, the sample as a whole will not reflect the population. If one wanted to estimate, for example, the population mean, a weighted mean (see Section 2.2) would be used with the weights equal to the size of the population in each of the strata.

A sampling method similar to the stratified random sample, and commonly used in opinion polls and market research, is the *quota sample*. This, however, is not a random sample in the true sense of the word and the method should be avoided. In quota sampling, the main objective is to fill certain quotas of individuals in well-defined groups, such as males aged 25 to 34 years. The quotas are arranged so that the final sample mirrors the population exactly in relation to, say, age and sex groups, and to that extent a quota sample is similar to the stratified sample. However, one is free to choose anyone who will fit the require-ments of the quotas, and obviously only co-operative individuals and easily contactable persons would be included. There is no guarantee that the persons chosen within a particular group are representative of the population in that group as regards the factors being studied, and large unquantifiable biases may occur. In a stratified random sample however, every person in a particular stratum has the same probability of inclusion in the sample, and this ensures, in a probability sense, representativeness in terms of other variables.

The *multistage random sample* is another sampling technique, which has the advantage that a full list of the population to be surveyed is not required. Suppose that primary school children in a certain area are to be sampled. Rather than obtaining (with great difficulty) a full list of all such children and taking a simple random sample of these, a list of the different schools in the area could be obtained, and a simple random sample taken of the schools. A simple random sample could then be taken from a list of the children in these schools only (much smaller than the full list of children in the population). The sampling would, thus, be accomplished in two stages with a large reduction in the practical work involved. There are potential difficulties in multistage samples however, and a statistician should be consulted before undertaking such a task. A variant on the multistage sample is the *cluster sample*, where a simple random sample of groups (e.g. schools) is taken, and everyone in the chosen group is studied. This method too should be used only with professional advice.

An approximation to the simple random sample which, though requiring a list of the population is much easier in practice, is the *systematic sample*. In such a sample every nth person is chosen, where n depends on the required sample size and the size of the population. One starts at random in the list, somewhere among the first n members; thus, if every 10th member of a population is to be chosen, one would start by choosing a random number from 1 to 10 — say 7 — and include the 7th, 17th, 27th, etc., persons on the list. Such a method could be used advantageously for sampling hospital charts, for instance, when a simple random sample might prove very difficult indeed.

Sample surveys of defined populations have an important part to play in medical research, and should be characterized by the care taken in choosing the sample correctly. Random samples refer to very specific techniques and should not be confused with haphazard sampling, when anyone and everyone can be included in the sample on the researcher's whim. The importance of a random sample is threefold: it avoids bias, most standard statistical inferential methods assume such sampling and, as is seen in the next chapter, precise statements concerning the likely degree of accuracy of a sample result can be made.

Apart from bad sampling, there are two main sources of bias in any sample survey. The first is that of non-response. To conduct any survey of people, one must eventually contact the individuals actually sampled. If some are unco-operative or impossible to trace, these exclusions from the sample may affect its representativeness. Non-response rates higher than $15 - 20\%$ may throw doubts on any conclusion drawn from a particular study. The second source of the bias in a sample survey relates to the inference actually made. It is very important not to draw conclusions about a different population to that actually sampled. It is always necessary to check the adequacy of the sampling frame (the population list) in terms of its coverage of the population, and care should be taken in not over-generalizing the results. For instance, a medical researcher may sample rheumatoid arthritis patients who attended a particular teaching hospital, but would be in error to generalize any of the results to a target population of all rheumatoid arthritis patients. Rheumatoid arthritis does not necessarily lead to hospitalization, and in a teaching hospital in particular, a more severe type of arthritis may be seen. At best, the results of such a study should be generalized to rheumatoid arthritis patients in hospital.

A major problem of medical research however, is that in many situations random sampling is impossible because the population of interest is not strictly definable. Many studies are performed on what are known as samples of con-venience, or *presenting samples*. Typically, a doctor may decide to study 100 consecutive hospital admissions with a particular condition. There is no sense in which such individuals could be considered a random sample from a particular population, but it can be reasonably hoped that information on such patients might provide insight into other similar patients who may be diagnosed some time in the future. The best approach is to ask from what population the patients actually in the study could be considered a random sample, and to make a statistical inference about that hypothetical, and possibly non-existent, population. There are large departures from the theoretical assumptions underlying statistical analysis with this approach, but it still seems the only solution to the problem of definite non-random samples often met with in the medical situation.

3.7 The normal distribution

In this section, one of the most important theoretical distributions in statistics — the *normal*, or as it is often called, the *Gaussian distribution* — is introduced. The importance of this distribution is seen in the next chapter, where its use in statistical estimation is examined but, for the moment, it is considered in its own right. The term 'normal' applied to this particular distribution should not be taken to mean that the distribution is common or typical. In fact, many variables in medical research are non-normal (not abnormal!) but there is nothing wrong with them. It should also be mentioned that a normal distribution for a variable is not a prerequisite for many forms of statistical analysis, although it can be a great help.

The normality of a distribution always refers to the distribution of a variable in a population, so that the mean and standard deviation of such distributions are denoted by μ and σ respectively. The normal distribution has certain definite features: it is unimodal, symmetrical, and bell-shaped, but this is not to say that all unimodal, symmetrical, bell-shaped distributions are normal. Since normal distributions are unimodal and symmetrical, the mean, median and mode are equal in value. A normal distribution is characterized completely by its mean and standard deviation; that is to say, two normal distributions with the same means and standard deviations are identical. Normal distributions can, of course, have different means and different standard deviations. Figure 3.5 illustrates (a) normal curves with the same standard deviations but different means and (b) normal curves with the same means but different standard deviations. What distinguishes normal distributions from other unimodal, symmetrical, bell-shaped distributions are their area properties, or more precisely, specific relationships between their percentile values and their means and standard deviations.

What are some of these properties? Figure 3.6 shows a typical normal distribution with a mean μ and standard deviation σ. Obviously, 50% of the area lies above the mean and 50% lies below the mean. Now, in a normal distribution it is also true that 68·27% (just over two-thirds) of the area lies between the values obtained by subtracting and adding the value of the standard deviation to the value of the mean i.e. between $\mu - \sigma$ and $\mu + \sigma$ or within $\mu \pm \sigma$. Also, 95% of

(a)

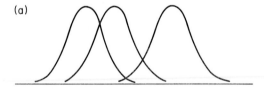

(b)

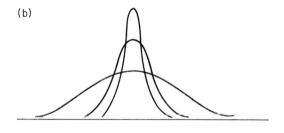

Fig. 3.5. Normal distributions: (a) same standard deviations, different means (b) same means, different standard deviations.

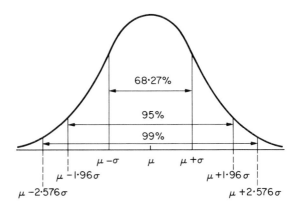

Fig. 3.6. Area properties of the
normal distribution.

the area of a normal curve lies within $\mu \pm 1.96\sigma$. (The figures 68·27% and 1·96 in these relationships arise from the normality of the distribution and are specific to such distributions.) The area within which all (100%) of the area is contained cannot be stated since the two tails of the distribution continuously approach, but never reach, the horizontal axis.

Suppose, for example, systolic blood pressure is known to follow a normal distribution with a mean of 125 mmHg and standard deviation of 12 mmHg in males aged 35−39 years. Remembering that any area under a distribution curve can be interpreted as a proportion or percentage of the possible observations, it can be said that 68·27% of the blood pressures of the persons in this population will lie between 125 − 12 and 125 + 12 mmHg, that is to say, between 113 and 137 mmHg. Similarly, it could be said that 95% of the blood pressures will lie within 125 ± 1·96(12) or between 101·48 and 148·52 mmHg (Fig. 3.7). These results can, of course, be taken to mean that if one person in this population is randomly chosen, there is a 68·27% chance that the blood pressure of this person will lie between 113 and 137 mmHg. These area properties are, of course, true for any normal distribution of a given mean and standard deviation, and essentially, are statements concerning percentiles of such distributions. For instance,

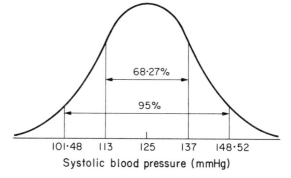

Fig. 3.7. Population distribution of
systolic blood pressure in males
aged 35−39; a normal distribution
with mean 125 mmHg and
standard deviation 12 mmHg
(hypothetical example).

$\mu + 1 \cdot 96\sigma$ gives the $97\frac{1}{2}$th percentile of a normal distribution because 95% of the area is between $\mu \pm 1 \cdot 96\sigma$, leaving 2·5% in each of the two tails. $\mu - 1 \cdot 96\sigma$ gives the $2\frac{1}{2}$th percentile. In fact, any percentile of a normal distribution can be calculated by adding or subtracting a particular multiple of the standard deviation to or from the mean. Tables of these multiples are widely available, and a very abbreviated table is to be found in Appendix B (Table B.2). These properties, of course, are valid only for normal distributions.

Since the multiplying factors are independent of the mean and standard deviation of the distribution, the table conveniently gives the factors for a particular normal distribution of mean zero and standard deviation unity. This is called the *standard normal distribution*. For such a distribution, 68·27% of the observations lie between $\pm 1 \cdot 0$; 95% are within $\pm 1 \cdot 96$, and 99% are within $\pm 2 \cdot 58$ (e.g. with $\mu = 0$, and $\sigma = 1$, $\mu \pm 1 \cdot 96\sigma$ becomes $\pm 1 \cdot 96$). Table B.2 gives these factors (denoted z_c) for specified areas in both tails and also in the upper tail of the standard normal distribution. The table is given in terms of areas in the tails for later application, and much more extensive tables are to be found in most statistical textbooks. (It is worthwhile becoming familiar with one particular table of the normal distribution, since the layout and notation tend to change from book to book.)

To find the z value, which cuts off a particular area in both tails of a standard normal distribution, look at the areas in the top row. (Ignore for the moment the alternative description — two-sided significance level, etc.) The area is given as a proportion rather than as a percentage, thus 0·05 means 5%. The z value corresponding to each area is given in the last row. For example, in the standard normal curve, the values given by $\pm 2 \cdot 326$ cut off a total area of 2% in the two tails. For a normal distribution of mean μ and standard deviation σ, the figures which encompass 98% of the area are $\mu \pm 2 \cdot 326\sigma$. Note that since the normal distribution is symmetrical, only the $+ z$ value is given in the table. The table also gives the z values which cut off particular areas in the upper tail of the normal distribution; thus, for example, 0·5% or 0·005 of the area is above 2·576 in the standard normal curve, or in a normal distribution of mean μ and standard deviation σ, 0·5% of the values will lie above $\mu + 2 \cdot 576\sigma$.

The standard normal curve is obtained by a transformation of the observations in a general normal distribution. This is akin to changing the measurement unit, as for example, from inches to centimetres in measuring height, or from degrees Fahrenheit to degrees Centigrade in measuring temperature. If x has a normal distribution with mean μ and standard deviation σ, then $x - \mu$ has a normal distribution with mean zero and standard deviation σ, while $(x - \mu)/\sigma$ has the standard normal distribution of mean 0 and standard deviation 1. Often,

$$z = \frac{x - \mu}{\sigma} \tag{3.5}$$

is written as the equation for transforming a variable with a normal distribution to a variable with the standard normal distribution. $x - \mu$ measures how far the observation is from the mean and division by σ converts this to multiples of the standard deviation. Rather than being measured in the original units, each value is thus assigned a number which measures how many standard deviations it is away from the mean. z is often referred to as a *standard normal deviate*.

3.8 Summary

In this chapter some background material, necessary for a complete grasp of the chapters to follow, has been introduced. A basic understanding of probability and its relationship to frequency distributions is central to most statistical inference. The distinction between populations and samples and the notion of making an inference about a population on the basis of a sample from that population is, of course, the core idea in statistical analysis, while from the practical point of view, the different techniques which can be used in actually taking a random sample from a population are important. The normal distribution was introduced here as a theoretical population distribution which will play a central role in many of the analytical techniques which are discussed in the remainder of the book.

4

Estimation: Confidence Intervals for Means, Proportions, Counts and Rates

4.1 Introduction

The first two chapters of this book discussed various methods available to organize, present and summarize data obtained in a particular study, and as has been said, such descriptive statistics form the basis of any statistical analysis. The third chapter considered the notion of probability or chance, and discussed the various methods of choosing samples from a population, leading to the idea of statistical inference. The normal distribution was also discussed. This chapter considers statistical inference in the context of estimating population parameters on the basis of sample statistics. The estimate of a single population mean is discussed in detail, and the extension of the method to estimate population proportions, counts and rates is described. Statistical estimation using confidence intervals is now accepted as the preferred approach to the analysis of medical research and the presentation of results.

Prerequisites for this chapter are an understanding of frequency distributions and, in particular, the normal distribution.

4.2 Sampling variation

Some of the concepts are illustrated in this chapter using a simple example. The length of survival of 100 lung cancer patients on a particular new therapy is determined. Overall, these patients are observed to have a mean survival of 27·5 months with a standard deviation of 25·0 months. From these sample statistics, the researcher wants to estimate the true (population) mean survival of such patients. Assume for the moment that the standard deviation in the population, σ, is actually 25·0 months even though, in reality, this is only the sample estimate. Assume also (see discussion in the last chapter) that it is meaningful to talk about a population of all such lung cancer patients from which this particular random sample was taken.

The sample mean, $\bar{x} = 27\cdot5$ months, could of course be used as an estimate of the population mean μ. This is called a point estimate and is the best single estimate available. It cannot be said that the population mean is exactly equal to this particular sample mean. Intuitively, however, it seems reasonable to assert that the true unknown mean is *fairly likely* to be *somewhere around* the sample mean, or that the true mean survival is somewhere around 27·5 months. The theoretical considerations in the remainder of this chapter are purely to make it possible to quantify (put figures on) the vague terms 'fairly likely' and 'somewhere around' and lead to the definition of a confidence interval.

The problem is, however, that the sample obtained is one of many (an infinite number of) possible samples; a different sample would, most probably, give a different sample mean. Thus, the sample mean itself, on which the estimate of the population mean is based, is one of many possible sample means. *Sampling variation* refers to the fact that the sample mean can vary with the particular sample chosen. Can then the single sample mean actually obtained reveal anything about the population mean, since another sample would have given a different result?

At this stage, it is necessary to do a 'thought' experiment, which is basically the consideration of a 'what if' situation. It is important to realize that this experiment is never carried out in reality — one sample only is taken to estimate a population parameter. What would happen though if very many different samples, all of the same size, were taken from the population? Many different sample means would be obtained. If these means were then considered as a collection of quantitative data, a frequency distribution of these means could be produced and a frequency polygon formed from the histogram in the usual manner. If a large enough number of samples (an infinite number) was taken, the frequency polygon would become a smooth frequency curve, and it would be possible to talk about the underlying frequency distribution of these means.

This is, perhaps, where most of the confusion in the interpretation of statistical results arises. To recap in the context of the example already mentioned: a particular sample of 100 lung cancer patients have survival times which may be formed into a frequency distribution whose mean, $\bar{x}$, happens to be 27·5 months. There is also the underlying distribution of survival times in the population of all such patients; it is not known what this distribution looks like and it is necessary to estimate its mean μ. The third distribution of interest is a theoretical one, based on the 'thought' experiment. It is not, however, a distribution of survival times; it is a distribution of mean survivals, calculated from repeated samples sized 100, taken from the population of lung cancer patients. For obvious reasons, this distribution is called the *sampling distribution of the mean*. Again, it must be emphasized that the only distribution which can actually be formed is the distribution of survival times in the sample and that the sampling distribution of the mean, in particular, is a theoretical distribution which exists only in the mind of the statistician, but exists nonetheless. Figure 4.1 summarizes the properties of these three distributions.

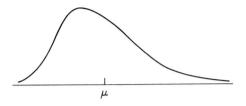

Original (underlying) distribution of a variable x in the population, with a mean μ and standard deviation σ (not necessarily normal).

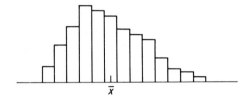

Distribution of the variable in a sample sized n from this population with a mean of $\bar{x}$.

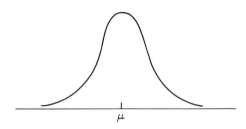

Distribution of all possible means from samples sized n — a normal distribution with mean μ and standard deviation $\sigma/\sqrt{n}$ (the sampling distribution of the mean).

Fig. 4.1. The sampling distribution of the mean.

4.3 Properties of the sampling distribution of the mean

It was seen in Chapter 2 that any frequency distribution could be summarized by describing its shape, and giving its mean and standard deviation. Now, the theoretical sampling distribution of the mean also must have a shape, must itself have a mean and must also have a standard deviation. From studies in theoretical statistics, certain facts can be deduced about these quantities. Proofs are not given here.

Firstly, the sampling distribution of the mean turns out to be a normal distribution. This is always true if the underlying distribution of the variable (survival time in the example) is itself normal; but even more importantly, it is approximately true as long as the distribution of the original variable is not very skewed, and the approximation improves as the sample size (n) increases. This is called the *central limit theorem* and explains the important role of the normal distribution in statistics. Note that non-normality of the distribution of the variable under examination does not invalidate this very important result, except with small sample sizes. Unless the distribution of the variable is very skewed, sample sizes of over 30 are likely to be adequate for application of the central limit theorem. If the distribution of values in the sample is very skewed then a transformation of the data might reduce the degree of skewness, allowing application of the techniques discussed below (see Section 1.7).

The second result which is of concern relates to the mean of all the sample means in the sampling distribution of the mean. Fairly reasonably it turns out that the mean of all these means is nothing more than the mean (μ) of the population from which the samples were chosen (in the 'thought' experiment). Thus, sample means are distributed normally about the unknown population mean which is being estimated. This justifies the intuitive notion that most of the possible sample means should be fairly near this population value.

Finally, the question arises of how near is fairly near, which, of course, relates to the dispersion of the sample means around the population mean. It can be shown that the standard deviation of the sampling distribution of the mean is given by $\sigma/\sqrt{n}$, where σ is the standard deviation of the original population, and n is the sample size. The standard deviation of the sampling distribution of the mean is, more usually, called the *standard error of the mean*, or, when there is no ambiguity, the standard error. It is often denoted SE or SE ($\bar{x}$). This name arose from the historical context in which the parameter was introduced, and 'error' has nothing at all to do with a mistake.

$$\text{SE} (\bar{x}) = \sigma/\sqrt{n}. \tag{4.1}$$

This formula for the standard error of the mean may seem strange, but it is possible to justify it if one is willing to take some liberty and not question the explanation too much. If, for instance, samples sized one were taken from the population, the mean of each of these would be nothing more than the value of the observation on the individual unit chosen in the sample. The distribution of all possible means from different samples sized one would then be identical to the distribution of the variable in the original population. Thus, with a sample size of one, the standard deviation of the sampling distribution of the mean would be equal to the standard deviation in the population itself — σ. This agrees with Eqn. 4.1 when n is set equal to one. If now it is imagined that samples are taken whose size is the size of the original population, the mean of each of these samples (all identical) would be necessarily equal to the population mean μ. In this case, there would be no spread of sample means around μ and the standard deviation of the sampling distribution of the mean, for sample sizes equal to the

---

* For infinite populations; the finite population case is not considered.

size of the population, would be zero. For an infinite population, the sample size n would be infinite also and Eqn. 4.1 would give the standard error as zero also. This serves to explain the reasonableness of Eqn. 4.1 as representing the standard deviation of the sampling distribution of the mean. The standard error increases with increasing variability in the original population and decreases with sample size. The fact that the divisor is the square root of n rather than n itself (or any other function of n) is best accepted on faith.

In this section then, it has been seen that the distribution of the means from all possible samples of a given size is normal, with a mean equal to the mean of the population from which the samples were taken, and a standard deviation (called the standard error of the mean) equal to the standard deviation of the population divided by the square root of the sample size. This result and variants on it form the basis of much of statistical inference.

4.4 Confidence intervals for a mean using the normal distribution

Having looked at the theoretical properties of the sampling distribution of the mean, it is now possible to return to the example of the 100 lung cancer patients whose mean survival is $\bar{x} = 27 \cdot 5$ months and whose population standard deviation σ, as mentioned, is known to be $25 \cdot 0$ months. It can now be said that the sample mean actually obtained is one random observation from all the possible means which could have been obtained with different samples of 100 patients. These possible means have a normal distribution, whose mean is equal to the unknown population mean, μ, which is being estimated, and whose standard deviation (the standard error) is equal to

$$\sigma/\sqrt{n} = 25/\sqrt{100} = 2 \cdot 5.$$

From the properties of the normal distribution discussed in Chapter 3, it can be said that there is a 95% chance that

$$27 \cdot 5 \text{ is within } \mu \pm 1 \cdot 96 \ (2 \cdot 5)$$
or
$$27 \cdot 5 \text{ is within } \mu \pm 4 \cdot 9.$$

Note that $2 \cdot 5$ is the standard error of the mean, which is the standard deviation of the sampling distribution of the mean from which the observation of $27 \cdot 5$ was taken. This statement can now be switched around to say that the following expressions have a 95% chance of being correct:

$$\mu \text{ is within } 27 \cdot 5 \pm 4 \cdot 9$$
or
$$\mu \text{ is between } 22 \cdot 6 \text{ and } 32 \cdot 4.$$

Alternatively, it could be said that the level of certainty or confidence about the truth of either of these statements is 95%. The range 22·6 to 32·4 is called a 95% *confidence interval* for the unknown population mean μ, and the figures 22·6 and 32·4 are called the *confidence limits*.

It was stated earlier that, intuitively, the unknown population mean is fairly likely to be somewhere around the sample mean. In the example above, 'fairly likely' has been quantified as 95% likely and 'somewhere around' as ± 4·9. Note that the confidence interval is not a statement concerning the bounds within which a proportion of the survival times in a population can be found; rather, it is a statement which gives a range within which the unknown population mean survival is likely to be. The bounds for proportions of the population should be estimated using percentile indices.

In terms of a formula, a 95% confidence interval for an unknown population mean is given by

$$\bar{x} \pm 1 \cdot 96 \; \text{SE} \, (\bar{x}) \tag{4.2}$$

or
$$\bar{x} \pm 1 \cdot 96 \; \sigma/\sqrt{n}. \tag{4.3}$$

What if a higher level of confidence is desired — say 99%? What you gain on the roundabout, you lose on the swings; a 99% level of confidence would mean that the width of the confidence interval would be wider than that for 95% confidence. In Eqns. 4.2 and 4.3 the value 1·96 would be replaced by 2·576 (in a normal distribution 99% of observations are within ± 2·576 standard deviations of the mean) obtaining for a 99% confidence interval

$$\bar{x} \pm 2 \cdot 576 \; \sigma/\sqrt{n} \tag{4.4}$$

which, in the example, would give confidence limits of 21·06 and 33·94. Usually, only 99% or 95% confidence intervals are used, but with tables of the normal distribution it is obviously possible to calculate confidence limits for any specified level of confidence. Appendix C (Section C.2) summarizes these calculations.

4.5 Standard deviations and standard errors

There is often much confusion between a standard deviation and a standard error in the medical literature. The standard deviation is a measure of the spread of a particular population, and is a descriptive statistic for a sample. If one wanted to describe or summarize sample results, then the standard deviation should be presented. Often figures such as 44·3 ± 17·0 are seen where it may be stated in the text that this represents a mean plus or minus a standard deviation. If the distribution of the variable is normal, then it can be concluded that just over two-thirds of the observed values lie within these bounds. If the distribution is not normal, as will often be the case, there is no immediate interpretation which can be put on such an expression.

If, on the other hand, one wanted to give an idea of how accurate a sample mean is as an estimate of a population mean, then the standard error is the more appropriate statistic to present. A mean ± a standard error ($\bar{x} \pm$ SE) gives a 68·27% confidence interval for the population mean. (Remember the properties of the normal distribution.) To get a 95% confidence interval, it is then necessary to add and subtract about two standard errors* rather than the one standard error usually presented.

Whether standard deviations or standard errors are presented depends on the purpose of the presentation. Just because they are smaller and therefore look better is not a sufficient reason to present standard errors. It is also worthwhile noting, when reading the medical literature, how many times a mean ± something is presented with no statement as to what that something is. After all, it could be one standard deviation, two standard deviations, one standard error or two standard errors, and its interpretation is impossible without knowing which.

4.6 The Student's *t* distribution

So far in this chapter it has been assumed that the population standard deviation σ was known. This, of course, is an unrealistic assumption in most cases, and what happens when σ is replaced by the sample standard deviation, S, in the formula for the standard error is now examined. Remember that a 95% confidence interval for an unknown population mean was given by

$$\bar{x} \pm 1·96 \ \sigma/\sqrt{n}, \qquad (4.3)$$

where $\bar{x}$ is the sample mean, σ is the population standard deviation, n is the sample size, and ± 1·96 are the values that include 95% of the area under the standard normal curve.

It was realized that the above formulation, based on the normal distribution, would be inaccurate whenever S, the sample standard deviation, was substituted for σ, the population value, and especially so for small sample sizes. (As an aside, the population variance σ^2, in a finite population of size N is correctly defined using a divisor of N rather than $N - 1$. The best estimate of this quantity from a sample sized n is given by S^2, however, with the $n - 1$ divisor. Hence this is the formulation used (see Eqn. 2.3).) It was not until 1908, however, that the solution to this problem was determined. In that year, a chemist-cum-mathematician, William Gosset, who was employed in the Guinness brewery in Dublin, published

---

* Usually, the standard error is not known exactly and 1·96 is a suitable multiplying factor only with an exact result. A value of 2 usually gives a good enough approximation (see Section 4.7 for the exact method).

a paper under the pseudonym 'Student', detailing the corrections which must be made in this situation. (Arthur Guinness Son & Co. did not allow Gosset to publish under his own name — possibly because they did not wish their competitors to realize just how useful statistics could be in sampling the quality of the brew!) Gosset's work essentially was to introduce what is now called the *Student's t* distribution, or the *t* distribution for short, for use in place of the normal distribution in the situation just described. The *t* distribution is, in fact, many different distributions, which are differentiated by their degrees of freedom (d.f.). Thus, there are *t* distributions with 1 d.f., 2 d.f., etc. Like the normal distribution, the *t* distribution is symmetrical, unimodal and bell-shaped, but it is more spread out, and has different area properties. The fact that this distribution is more spread out allows for the increased variability introduced into the calculation of confidence intervals when only the sample value of the standard deviation is known. The degrees of freedom increase with sample size in the applications considered, and the Student's *t* distribution with a large number of degrees of freedom is pretty well identical to the standard normal distribution (see below).

The *t* distribution with any particular number of degrees of freedom is akin to the standard normal distribution, and Appendix B (Table B.3) gives a table of this distribution for degrees of freedom from 1 to 30 and some higher values. The table is laid out similarly to that for the normal distribution in Table B.2. Take, for example, the Student's *t* distribution with 8 degrees of freedom. The critical values of *t*, t_c which cut off specified areas in the tail(s) of this distribution are found on the row marked with d.f. = 8. It is seen that, for instance, 2·5% of the area is above $t = 2\cdot306$ while 1% of the area lies outside the limits defined by $t = \pm 3\cdot355$. Figure 4.2 illustrates these values for the *t* distribution with 8 degrees of freedom. In the normal distribution, the corresponding values would have been 1·960 and ± 2·576 respectively, thus illustrating the extra spread of the *t* distribution. Looking at Table B.3 it can also be seen that as the degrees of freedom increase the *t* distribution becomes closer to the normal distribution, and that at about 60 degrees of freedom, for instance, the values tabulated are indeed fairly close to

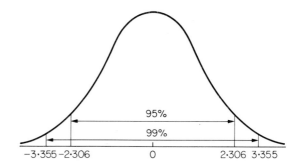

Fig. 4.2. The Student's *t* distribution with 8 degrees of freedom.

those given for the normal distribution. (The entry for degrees of freedom equal to ∞ refers to an infinite number of degrees of freedom when the t distribution and standard normal distribution coincide exactly.)

4.7 Confidence intervals for a mean using the t distribution

It was explained in the last section that when the population standard deviation is not available the sample standard deviation may be used in calculating confidence intervals provided that the t distribution is employed instead of the normal distribution. An alternative derivation of the confidence interval formulae (Eqns. 4.2 and 4.3) is to note that the standardized variable

$$z = \frac{\bar{x} - \mu}{\sigma/\sqrt{n}} \tag{4.5}$$

with the usual notation has a standard normal distribution. (See Eqn. 3.5 where the standard deviation of the sampling distribution of the mean is given by $\sigma/\sqrt{n}$.) Since 95% of the time z lies between $\pm 1\cdot96$, this can be reformulated to give the 95% confidence interval for μ as

$$\bar{x} \pm 1\cdot96\ \sigma/\sqrt{n} \tag{4.3}$$

which is the equation obtained before. Now, Student showed that

$$t = \frac{\bar{x} - \mu}{S/\sqrt{n}} \tag{4.6}$$

had a t distribution with $n - 1$ degrees of freedom, where $\bar{x}$ is the sample mean, μ is the population mean, S is the sample standard deviation and n is the sample size. (The degrees of freedom for the t distribution relate to the degrees of freedom for the sample estimate of the standard error. Since this is based on the sample variance, $n - 1$ d.f. are used.) From this a 95% confidence interval for the mean can be calculated as

$$\bar{x} \pm t_{\mathrm{c}}\ S/\sqrt{n} \tag{4.7}$$

where t_{c} is the t value on $n - 1$ degrees of freedom which cuts off 5% of the area in the two tails of the distribution (e.g. for d.f. $= 8$, $t_{\mathrm{c}} = 2\cdot306$). It can be seen that because the t distribution is more spread out the confidence interval is wider than would be obtained with normal theory when $1\cdot96$ would replace the $2\cdot306$ above. However, for large sample sizes ($n > 60$ is often suggested) the difference between the t value and that for the normal distribution is so small that the latter can be used with very little loss of accuracy.

Take a simple example. A research group studied the age at which nine children with a specific congenital heart disease began to walk. They obtained a mean figure of 12·8 months with a (sample) standard deviation of 2.4 months. What are the 95% and 99% confidence intervals for the mean age of starting to walk in all children affected with this disease? There are 8 degrees of freedom in this problem (one less than the sample size). The t value for a 95% confidence interval is, as noted above, 2·306. Thus, the researchers can be 95% sure that the mean age of walking for such children is

$$12·8 \pm 2·306 \ (2·4/\sqrt{9})$$

or

$$12·8 \pm 1·84$$

that is to say between 10·96 and 14·64 months. The 99% confidence interval is obtained by reading the t value corresponding to 1% of the area in both tails. For 8 degrees of freedom the t value is 3·355 so that the 99% confidence interval is

$$12·8 \pm 3·355 \ (2·4/\sqrt{9})$$

or

$$12·8 \pm 2·68.$$

This interval is, of course, wider than the 95% confidence interval. The quantity $S/\sqrt{n}$ is usually called the standard error, even though it is only an estimate of this quantity which is only known precisely when the population standard deviation σ is itself known. The formulae above (Eqns. 4.3 and 4.7) for the confidence interval for a mean both rely on the assumption that the population from which the sample was taken is not too skew, at least for small sample sizes. This must be checked on the sample data and if necessary a suitable transformation should be employed to reduce skewness (see Section 1.7). The confidence limits are calculated using the transformed data, and then converted back to the original scale. Section C.2 in Appendix C summarizes the calculations of confidence intervals for means in the one-sample situation.

4.8 Confidence intervals for a proportion using the binomial or normal distribution

In the previous sections the calculation of a confidence interval for an unknown population mean on the basis of sample statistics has been described. This method arose from a consideration of the sampling distribution of the mean, which was the frequency distribution of all possible means in samples of a particular size drawn from the parent or underlying population whose mean was being estimated. The standard error of the mean was defined as the standard deviation of this sampling distribution. In fact, any statistic calculated from a sample has a sampling distribution. The mean of this distribution is usually the population value of the specified statistic, and its standard deviation is called the standard error of the statistic and can be determined from theoretical considerations.

A parameter often of great interest in a population is the proportion of events or individuals with a given characteristic (e.g. the proportion of deaths due to coronary heart disease; the proportion of smokers among patients with a particular disease). As usual, the aim is to estimate a population proportion, denoted π (pi — the greek letter 'p'), on the basis of the proportion p observed in a sample sized n. As a practical example suppose that 23 histology slides of a sample of 40 were positive for a particular cancer. The sample proportion is $23/40 = 0.5750$ and a confidence interval for the population proportion of positive slides is required. If the population proportion is π then the proportion of positive slides in repeated samples of a given size has what is called a *binomial distribution*. The sampling distribution of a proportion is binomial just as the sampling distribution of the mean is normal.

The exact confidence limits for a proportion can be estimated from rather complex formulae based on the binomial distribution but Table B.11 in Appendix B gives the exact 95% and 99% confidence limits for all possible proportions in sample sizes ranging from $n = 2$ to $n = 75$. It saves confusion if all calculations on proportions are based on the decimal representation rather than on the percentage, which is the proportion multiplied by 100. Confidence limits for proportions are then transformed to percentages by multiplying the limits by 100.

The table is straightforward to use. If the observed number of events or units with a particular characteristic in a sample size n is x, then the sample proportion is $p = x/n$. The table is consulted for the sample size (n) at the top of the leftmost column, and the observed number of events (x) in the next column. The third column gives the proportion of events (p) and the next two columns give the lower (p_l) and upper (p_u) 95% confidence limits for the population proportion. The final two columns give the 99% limits.

To calculate the confidence intervals in the histology example look up the table under $n = 40$. For $x = 23$ the proportion of positive slides is given as 0.5750, with a 95% confidence interval running from 0.4089 to 0.7296. On the basis of this sample of 40 slides, one can be 95% confident that the true percentage of positive slides in the population from which the sample was taken is between 40.89% and 72.96%. The 99% confidence interval is from 36.26% to 76.92%.

Table B.11 gives exact confidence intervals for proportions based on the binomial distribution for sample sizes up to 100. However approximate confidence intervals can be calculated from a simple formula in many situations. It so happens that as n (the sample size) increases, the binomial distribution approaches the normal distribution leading to what is called the normal approximation to the binomial. This holds so long as $n(\pi)$ and $n(1 - \pi)$ are both greater than 5, where n is the sample size and π is the proportion of units in the population with the required characteristic. Under these conditions, the sampling distribution of the proportion of individuals with the characteristic, in repeated samples sized n, is normal, with mean equal to the population parameter π and standard deviation (called the *standard error of the proportion*) equal to $\sqrt{\pi(1-\pi)/n}$. Whereas with means

$$SE(\bar{x}) = \sigma/\sqrt{n}, \tag{4.1}$$

for sample proportions

$$SE(p) = \sqrt{\pi(1-\pi)/n} \tag{4.8}$$

where $SE(p)$ is the standard error of a proportion. Using arguments similar to those in the last section, it can be said that

$$z = \frac{p-\pi}{\sqrt{\pi(1-\pi)/n}} = \frac{p-\pi}{SE(p)} \tag{4.9}$$

has a standard normal distribution, where p is the proportion of individuals with the characteristic in the sample, π is the unknown proportion in the population which is to be estimated and n, as usual, is the sample size.*

In practice, of course, π is being estimated, so that the standard error of the proportion must be approximated by

$$SE(p) \approx \sqrt{\frac{p(1-p)}{n}} \tag{4.10}$$

where the symbol $\approx$ is interpreted as approximately equal to, and p is the proportion observed in the sample. Even though this approximation is used for the standard error of a proportion, tables of the normal distribution are still used for calculating confidence intervals.

A 95% confidence interval for a proportion is then given by (using the properties of the normal distribution)

$$p \pm 1{\cdot}96\ SE(p) \tag{4.11}$$

or

$$p \pm 1{\cdot}96\ \sqrt{\frac{p(1-p)}{n}} \tag{4.12}$$

and a 99% confidence interval is given by

$$p \pm 2{\cdot}576\ SE(p). \tag{4.13}$$

---

* Some authors suggest that for $n\pi$ and $n(1-\pi)$ fairly close to 5 what is called the *continuity correction* should be employed in this formulation. This is, basically, a correction to allow for the fact that a discrete distribution (the binomial) is being approximated by a continuous distribution (the normal). The continuity correction is not used in this text.

The adequacy of the normal approximation is based on the value of the unknown population proportion π. In practice, since this is not known, the lower and upper confidence limits obtained with the normal approximation can be employed as a guide to the validity of the approximation instead. If these are denoted p_l and p_u respectively then the approximation is quite acceptable as long as all the following quantities are greater than 5: np_l, $n(1 - p_l)$, np_u and $n(1 - p_u)$. Even if the normal approximation is valid it will be more convenient and more accurate to use Table B.11 for samples sized 75 or less.

Taking the histology slide example the normal approximation for the 95% confidence interval is given by

$$0.5750 \pm 1.96 \sqrt{[(0.575)(0.425)/40]} = 0.5750 \pm 0.1532$$

which is from 0.4218 to 0.7282. These are quite close to the exact limits of 0.4089 and 0.7296 since the conditions for using the approximation hold. Section C.3, Appendix C summarizes the calculations of confidence intervals for proportions in the one sample situation.

4.9 Confidence intervals for a count or rate using the Poisson or normal distribution

The sampling distributions of means and proportions have been discussed in previous sections, and here the sampling distribution of counts is considered. This will allow confidence interval calculations for both counts and rates.

If one is counting the number of events over a period of time (number of attacks of angina in an individual over a 4-week period for instance) or the number of items distributed in space (bacterial colonies on a petri dish), the number of events or items will have a Poisson distribution (named after a French mathematician) under certain well-defined conditions, i.e. the sampling distribution of the count will be Poisson. This will happen only if the events or units have a random distribution and occur independently of each other.

Suppose that a patient is observed to have 18 attacks of angina over a 12-week period. This can be considered a sample in time of a 12-week period in the patient's history. Assuming that anginal attacks are random and independent (i.e. that one attack does not make the patient more liable to further attacks, or to the next attack being close in time to the initial one), what is the underlying or true number of anginal attacks per 12 weeks for this patient? In other words an estimate of the population number of anginal attacks per 12 weeks is required.

If the underlying number of anginal attacks in a 12-week period is μ (μ in this section denotes the number of attacks in a given period in the population and is not the population mean of a quantitative variable), then the number of attacks that would be observed in different periods of 12 weeks has a Poisson distribution with a mean of μ and a standard deviation of $\sqrt{\mu}$. In other words the sampling distribution of a count is Poisson with a mean equal to the population value and a standard error equal to its square root. If a variable has a Poisson distribution its variance is always equal to its mean, and this is one of the distinguishing features of the distribution.

Again, rather than detailing the somewhat complex calculations required for confidence intervals based on the Poisson distribution, Table B.12 in Appendix B gives the exact 95% and 99% confidence intervals for a count based on such calculations. Note that the confidence interval is calculated for a count in a given period, and the size of the period is irrelevant to the calculation. The count actually observed (not a figure converted to a count per week or whatever) must be used in the calculations. The table gives the observed count (denoted x) on the left-hand side ranging from zero to 100, and the 95% and 99% lower (x_l) and upper (x_u) confidence limits for that count. For the observed count of 18 anginal attacks in the example, the 95% confidence interval as given in the table is from 10·668 to 28·448. At a 95% level of confidence the underlying number of anginal attacks (in a 12-week period) is between 10·7 and 28·4.

When the count is large a normal approximation to the Poisson distribution is also available and the sampling distribution of the number of events or counts is normal with mean μ and standard deviation (the standard error for a count) $\sqrt{\mu}$. On this basis if x is an observed count the 95% confidence interval for the number of counts is given by

$$x \pm 1\cdot96 \sqrt{x}. \qquad (4.14)$$

Again this formula does not use the continuity correction and is only useful for large counts. Applying this to the angina example, a 95% confidence interval of

$$18 \pm 1\cdot96 \sqrt{18} \text{ or } 18 \pm 8\cdot316$$

which is from 9·684 to 26·316, is obtained. This is not a good approximation to the true interval of 10·668 to 28·448 because of the small count of 18. If the approximation is only used for counts above 100 (using Table B.12 for lower sample sizes), then the formula is reasonably accurate.

Although the discussion so far has been in terms of a count over a period of time, exactly the same principles hold if a count is made in a region of space. Suppose that a sample from a well-mixed suspension of live organisms were placed on a suitable nutrient in a petri dish, and the resulting number of bacterial colonies were counted. The count could be expected to follow a Poisson distribution and a confidence interval could be calculated for the number of colonies.

If one wished to express a count as a rate (e.g. the 18 anginal attacks in 12 weeks as a rate of 1.5 per week) the confidence limits for the observed count should be calculated and then converted to the rate. Using the exact limits, the

95% confidence interval for the weekly anginal rate is from 0·89 (10·688/12) to 2·37 (28·448/12) per week. Often in a follow-up study (see Chapter 10) an annual disease incidence rate is calculated by dividing the number of observed cases by the person-years of follow-up, or person-years at risk. (A person-year of follow-up is one person followed for one year; 10 person-years of follow-up could be achieved by following 10 persons for one year each, five persons for 2 years each, or one person for 10 years.) A confidence interval for such a rate is obtained by calculating the confidence limits for the number of cases and dividing these by the total person-years. This is also a useful approach for rates in vital statistics (see Chapter 13).

It is easy, using the normal approximation, to obtain a direct expression for the confidence interval for a rate. If the rate is denoted $r = x/\text{PYRS}$ where x is the number of observed cases and PYRS is the person-years at risk or of follow-up, then substituting this into Eqn. 4.14 gives

$$r \pm 1 \cdot 96 \sqrt{\frac{r}{\text{PYRS}}} \qquad (4.15)$$

as a 95% confidence for a rate based on the normal approximation to the Poisson distribution. Note that in this formula the rate must be expressed in the same units as the PYRS figure (e.g. if the rate is per 1000 person-years then PYRS should be given in thousands.)

The astute reader will note that the concept of a proportion is very similar to that of a rate, and that in vital statistics one talks about, for example, an annual death rate calculated as the number of deaths in a year divided by the total population. Without going into detail concerning the subtle distinctions between a rate and a proportion, it is easily shown that for a very small proportion the binomial distribution is approximated by the Poisson distribution. Equation 4.12 gave the 95% confidence interval for a proportion (using the normal approximation) as

$$p \pm 1 \cdot 96 \sqrt{\frac{p\,(1-p)}{n}}.$$

Now *if p* is very small, $1 - p$ in the expression above will be near to unity and the formula above becomes

$$p \pm 1 \cdot 96 \sqrt{\frac{p}{n}}$$

If the proportion p is based on x events out of a sample size of n ($p = x/n$) this formulation for the confidence interval of a small proportion is seen to be identical to Eqn. 4.15 obtained for a rate, showing the equivalence of the binomial to the Poisson approach in this case. Section C.4 in Appendix C summarizes the calculation of confidence intervals for counts and rates.

4.10 Summary

This chapter concentrated on the estimation of population parameters using statistics calculated on a single sample from the population. It was explained how theoretical considerations led to the concept of a sampling distribution of a statistic, which was the distribution of that statistic in repeated samples from a particular population. The important distinction between the standard error of the mean and the standard deviation was emphasized and the Student's t distribution was introduced. The estimation of confidence intervals was explained for means, proportions, counts and rates. The confidence interval is a range which, at a specified level of probability, is expected to contain the population parameter being estimated. If a normal distribution approximates the sampling distribution of a statistic a 95% confidence interval is given by

$$\text{statistic} \pm 1{\cdot}96 \text{ SE (statistic)}.$$

Table 4.1 summarizes the formulae for the situations considered.

Table 4.1. Summary of confidence intervals for a single parameter

Parameter	Confidence interval	(Eqn. no.)
Mean		
σ known	$\bar{x} \pm z_c\, \sigma/\sqrt{n}$	(4.3)
σ unknown	$\bar{x} \pm t_c\, S/\sqrt{n}$	(4.7)
Proportion	$p \pm z_c \sqrt{\dfrac{p\,(1-p)}{n}}$	(4.12)
Count	$x \pm z_c \sqrt{x}$	(4.14)
Rate	$r \pm z_c \sqrt{\dfrac{r}{\text{PYRS}}}$	(4.15)

The following chapter presents a non-mathematical introduction to the second area of statistical inference, that of hypothesis testing which, although distinct from, is closely related to the estimation of population parameters by confidence intervals.

5

Hypothesis Testing: Introduction to Statistical Tests of Significance

5.1 Introduction

In the previous chapter, the problems of estimating a population parameter using the information contained in a sample from that population were discussed. It was seen that confidence intervals provide a technique whereby it is possible to simultaneously express the degree of reliance and the degree of accuracy with which a sample result can be said to represent the true situation in a population. Although the confidence interval approach is gaining popularity in medical applications statistical inference is often carried out by hypothesis tests (significance tests) rather than by estimation via confidence intervals. The basic situation is the same — discovering something about populations on the basis of sampling — but the approach, although complementary, is quite different. This chapter introduces some of the concepts underlying hypothesis testing in the context of a specific clinical example, but avoids mathematical manipulations. The succeeding chapters examine hypothesis tests in more detail, and flesh out the skeleton introduced here. The concepts underlying hypothesis tests are central to a full understanding of the use of statistics in medicine, and the concept is far more general than the application of any specific test to a given set of data.

Prerequisites for this chapter include a knowledge of descriptive statistics and an acquaintance with the distinctions between samples and populations. A particular example will be taken to illustrate some of the ideas involved.

5.2 The example

A research group is interested in comparing the effects, on 5-year survival in breast cancer patients, of two different drug preparations, drug B, which is the standard therapy, and drug A which is potentially useful. They decide to put 25 patients on each of the two treatments and to follow the patients for 5 years to determine their mortality.

As described, such a study would fit into the category of a clinical trial, but as is seen in Chapter 11, the proper setting up of a clinical trial is more complex than outlined above. Postponing more detailed discussion to that chapter, however, assume for the moment that the two groups of patients (25 on drug A and 25 on

Table 5.1. Five-year outcome in a trial comparing drugs A and B

Treatment	Alive	Dead	Total
Drug A	17 (68·0%)	8 (32·0%)	25 (100·0%)
Drug B	12 (48·0%)	13 (52·0%)	25 (100·0%)

drug B) are similar as regards all factors which might affect overall mortality, such as age or the severity of their disease. The only factor which differentiates the two groups is assumed to be the particular treatment which they have been given. On this basis, a comparison between the two groups should be valid in determining the drug effects.

Suppose now, that at the end of the study the results shown in Table 5.1 are obtained. The 5-year survival rate with drug A is 68% compared to only 48% with the standard therapy, drug B. What can be concluded about the effects of the two drugs?

5.3 Medical importance

The first step in a statistical analysis of a particular study is to examine the results. As already seen in the example, the absolute survival advantage of drug A-treated patients over drug B-treated patients was 20% (68% − 48%). Examining the results of any study requires, usually, only the application of the simple methods of descriptive statistics and is a task which may be carried out with an absolute minimum of specialist statistical knowledge. Amazing as it may seem however, this task is sometimes overlooked by a researcher who mistakenly thinks that a statistical analysis in the form of a hypothesis test (considered in the next section) is all that is required. This point cannot be emphasized too strongly; examination of results, in terms of means, proportions, percentages or whatever, is a prerequisite for any formal statistical analysis.

In examining the results, the researcher must ask a question akin to 'Are my results medically important?' By this is meant − 'Do the results as they stand suggest that an important new finding has emerged that will perhaps change medical practice, or alter one's view of a disease process, or have a major impact of some sort?' Certainly a difference in mortality of 20%, as in the example above, would seem to be an important finding. On the other hand, if the two mortality rates had been 48% and 52% respectively, the medical importance of the finding would be questionable, since the difference between the two treatments is so small. The question of what size of result can be considered important however is one for the clinician and practising doctor and not for the statistician to answer. If the results of a particular study are not deemed to be medically important, little more can be done. No amount of mathematical or statistical manipulation can make a silk purse out of a sow's ear. A study, for instance, that shows only a very small difference between two groups in the variable under examination is of little interest unless it is carried out to show the equivalence of the groups in the first place. Such is not usually the case.

If the results of a particular study do seem medically important, then further analysis leading to a formal statistical hypothesis test must be performed. The purpose of such a test is to enable a judgement to be made on whether reliance can be placed on the (important) result obtained. The precise form of this hypothesis test will depend on, among other things: the sample size in the study, the number of groups being compared, how the groups were formed, the scale of measurement of the variable under analysis and the precise hypothesis being tested. Rather than examining at this stage the particular hypothesis tests which might be appropriate for the data in the above example, a more conceptual approach to the problem is now considered.

5.4 The null hypothesis

The medical hypothesis which the research group wish to test in the example is that in terms of 5-year survival drug A is better than drug B. There is no doubt, of course, that in the patients studied drug A is indeed better, but the basic question is whether or not it is legitimate to extrapolate from the particular situation of these 50 patients to the general situation of all patients. The problem is one of statistical inference and requires a decision to be made concerning drug effectiveness on the basis of a small group of patients.

The notion of making a decision on the basis of a sample, and thus on incomplete evidence, is not unique to statistics. The holding of an examination to decide if an individual should obtain a degree is but one example. Performance in a particular examination will not necessarily reflect true ability — the person may have an off-day; the questions asked may be in his/her one weak area — or, of course, the opposite could occur with a bit of luck (chance). The decision however is made on the basis of the examination taken. The decision may be fair or it may not and an element of doubt always remains. This element of doubt is the price paid for incomplete information, and is the only reason that statisticians have a part to play in medical, or any other, research.

The first step in performing a statistical hypothesis test is to reformulate the medical hypothesis. In many situations, it is far easier to disprove a proposition than to prove it. For instance, to prove that (if it were true) all cows were black would require an examination of every cow in the world, while one brown cow disproves the statement immediately. In branches of mathematics, such as geometry, many proofs commence with the supposition that the required result is not true.

When a consequent absurdity occurs the supposition is rejected and the result required is thus proved. In statistical analysis, a very similar approach is used. Rather than trying to 'prove' the medical hypothesis (drug A is better than drug B) an attempt is made to 'disprove' the hypothesis that drug A is the same as drug B. This reformulation to what is essentially a negative hypothesis is central to an understanding of hypothesis tests. In fact, the reformulated hypothesis is generally referred to as a *null hypothesis* and in most cases the researcher wants to disprove or reject it. In general, such hypotheses refer to no differences being present in groups being compared. Although in many situations the null hypothesis may not be explicitly stated, it is the cornerstone of every statistical test.

Having reformulated the original medical hypothesis in the form of a null hypothesis, the further premise that it can be 'proved' or 'disproved' in some way must be examined. Unfortunately real life is not like geometry, and when dealing with biological variability and the uncertainty introduced by not being able to study everybody, proof or disproof of a proposition can never be absolute. This is why rejection or acceptance of a null hypothesis is referred to, rather than the proof or disproof of it. In fact, for reasons discussed later, it is preferable to refer to the non-rejection of a null hypothesis rather than to its acceptance.

An interesting analogy may be drawn with the judicial process. An individual is assumed innocent until proved guilty. The assumption of innocence corresponds to the null hypothesis and 'proven guilty' (which corresponds to rejection of this hypothesis) does not refer to absolute truth but to the decision (possibly fallible) of a jury on the basis of the (possibly incomplete) evidence presented. Absolute truth is no more discernible in statistics than in a court of law.

The first step then in hypothesis testing requires that a hypothesis of medical interest must be reformulated into a null hypothesis which, on the basis of the results of a particular study, will or will not be rejected, with a margin of error in whatever conclusion is reached.

A null hypothesis always makes a statement about reality, or in more technical terms, about a population or populations. The results of a study are based on a subset of (or sample from) the population(s) of interest. In medical situations, however, it is sometimes very difficult to identify the precise population(s) referred to in a null hypothesis, as in many situations the study groups are not random samples from fully specifiable populations. In the example, the null hypothesis that drug A has the same effect on 5-year survival as drug B refers, in a vague sense, to all patients similar to those included in the study. In some way, however, the results are important only insofar as they can be applied to patients in the future, while the study groups themselves are based on patients already diagnosed and treated in the past. As is discussed in Chapter 11, hypothesis testing in the context of a clinical trial such as this requires a slight alteration in the interpretation of the null hypothesis, but for clarity at this point it will be assumed that the two treated groups (drug A and drug B) are representative of two populations. The 25 persons on drug B are representative of the population of all patients with breast cancer if they had all been given the standard treatment, and the 25 persons on drug A are representative of the population of patients if they had all been treated with that particular drug. The fact that the populations do not exist in reality does not detract from the approach, and the conclusion of the study will relate to the question — 'What would happen if all patients were treated with either one of the preparations?'

The above discussion may seem somewhat convoluted, but it is important to realize that the results of any study are useful only insofar as they can be generalized and that for statistical analysis the existence of certain populations may have to be postulated for valid application of the techniques.

5.5 Testing the hypothesis

Figure 5.1 illustrates the two states of reality referred to in the hypotheses. Reality, according to the null hypothesis, is that the two drugs are equivalent (in terms of 5-year survival). Corresponding to any null hypothesis there is always an alternative hypothesis which includes all possible realities not included in the null hypothesis itself. In this example, reality according to the alternative hypothesis is that drugs A and B have different effects.

Of course, it can never be known what actually corresponds to reality, and the whole purpose of hypothesis testing is to enable a decision to be taken as to which of the two alternatives (a null hypothesis or the alternative hypothesis) should be

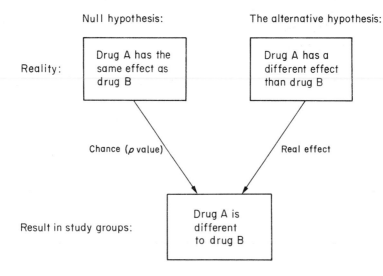

Fig. 5.1. Reality and results in hypothesis testing.

decided upon. Important results, of course, immediately suggest that the alternative hypothesis is more tenable than the null hypothesis (which states there is no difference between the two groups). The main problem however is whether or not enough reliance can be placed on the results to actually reach such a conclusion. The question which should be asked is whether or not the results are spurious (due to chance and sampling variation) or whether they reflect a real difference between the effects of the two drugs. What is meant by spurious is best illustrated by examination of Table 5.2. This shows the number of heads and tails obtained by tossing a 50p coin and a 10p coin 25 times each. The figures are identical to those obtained in the clinical trial example (Table 5.1) with the coins replacing the two treatments and heads and tails replacing the outcomes of 'alive' and 'dead'.

Because the two coins were unbiased, a large number of tosses would in the long run have resulted in 50% tails (approximately). The results in Table 5.2 did, however, actually occur. Knowing how the results were obtained, it can be said with hindsight that the percentages of heads and tails do not indicate differences between the two coins and in that sense it may be said that the observed result is spurious or due to chance. Since the figures obtained in the clinical trial are, however, identical to those of the coin-tossing experiment it can only be concluded that they can throw no light on the efficacy of the drugs in question and that interpretation of the results is difficult. Drug A could be better than drug B, but it could also have an identical effect. In statistical terms, there is no firm evidence to reject the (null) hypothesis that the two drugs are the same.

As well as illustrating the two possible states of reality, Fig. 5.1 also shows the sample results and how they might be achieved. If the null hypothesis were true it would be expected that the results in the two groups would be fairly close, and if it were false the observed results would be expected to reflect the true actions of the drugs. It is, of course, necessary to work backwards from the results to reality. If there is a large (important) difference between the groups then either the null hypothesis is false, or it is true, and, in the latter case, sampling variation is the explanation for the observed spurious result. Hypothesis testing provides a method whereby it is possible to differentiate between these two alternatives.

The approach taken is to calculate (as described in the next chapter) the probability of obtaining the observed result or one even more at variance with the null hypothesis if, in fact, the null hypothesis were true. In the example, the

Table 5.2. Results of tossing two coins 25 times each

Coins	Heads	Tails	Total
10p	17 (68·0%)	8 (32·0%)	25 (100·0%)
50p	12 (48·0%)	13 (52·0%)	25 (100·0%)

probability of getting a mortality difference between drugs A and B of 20% or greater, in a study of two groups of 25 patients on two similar drugs, is calculated. If the size of this probability is large (often arbitrarily set at 5% or greater), it is accepted that the result could be spurious and due to chance and that, therefore, the null hypothesis cannot be rejected. In the example, it was seen that the results of the trial could have been obtained in practice by tossing two coins, and it might therefore be predicted that there is a fairly large probability of this result being spurious. (The actual probability is, in fact, greater than 10%.)

If, on the other hand, the magnitude of this probability is small, it may be decided that, since the result is unusual, there is evidence to reject the null hypothesis and to accept the alternative hypothesis. Of course, to reject the null hypothesis could be wrong, but the smaller the calculated probability, the less the chance of making a wrong decision. Going back to the analogy with the judicial process, the jury must decide whether the evidence (corresponding to the observed result) is consistent with the accused being innocent (the null hypothesis). If the evidence is such that it is difficult to explain its existence if the person is innocent, then the jury will probably declare a verdict of guilty (rejecting the null hypothesis).

It has already been pointed out that when the probability of a spurious result is large, it is not possible to distinguish between the realities postulated by the null and alternative hypotheses (between spurious and real results). Because of this ambiguity the statement 'do not reject the null hypothesis' is generally used instead of the clearer 'accept the null hypothesis'. This corresponds to the possible judicial verdict in Scottish law of 'not proven' rather than 'not guilty'. Rejection or non-rejection of a null hypothesis depends on the magnitude of the probability of getting the observed result, or one even more discordant, if the null hypothesis were true. If the probability is small, the null hypothesis is rejected and the alternative hypothesis accepted. The value for this probability is often called the p value for the significance test. The purpose of every statistical hypothesis test is to enable calculation of a p value under a specified null hypothesis and, in a sense, it is far more important to understand the meaning of a p value than to know how to calculate it. This p should not be confused with the p used in the last chapter to denote a sample proportion.

The rule of thumb mentioned above, i.e. that a value of p less than 5% ($p < 0.05$) leads to a rejection of the null hypothesis, is fairly arbitrary but universally used. Cut-off points other than 5% can be taken and whichever is chosen is called the significance level of the test. Sometimes, a significance level of 1% is taken, in which case the p value (chance of a spurious result) must be less than 1% before the null hypothesis can be rejected. The smaller the p value, the more reliance can be placed on the sample results as reflecting reality, but when a p value very close to 5% is calculated it is obviously nonsense to reject a null hypothesis at, say, a *p* of 4·99% and to fail to reject it at a *p* value of 5·01%. The 5% level is purely a guideline.

In a statistical analysis, rejection of a null hypothesis is often referred to as a *significant result*. Thus, a significant result is a result which is not likely to have occurred by chance. Although the significance level should be stated explicitly, usage often takes a 'significant result' to imply the rejection of a null hypothesis at a 5% level and a 'highly significant result' to imply a 1% level of significance. A non-significant result means that the null hypothesis is not rejected (usually with $p > 5\%$). Table 5.3 lists the various meanings or descriptions which could be put on a significant result.

For those persons unhappy about postulated populations to which the null hypothesis refers, an alternative interpretation of hypothesis tests can be suggested. As has been said, the reason for any statistical analysis in the first place is the problem of sampling variation or the uncertainty introduced into results due to the small number of subjects studied. If any given study was repeated on millions of subjects and showed the same results as obtained on the smaller, actual number studied, no statistical analysis would be necessary, since (apart from problems due to bad study design or implementation) the results would speak for themselves. In this light, a significant result can be interpreted to mean that if large numbers were, in fact, studied, similar results to those obtained in the smaller study actually carried out would be expected. A non-significant result, on the other hand, would mean that if a study were to be performed on a very large number of subjects, there could be no certainty that the actual sample results would be observed in the larger study. For instance, if the two coins were tossed millions of times, the percentage of tails in each coin would be very close to 50%, unlike the percentages obtained in the small number of tosses in the example.

At this point, the difference between a statistically significant result and a medically important result must be reiterated. Medical importance relates to the magnitude of the observed effect while significance refers to the statistical question of whether or not the result is spurious. What is ideal in any situation is an

Table 5.3. Equivalent descriptions of a statistically significant result

Reject the null hypothesis
Accept the alternative hypothesis
There is strong evidence to doubt the null hypothesis
The chance of the result being spurious is small
$\quad p < 5\%$ or $p < 0.05$
The observed result is not compatible with the null hypothesis
Sampling variation is not sufficient to explain the observed result
Result is unlikely to be due to chance

important result that is also significant. An important result that is non-significant (as in the example discussed above) may provide some grounds for optimism but no reliance may be placed on the results. Non-important results, statistically significant (as they can be) or not, usually give very little information to the researcher.

5.6 Summary

The general form of a hypothesis or significance test thus runs as follows: a null hypothesis is postulated, and it is usually hoped to be able to reject it, the results of the particular study are examined and, if medically important, are subjected to further mathematical manipulation which depends on the type of study, the measurements made and other relevant factors. This eventually leads to the calculation of a p value, which is the probability of the observed results (or results even more at variance with the null hypothesis) being spurious if the null hypothesis were true in the first place. If the p value is small (usually with $p < 5\%$), the null hypothesis is rejected and the result declared statistically significant. If the p value is large, it is concluded that the result is non-significant, and that no decision can be made about whether or not there is a real effect. Therefore, the null hypothesis cannot be rejected.

The following chapter considers hypothesis testing from a more mathematical viewpoint, examining one specific test in some detail. In particular, points not considered above, relating to the interpretation and further examination of non-significant results and different forms of the null hypothesis, are considered.

6

Hypothesis Testing: General Principles and One-Sample Tests for Means, Proportions, Counts and Rates

6.1 Introduction

In the previous chapter, some of the concepts underlying *hypothesis testing* or, as it is often called, significance testing were considered. The null hypothesis was introduced in the context of a specific example and the important distinction between medical importance (based on the magnitude of an observed result) and statistical significance (based on a *p* value) was made. In this chapter it is described how the *p* value is calculated in a particular situation, and some of the concepts underlying this approach to statistical analysis are considered in more detail. The problems of negative results and appropriate sample sizes are also raised.

The examples considered are based on hypotheses concerning population parameters in studies consisting of one sample only, although most practical applications of hypothesis testing in medical statistics involve two samples. However, at this stage, the theory is best illustrated in the one-sample situation.

Prerequisites for this chapter, apart from the previous chapter, include knowledge of the sampling distributions of means, proportions and counts.

6.2 The null and alternative hypotheses

The example which is taken has already been considered in Chapter 4 in the context of statistical estimation using confidence intervals. A sample of 100 lung cancer patients on a new drug are observed to have a mean survival of 27·5 months with a standard deviation of 25·0 months. Suppose now, that from previous studies it is known that the mean survival of such patients (before the new drug was introduced) is 22·2 months. The investigators want to know if, on the basis of these data (the adequacy of which will be discussed in Chapter 11), they can conclude that the new drug prolongs survival.

The investigators' first step is to form a null hypothesis — in this case, stating that the new drug has no effect on survival. This is equivalent to saying that the population mean survival with the new drug is 22·2 months, the same as observed in a large series of patients who did not have this particular treatment. Another way of looking at the null hypothesis is that it states that the 100 patients are a random sample from the population of all lung cancer patients who, because the drug has no effect, have a mean survival of 22·2 months. Notationally, this may be written

$$H_0: \mu_D = 22·2 \text{ months,}$$

where H_0 means 'the null hypothesis is', and μ_D represents the mean survival in the population of patients treated with the new drug.

Having stated the null hypothesis the investigators must then specify what the alternative hypothesis is. Without prior knowledge, they cannot be sure that the new drug does not actually reduce survival, so their alternative hypothesis is that the survival of patients with this drug is different from that of patients not so treated, and

$$H_A: \mu_D \neq 22·2 \text{ months,}$$

where H_A refers to the alternative hypothesis and $\neq$ means 'not equal to'. In most situations in medicine, the alternative hypothesis is stated in this simple way unless prior knowledge outside of the study data suggests otherwise (see below). The alternative hypothesis is vague or diffuse in that all survival times not equal to 22·2 months are included. As with the null hypothesis, the alternative hypothesis may be interpreted as implying that the 100 patients were a random sample from a population of treated lung cancer patients whose mean survival was not 22·2 months. Since these 100 patients may have been the only group ever treated on the drug, a slight modification of the theory is required in that they should be considered to be a sample from a hypothetical population of lung cancer patients treated with this drug. The fact that the population only exists in the mind of the investigators does not matter, since the sample was treated and, of course, the inference is being made to a population of potentially treatable patients.

6.3 The significance test

It was said in the last chapter that for a significance test one must calculate the probability (p) that a result, such as the one obtained, or one even more unlikely, could have arisen if the null hypothesis were true. If this probability is less than the significance level, the hypothesis is rejected. This significance level should be stated before the test and it will be assumed here that it is set at the 5% level. The p value for this example can now be calculated.

From the results of Chapter 4, it is known that 95% of all possible sample means, sized $n = 100$, from a population of mean $\mu_D = 22·2$ (as specified by the null hypothesis) and standard deviation $\sigma = 25·0$ will lie between

$$\mu_D \pm 1·96 \, \sigma/\sqrt{n}$$

where $\sigma/\sqrt{n}$ is the standard error of the mean, and is equal to $25/\sqrt{100} = 2{\cdot}5$. (Note that it is assumed that σ is known exactly.) Thus, there is a 95% chance that a particular sample mean will lie between these limits, i.e.

$$22{\cdot}2 \pm 1{\cdot}96 \ (2{\cdot}5)$$
or
$$22{\cdot}2 \pm 4{\cdot}9$$

that is, between 17·3 and 27·1. Alternatively, it could be said that there is only a 5% chance that the mean of such a sample is greater than 27·1 or less than 17·3, or equivalently more than 4·9 months away from the hypothesized mean. (Note that the addition law of probability (see Chapter 3) was used in making this statement.)

Now, the sample mean happens to be 27·5 (5·3 months above the hypothesized mean of 22·2) and thus it may be said that if the null hypothesis were true the chances of getting a sample result more than 5·3 months above or below 22·2 are less than 5%. But by definition this is the p value, so that as a result of the calculation it can now be stated, for this example, that p is less than 5% or $p <$ 0·05. Thus, statistical significance at a 5% level can be declared and the null hypothesis rejected, leading to the conclusion that sampling variation is an unlikely explanation of the observed sample result. In more medically meaningful terms it might be said that the new drug gave a statistically significant increased survival in lung cancer patients compared with that of previously available treatments.

If instead of a 5% level of significance the researchers had decided to declare a significant result only if the p value was less than 1%, they could not have rejected the null hypothesis. Again, using the properties of the normal distribution, it is known that if the null hypothesis were true only 1% of possible sample means would lie outside

$$\mu_D \pm 2{\cdot}576 \ \sigma/\sqrt{n}$$
or
$$22{\cdot}2 \pm 2{\cdot}576 \ (2{\cdot}5)$$

and be less than 15·8 or greater than 28·6 months. The observed sample mean of 27·5 months does not lie outside these limits, and therefore by definition p must be greater than 1%. Thus, the null hypothesis cannot be rejected at a 1% level of significance and a non-significant result must be declared at that level. It can be seen from this that a result which is significant at one level may not be significant at a higher level. (A 1% significance level is usually referred to as a higher significance level than 5%.) To be more certain of the result, a more stringent criterion for rejecting the null hypothesis is necessary. On the other hand, a result which is significant at the 1% level is obviously also significant at the lower 5% level.

Values such as 17·3 and 27·1 as obtained in the example for the 5% significance level are referred to as the *critical values* (lower and upper respectively) for the test. Obviously, they depend on the actual study situation and the chosen significance level. If the test statistic, which for this formulation is the sample mean, falls between the two values, the null hypothesis is accepted at the defined significance level, and the interval from 17·3 to 27·1 is called the acceptance region for the test. The *critical region* for the test comprises all values below and including the lower critical value (17·3) and all values above and including the upper critical value (27·1). If the test statistic falls in the critical region, the null hypothesis can be rejected.

6.4 Relationship with confidence intervals

In the one-sample hypothesis test for a mean it was stated that a result significant at the 5% level would be obtained if the sample mean ($\bar{x} = 27\cdot5$) lay outside the critical values given by

$$\text{Hypothesized mean } \pm 1\cdot96 \text{ standard errors} \tag{6.1}$$

which, in the example, were 17·3 and 27·1. When, in Chapter 4, the estimation of the population mean survival of all lung cancer patients that could have been treated with the new drug was considered, a 95% confidence interval was calculated as (see Eqn. 4.3)

$$\text{Sample mean } \pm 1\cdot96 \text{ standard errors} \tag{6.2}$$

which was from 22·6 to 32·4. This was interpreted to mean that it is 95% certain that the unknown mean survival lies between these values.

It is seen immediately that if the population mean specified by the null hypothesis is outside the 95% confidence interval the sample mean is outside the limits given by Eqn. 6.1 and, thus, an alternative approach to hypothesis testing is to declare a statistically significant result at the 5% level if the hypothesized mean is outside the 95% confidence interval. This is quite logical and in many cases provides an acceptable alternative method of testing hypotheses. Note, however, that the confidence interval approach and the significance test approach are not equivalent in all situations (comparing proportions for instance) and the usual approach for significance testing is that outlined in Section 6.3. To reiterate the distinction, the hypothesis test is performed by seeing if the observed sample mean is further than $\pm1\cdot96$ SE away from the hypothesized mean (Eqn. 6.1). The confidence interval approach, on the other hand, is based on whether or not the hypothesized mean is more than $\pm1\cdot96$ SE away from the sample mean. The two approaches happen to give identical results for the one-sample test given here; but this is not true in general (see Section 6.12 for further discussion).

6.5 One-sided and two-sided tests

The example which has been considered so far of a sample of 100 lung cancer patients has been analysed with a null hypothesis of

$$H_0: \mu_D = 22 \cdot 2 \text{ months}$$

and an alternative hypothesis of

$$H_A: \mu_D \neq 22 \cdot 2 \text{ months.}$$

This alternative hypothesis does not distinguish between the situations where the new drug has a beneficial as opposed to a deleterious effect on survival. Consequently, the criterion for a significant result is whether or not the sample mean is further away from 22·2 months *in either direction* by 1·96 standard errors or 4·9 months. The ± 1·96 SE is based on the areas in both tails of the normal distribution, adding up to the chosen significance level of 5% (see Fig. 6.1). For this reason, the test as described above is referred to as a *two-tailed* or *two-sided* significance test.

The two-sided significance test as outlined is appropriate to most medical applications when the direction of the anticipated results (i.e. greater or less than the value specified by the null hypothesis) cannot be determined beforehand. In the example, for instance, it would be dangerous if the researchers assumed, prior to the study, that the drug could only have a beneficial effect on survival. They were, therefore, correct in using a two-sided test, allowing for either increased or decreased survival compared with the hypothesized population value of 22·2 months. One-sided tests (to be discussed below) may be legitimate, however, when either a result in one particular direction is of no interest to researchers, or they are sure that the true result will be in one direction only.

Suppose that in the general male population the mean cholesterol level is known to be 6·5 mmol/l with a standard deviation of 1·2 mmol/l. If researchers are interested in studying cholesterol levels in male agricultural labourers, and

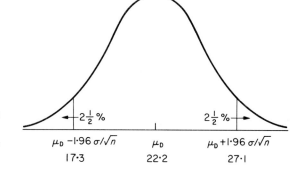

Fig. 6.1. Sampling distribution of the mean for samples sized $n = 100$ taken from a population of mean $\mu_D = 22\cdot2$ and standard deviation $\sigma = 25\cdot0$.

$2\frac{1}{2}\%$ $2\frac{1}{2}\%$

$\mu_D - 1\cdot96\,\sigma/\sqrt{n}$ μ_D $\mu_D + 1\cdot96\,\sigma/\sqrt{n}$

17·3   22·2   27·1

know that whatever the mean level may be it cannot be below 6·5, they might decide on a one-sided significance test for the study. In such a case, the alternative hypothesis would be expressed as

$$H_A: \mu_L > 6·5$$

where μ_L refers to the population mean cholesterol level in agricultural labourers. If the null hypothesis is rejected, only the alternative of mean cholesterol levels being greater than 6·5 mmol/l can be accepted. To continue with this example, suppose that the researchers studied 25 agricultural labourers and discovered a mean cholesterol level of 6·9 mmol/l; what can they conclude? In such a situation, it has been asserted beforehand that observed mean results less than 6·5 are due to chance and, therefore, spurious. It is only of interest to decide if mean values greater than 6·5 could be spurious or if they reflect a real difference in cholesterol levels of agricultural labourers. Again, using the properties of the sampling distribution of the mean, it can be asserted that if the population mean cholesterol of agricultural labourers is 6·5 mmol/l only 5% of possible sample means will lie above

$$\mu_L + 1·645 \; \sigma/\sqrt{n}$$

or
$$6·5 + 1·645 \; (1·2/\sqrt{25}) = 6·89$$

(see Fig. 6.2 and Table B.2).

For a one-sided significance test, there is only one critical value. In this case, with the sample mean as the test statistic, it is the upper critical value of 6·89. The observed result obtained by the researchers was a sample mean of 6·9 mmol/l, which is just above the critical value, so that the null hypothesis may be rejected at a 5% one-sided level of significance. Agricultural labourers may be said to have statistically significant higher cholesterol levels than those observed in the general male population.

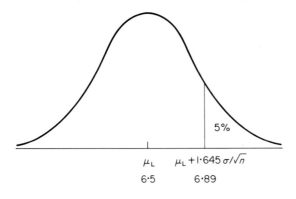

5%

μ_L $\mu_L + 1·645 \, \sigma/\sqrt{n}$
6·5   6·89

Fig. 6.2. Sampling distribution of the mean for samples sized $n = 25$ taken from a population of mean $\mu_L = 6·5$ and standard deviation $\sigma = 1·2$.

Note that if a two-sided test had been specified, the observed mean cholesterol level of agricultural labourers would have had to lie outside

$$\mu_L \pm 1\cdot96 \ \sigma/\sqrt{n}$$

and be greater than or equal to 6·97 or less than or equal to 6·03. The observed sample value of 6·9 mmol/l is inside the acceptance region, so the result would be non-significant for a two-sided significance test. In general, two-sided tests are more conservative than one-sided tests and make it harder to reject the null hypothesis. If in doubt, however, two-sided tests should always be employed, since definite prior information is required before the one-sided test is legitimate. The decision to perform a one-sided test must be made on *a priori* grounds before the data are examined. In medical applications a one-sided test is rarely indicated. Note that if the null hypothesis for the one-sided test had specified a difference in the opposite direction to that discussed above, the plus sign should be replaced by a minus sign and the critical region would be below the point defined by $\mu_L - 1\cdot645 \ \sigma/\sqrt{n}$.

6.6 General structure of a significance test: the one-sample z test for a mean

So far, two examples have been worked through in detail, showing how a particular null hypothesis could be accepted or rejected at a specified significance level. The examples taken dealt with the one-sample situation, and hypotheses concerning means. As has already been stated, the particular hypothesis test used in a specific situation will depend on many factors, but the underlying approach is the same. The one-sample test described in the previous sections will now be reformulated into a format that will be generally applicable in nearly all situations. This is achieved by changing the scale of measurement used in the example. It was seen in Chapter 3 that a normal variable with a given mean and standard deviation can be transformed so that the resulting variable has a mean of 0 and standard deviation of 1. This is achieved by using the equation

$$z = \frac{\text{Value of variable} - \text{mean}}{\text{Standard deviation}}, \tag{6.3}$$

where z is the transformed or standardized variable (see Eqn. 3.5).

In the example of the lung cancer patients, the sampling distribution of the mean under the null hypothesis had a mean of $\mu_D = 22\cdot2$ and a standard deviation (called the standard error of the mean) of 2·5 calculated from $\sigma/\sqrt{n}$ with $\sigma = 25$ and $n = 100$. If instead of looking at the distribution of possible sample means ($\bar{x}$) the distribution of

$$z = \frac{\bar{x} - \mu_D}{\sigma/\sqrt{n}} \tag{6.4}$$

is examined, it could be said that it follows a standard normal distribution of mean 0 and standard deviation 1. Thus, 95% of the time the value of z should lie between $-1\cdot96$ and $+1\cdot96$. In 5% of samples, z, calculated from Eqn. 6.4, would lie outside these limits. The z value corresponding to the sample mean of $27\cdot5$ is

$$z = \frac{27\cdot5 - 22\cdot2}{2\cdot5} = 2\cdot12$$

which is greater than $1\cdot96$. Thus, if the null hypothesis were true, a value of z as extreme as $2\cdot12$ would occur less than 5% of the time, so that the p value for the test is less than 5%. This is, therefore, a significant result and the null hypothesis that a population of patients treated with this new drug would have the same survival as all previous patients can be rejected. This, of course, is the conclusion that was reached before, using a slightly different but equivalent mathematical approach. In general for a one-sample two-sided hypothesis test on a mean, the null hypothesis specifying the mean of a population to be μ_0 (a particular numerical value) may be rejected at a 5% level if

$$z \geqslant 1\cdot96 \text{ or } z \leqslant -1\cdot96$$

where

$$z = \frac{\bar{x} - \mu_0}{\text{SE}\,(\bar{x})} \tag{6.4}$$

is the test statistic for this formulation of the test. Tests which employ the standard normal deviate (z) as a test statistic are generally called z tests. The critical and acceptance regions for this test are illustrated in Fig. 6.3. If $z \geqslant 1\cdot96$ it can be concluded that the true population mean is greater than that specified by

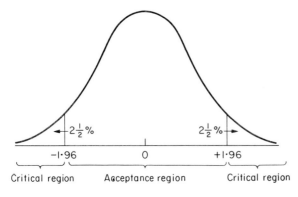

$2\frac{1}{2}\%$ $2\frac{1}{2}\%$

$-1\cdot96$ 0 $+1\cdot96$

Critical region   Acceptance region   Critical region

Fig. 6.3. The standard normal curve showing the critical region for rejection of H_0 and the acceptance region for non-rejection of H_0 for the z test at a two-sided significance level of 5%.

the null hypothesis, while if $z \leqslant -1 \cdot 96$ it can be concluded that the population mean is, in fact, less than that specified by the null hypothesis.

Going back to the properties of the standard normal distribution, it is known that $\pm 1 \cdot 96$ cuts off 5% of the area in the two tails. If a significance test at a 1% level is required $1 \cdot 96$ would be replaced by $2 \cdot 576$ which corresponds to 1% of the area in both tails of a standard normal curve. Similarly, for a one-sided test, where the alternative hypothesis states that the population mean should be greater than that specified by the null hypothesis, a significant result at a 5% level would be obtained if $z \geqslant 1 \cdot 645$ where $1 \cdot 645$ corresponds to a 5% area in the upper tail of the standard normal distribution. Table B.2 in Appendix B gives the critical values for various significance levels of one- and two-sided z tests. The table does not, however, allow for the calculation of an exact p value. In the example, for instance, with a z of $2 \cdot 12$ it was calculated that p was less than 5%. Obviously, if the area in the tails of the distribution outside $\pm 2 \cdot 12$ could be calculated, the exact p value could be calculated. In fact, extensive tables of the standard normal distribution are available which would enable such an exact calculation, but the fact that p is less than 5% is sufficient for most practical purposes. Note that the higher the absolute value of the test statistic, z, the smaller are the corresponding areas in the tails of the distribution and, thus, the greater the level of statistical significance achieved. Often, the results of a significance test may be expressed by giving a range within which the p value lies. Thus, using the table, if z was $1 \cdot 72$, the two-sided p value would be given as greater than $0 \cdot 05$ but less than $0 \cdot 10$. This would be written: $0 \cdot 05 < p < 0 \cdot 10$ which, of course, is not a significant result at the 5% level. The highest significance level achieved should be given if p happens to be less than 5%; thus 'p less than 1%' would be quoted rather than 'p less than 5%'. On the other hand, most researchers just write down NS (for non-significant) for all values of p above 5%, although it might perhaps be better if a more exact range were given. The results of a significance test are often written as $z = 2 \cdot 12$; $p < 0 \cdot 05$ or $z = 1 \cdot 72$; NS. Use of the one-sample z-test is summarized in Section C.2 of Appendix C.

As shall be seen later, many test statistics are also formulated in a similar manner to the one-sample z test as

$$\frac{\text{Sample estimate}}{\text{Standard error of the estimate}} \tag{6.5}$$

and the format of the one-sample z test has general applicability to most statistical tests of significance (see Table 6.1). A null hypothesis is postulated, a significance level is set and a one- or two-tailed test chosen. A test statistic is calculated on the basis of the sample data and null hypothesis. The particular statistic will, of course, depend on the data, the type of study and many other factors, but whatever the statistic, it is known from theoretical considerations to have a

Table 6.1. General structure of a significance test

General test	Example of one-sample z test
State the null hypothesis (H_0)	$\mu_D = 22{\cdot}2$
↓	
Set the significance level	5%
↓	
One- or two-sided test?	Two-sided
↓	
Calculate the test statistic	$z = \dfrac{\bar{x} - \mu_D}{\sigma/\sqrt{n}} = 2{\cdot}12$
↓	
Find the critical values of the distribution of the test statistic for the given (one- or two-sided) significance level	Critical values are $-1{\cdot}96$ and $+1{\cdot}96$
↓	
If the test statistic lies within the acceptance region do not reject H_0. If the statistic lies in the critical region reject H_0 and claim a significant result	Acceptance region: $-1{\cdot}96 < z < 1{\cdot}96$ Critical region: $z \leqslant -1{\cdot}96$ or $z \geqslant 1{\cdot}96$ So H_0 rejected with $z = 2{\cdot}12$

specific distribution if the null hypothesis is true. Tables of this distribution are examined to see if the statistic lies in the acceptance region or inside the critical region for the particular test chosen. The critical region usually corresponds to areas in the tail or tails of the distribution in question. If the test statistic lies within the critical region, a significant result may be claimed. In practice, what is often done is to calculate the highest level of significance for the given statistic without prior setting of the level required. By convention however, a significance level of 5% is usually assumed to be necessary for rejection of the null hypothesis.

6.7 Power considerations, sample size, type I and type II errors

Having looked in detail at the calculation of significance levels and their interpretation in the context of the one-sample z test, the interpretation of non-significant results is now considered. This is sometimes referred to as 'the other side of significance testing' and leads on to the important question of determining adequate sample sizes for specific studies.

The example of the 100 lung cancer patients and the one-sample z test will again be used to illustrate the ideas. As was seen, the level of statistical significance attained depends on the magnitude of the test statistic

$$z = \frac{\bar{x} - \mu_0}{\sigma/\sqrt{n}} \tag{6.4}$$

where $\bar{x}$ is the observed sample mean, μ_0 is the hypothesized mean, σ is the standard deviation in the population, and n is the sample size. The larger the value of z, the greater the level of statistical significance achieved, and the less likelihood that the observed result is spurious. What, then, are the factors which lead to statistically significant results? Firstly, the magnitude of $\bar{x} - \mu_0$ is important; all else being equal, sample means far away from the hypothesized population value will give significant results more readily than values close to it. This is an intuitively obvious result, in the sense that a sample with a mean very much larger (or smaller) than what was hypothesized tends to throw doubt on the hypothesis. So the degree of statistical significance depends on the true (unknown) population value when the null hypothesis is false. The second factor which will affect the likelihood of a significant result is the population standard deviation σ. Statistically significant results are more likely with small values of σ. Again this is reasonable, since if the spread or variation in the population is small it should be easier to detect samples not originating from that population. The third and perhaps most important factor which will determine whether or not significance may be achieved is the sample size, n. For a given observed difference, $\bar{x} - \mu_0$, and given σ, larger sample sizes will more easily give significant results. In fact, it is easily seen that any difference (no matter how small or unimportant) can be made statistically significant if the sample size is large enough. This highlights the distinction made in the last chapter between medically important and statistically significant results, and also justifies the claim that with an important result based on large enough numbers statistical analysis is almost entirely redundant.

From the opposite point of view, a non-significant result can be due to the true population mean lying very near the hypothesized value, too large a spread in the population, too small a sample size or any combination of these three factors. Although illustrated in the context of the one-sample z test, the above points may be taken as being generally applicable to most statistical tests of significance.

Figure 6.4 illustrates the main elements of the decision process involved in hypothesis testing, using the one-sample drug trial as a practical example. On the top of the figure two possible states of 'reality' are shown; either the null hypothesis is true, and the mean survival of patients treated with the drug is 22·2 months, or the null hypothesis is false. On the left side of the figure are noted the two possible decisions which can be made — rejection or acceptance of this null hypothesis. In the body of the figure are the implications of any particular decision for either of the two realities.

If the null hypothesis is true and a non-significant result is obtained everything is fine and the correct decision has been made. If, however, the null hypothesis is true and a significant result is obtained, the decision to reject the hypothesis is incorrect and an error has been made. This form of error is called an alpha (α — the Greek letter 'a') error or type I error. The probability of making a type I

REALITY

	Null hypothesis true	Null hypothesis false (alternative hypothesis true)
	$H_0: \mu_0 = 22 \cdot 2$	$\mu_0 \neq 22 \cdot 2$
Do not reject H_0 (non-significant result)	Correct decision	β or type II error
Reject H_0 (significant result)	α or type I error	Correct decision

DECISION

Fig. 6.4. Type I and type II errors in hypothesis testing.

error, denoted by α, is by definition the probability of rejecting the null hypothesis when it is in fact true. This, of course, is nothing more than the significance level of the test. (Remember — a significant result obtains if, traditionally, p is less than 0·05 and, by definition, p can be less than this value for 5% of the possible samples when the null hypothesis is true.) The p value for any result can be alternatively interpreted as the chance of making a type I or alpha error (see Table 6.2). Returning to Fig. 6.4: if the null hypothesis is false a statistically significant result leads to a correct decision. If, however, in this situation a non-significant result is obtained, a decision error has again been made, and this is called the beta (β — the Greek letter 'b') or type II error. For non-significant results, it is, therefore, necessary to calculate the probability of making this error. It has already been mentioned that a non-significant result should be expressed as a non-rejection of the null hypothesis rather than an acceptance of it since, in this case, the two states of reality cannot be distinguished. The problem is, of course, that the alternative hypothesis (in the example for instance) encompasses every possible mean survival not exactly equal to 22·2 months. If, in fact, the mean population survival of the drug-treated group was 22·3 months (3 days greater than in the group without the drug) it would be technically wrong to fail to reject the null hypothesis. Such an error, however, would not be very important, since an increase of mean survival of this magnitude would be irrelevant in cancer therapy. Obviously, if the true mean survival was as close to 22·2 months as

Table 6.2. Definition of type I and type II errors

α	β
Probability of making a type I error	Probability of making a type II error
Probability of rejecting H_0 when it is true	Probability of not rejecting H_0 when it is false
Significance level of the test	

above, it would be very difficult to obtain a significant result (the sample mean $\bar{x}$ would most likely be very close to the hypothesized mean of 22·2) and there would be a high chance of a beta or type II error. On the other hand, if the true survival was much greater or less than 22·2 the chances of a type II error should decrease. This illustrates one of the important facts concerning type II errors — the chances of their occurrence depend on the true value of the population mean. The actual size of the β probability depends on the overlap between the sampling distributions of the mean under (a) the null hypothesis, and (b) a specific alternative hypothesis for which the type II error is to be calculated. Figure 6.5 shows the sampling distribution of the means for the reality specified by the null hypothesis, and a reality specified by an alternative hypothesis, suggesting a mean drug group survival of 30 months. It has already been shown that the null hypothesis would not be rejected at the 5% level if the sample mean was less than 27·1 months, or did not lie in the shaded area of the upper distribution. If, however, the real population mean was 30·0 months (and thus the null hypothesis was false) a mean value of less than 27·1 could arise in a sample from this population. The probability (denoted β) that it would arise with a consequent type II error is given by the shaded area in the second curve. This can be calculated to be about 0·12 or 12%. The calculations are not detailed in this text.

Figure 6.6 shows a graph of calculated β values for various alternative survival times in the drug-treated population, with a sample size of 100 and a two-sided significance level of 5%. Such a graph is called the *operating characteristic curve* for a test. From this it can be seen that if, for example, the true mean survival is 24 months, then β equals 0·9 and thus there is a 90% chance of making a type II

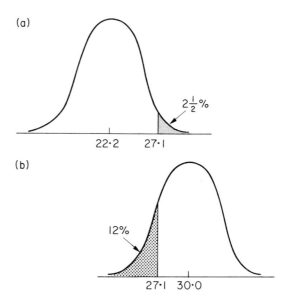

(a)

$2\frac{1}{2}\%$

22·2   27·1

(b)

12%

27·1   30·0

Fig. 6.5. Sampling distributions of the mean for (a) the null hypothesis $\mu_D = 22·2$ and (b) a specific alternative hypothesis $\mu_D = 30·0$.

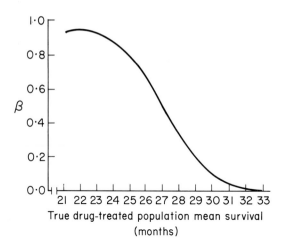

Fig. 6.6. Operating characteristic curve for a two-sided 5% test of significance of the null hypothesis that the mean survival in the treated group is 22·2 months for samples sized 100 and population standard deviation of 25·0 months.

error. For a mean survival of 30 months however, the probability of a type II error reduces, as was said above, to about 12%. Sometimes, the value of $1 - \beta$ is quoted rather than the value of β itself. $1 - \beta$ is called the *power* of the test. For a true mean survival of 30 months, the power of the test is $1 - 0·12 = 0·88$ or 88%. The power of a test increases as the difference between the hypothesized value of the mean and the real value increases, and a high power means a low chance of a type II error, or alternatively, a large chance of detecting (significantly) a particular result.

How, then, can the probability of a type II error be reduced? Looking at Fig. 6.5, it can be seen that there are two main possibilities. Firstly, the significance level could be reduced to greater than 5%, thus increasing the shaded area in the upper curve. This, in turn, will decrease the shaded area in the lower curve, corresponding to the β probability. This is a fairly general result: for a given sample size and a specified difference between the true population mean and the hypothesized mean, increases in α will decrease β and vice versa. What you lose on the roundabout, you gain on the swings. However, since the α value or p value of the test is usually specified beforehand, decreasing the type II error in this manner is not to be encouraged. The other way of reducing β is by reducing the spread of the sampling distribution of the mean, thus reducing the overlap of the two curves. Now, remember that the spread of the sampling distribution of the mean is determined by the standard error of the mean or $\sigma/\sqrt{n}$. The population standard deviation, σ, cannot be controlled, but the sample size can be increased, thus reducing the standard error. This is a second important result: for a given significance level and specified difference between the hypothesized population mean and the true population value, the β error may be reduced by increasing the sample size.

The further analysis required for negative or non-significant results can now be explained. So far, the interdependence of four quantities has been seen — the significance level (α); the probability of a type II error (β); the sample size (n); and the difference between the hypothesized mean μ_0 and that actually obtaining in the population sampled. Given three of these factors, the fourth may be calculated, assuming that the population standard deviation is known.

If the study gives a significant result, then quoting the significance level is sufficient, since it gives the probability of the only error which could have been made — the type I error (see Fig. 6.4). If the study, however, gives a non-significant result at a specified level (usually 5%) the reader should be told what the chances of missing a real result were, i.e. the β probabilities should be presented for a range of possible values for the mean of the population from which the sample was taken. This may show that, in fact, the chances of missing a result where the true mean lay a fair distance from that given by the null hypothesis were quite high, and that from the beginning the study could have been judged inadequate to detect important medical findings. This is often expressed by saying that the power ($1 - \beta$) of the study was too small. With non-significant results the presentation of a confidence interval indicates clearly the precision achieved by a study, and whether the sample size was adequate as determined by the width of the interval.

The usual reason for missing important results is that the sample size is too small, and investigations have shown that many medical studies with non-significant results were too small to detect anything but the most marked departures from the null hypothesis. When the sample size is too small, it is impossible to distinguish between real and spurious results. The solution, of course, is to estimate the required sample at the beginning of a study, in the planning stages. In certain situations this is relatively easy, and Appendix D gives some sample-size formulae which may be useful in certain simple situations. In general, however, professional statistical advice should be obtained at the planning stages to determine how large a study is required. Usually, the requirements needed to calculate a sample size are a specification of the significance level, the chance one is willing to take in making a type II error (β), the size of the effect one does not want to miss (i.e. the magnitude of what would be considered an important result in terms of departure from the null hypothesis) and an estimate of the population variability σ. (This last requirement is not necessary when estimating sample sizes for comparing proportions.) From these factors, a required sample size can usually be calculated. Unfortunately, sample sizes often turn out to be much larger than expected by the investigator, and the final size of the study is often a compromise between the numbers required from the statistical point of view and the practical situation relating to the resources available. In this situation at least, whatever sample size is chosen the investigator can know what the chances are of detecting an important result, and if these prove to be too low the study should probably not be undertaken in the first place.

6.8 The one-sample t test for a mean

So far in this chapter, it has been assumed that the population standard deviation σ is known, and this led to the derivation of the one-sample z test. The other assumptions underlying this test were that a random sample in the population of interest had been taken and that this parent population was not very skewed (see Section 4.4 also). As discussed in Section 4.6 in the context of confidence intervals, the Student's t distribution should be used in place of the normal distribution (z) when the sample standard deviation S is used instead of the population standard deviation σ for sample sizes of less than 60 or so. In this more realistic situation, the appropriate one-sample test statistic is, instead of Eqn. 6.4,

$$t_{n-1} = \frac{\bar{x} - \mu_0}{S/\sqrt{n}} \tag{6.6}$$

where $\bar{x}$ is the sample mean, μ_0 is the hypothesized population mean, n is the sample size and S is the sample standard deviation. The t_{n-1} indicates that it is necessary to look up a table of the t distribution on $n - 1$ degrees of freedom, rather than the table of the normal distribution, for obtaining the critical values. The resulting significance test is called the t test.

The one-sample t test will be illustrated using the example already discussed in Chapter 4. In that example, a researcher studied nine children with a specific congenital heart disease, and found that they started to walk at a mean age of 12·8 months with a standard deviation of 2·4 months. Assume now that normal children are known to start walking at a mean age of 11·4 months. Can the researcher conclude that congenital heart disease delays the age at which children begin to walk? Since the sample size is much less than 60, and only a sample estimate of the standard deviation is available, a t test must be employed. The null hypothesis is that children with congenital heart disease start to walk at a mean age of $\mu_W = 11\cdot4$ months, and a two-sided significance level of 5% is chosen. The test statistic is from Eqn. 6.6

$$t = \frac{12\cdot8 - 11\cdot4}{2\cdot4/\sqrt{9}} = 1\cdot75$$

on 8 degrees of freedom. Looking up Table B.3 for the Student's t distribution, it is seen that the critical values for a two-sided 5% level of significance are $\pm2\cdot306$. The calculated t of 1·75 falls within the acceptance region for the test and thus the null hypothesis cannot be rejected. The effect of the congenital heart disease on mean age at starting to walk is non-significant ($t = 1\cdot75$; d.f. $= 8$; NS). The one-sample t test is summarized in Section C.2 of Appendix C.

6.9 The one-sample z test for a proportion

The significance test for comparing an observed sample proportion with some hypothesized value is similar in form to the one-sample z test for means. If the population proportion specified by the null hypothesis is called π_0 and the proportion observed in the sample is denoted by p, then an appropriate test statistic which has the standard normal distribution is

$$z = \frac{p - \pi_0}{\mathrm{SE}(p)} \tag{6.7}$$

where $\mathrm{SE}(p)$, the standard error of the sample proportion, is given by Eqn. 4.8. Thus,

$$z = \frac{p - \pi_0}{\sqrt{\dfrac{\pi_0 (1 - \pi_0)}{n}}} \tag{6.8}$$

where n is the sample size. Note that, assuming the null hypothesis is true, an exact expression for the standard error of the sample proportion can be given, rather than the approximation with the confidence interval approach, where Eqn. 4.10 was used instead. Note that the restriction mentioned in Chapter 4 on the adequacy of the normal approximation to the binomial distribution applies here as well. Both $n\pi_0$ and $n(1 - \pi_0)$ must be greater than 5 for the valid use of the z test on proportions.

Take as an example a study of 200 death certificates of which 32% or 0·32 recorded coronary heart disease as the cause of death. Are these data compatible with a null hypothesis stating that the proportion of deaths due to coronary heart disease is actually 0·4 in the population? The test statistic is, from Eqn. 6.8,

$$z = \frac{0\cdot32 - 0\cdot4}{\sqrt{\dfrac{0\cdot4\,(0\cdot6)}{200}}} = -2\cdot309.$$

Since the two-sided 5% critical values for the z test are $\pm 1\cdot96$, the hypothesis may be rejected at a 5% level of significance. Note that the hypothesis cannot be rejected at a 1% level since the critical values in this case are $\pm 2\cdot576$. The one-sample z test for a single proportion is summarized in Section C.3 of Appendix C.

6.10 The one-sample χ^2 test for many proportions

Sometimes researchers may have sample values of a qualitative variable taking on more than two values which they wish to compare with a known population distribution. For instance, a survey of the smoking habits of 250 female nurses gave 108 (43·2%) current smokers, 24 (9·6%) ex-smokers and 118 (47·2%) non-smokers. Are these percentages significantly different from those obtained in females in the general population — 36·4, 15·7 and 47·9% respectively? (Assume that these define the population distribution exactly. See Table 1.1.) Since this smoking variable has more than two categories, the test described in the last section for single proportions cannot be applied. A special test is available for this situation however. It is called the chi-square test and is denoted χ^2 (χ, chi — the Greek letter corresponding to 'ch'). The formulation of this test is quite different from anything encountered so far. The test is based on calculating expected numbers in the different categories of the variable if the null hypothesis were true, and comparing these with the numbers actually obtained (the observed frequencies).

In the example, the null hypothesis would specify that the percentages in the nursing population of current, ex- and non-smokers were 36·4, 15·7 and 47·9% respectively. Of the 250 nurses sampled, it would therefore be expected that 36·4% or 91·0 (250 × 0·364) would be current smokers, 15·7% or 39·25 (250 × 0·157) would be ex-smokers, and 47·9% or 119·75 (250 × 0·479) would be non-smokers. These are called the expected numbers. (In statistics, fractions of people are often allowed to end up in different categories, and this should not worry you!) Table 6.3 shows these expected numbers (E) and the numbers actually observed in the sample (O). The expected numbers will add up to the total sample size. The hypothesis test is now based on the discrepancy between the observed and expected values. If the observed and expected values are close, it would be reasonable to think that there would be little evidence to reject the null hypothesis. On the other hand, large discrepancies may make it possible to reject it. In fact, it is the relative differences which are perhaps more important, and the test statistic that compares these quantities and has a known theoretical distribution is χ^2. χ^2 is obtained by subtracting each expected quantity from each observed

Table 6.3. Calculations for the one-sample χ^2 test

Smoking category	Observed numbers (O)	Hypothesized proportions	Expected numbers (E)	($O - E$)	($O - E$)^2/E
Current smokers	108	0·364	91·00	17·00	3·176
Ex-smokers	24	0·157	39·25	−15·25	5·925
Non-smokers	118	0·479	119·75	− 1·75	0·026
Totals	250	1·0	250·00	0·00	9·127

$\chi^2 = 9·127$; d.f. = 2; $p < 0.05$

quantity, squaring the answer, dividing by the expected number and adding the result over the categories of the variable.

$$\chi^2 = \sum \frac{(O - E)^2}{E} \qquad (6.9)$$

This calculation is illustrated in Table 6.3 where a χ^2 value of 9·127 is obtained. Note that the $O - E$ quantities themselves always sum to zero.

The critical values of the chi-square distribution must now be looked up in tables, just as for the z and t tests in previous sections. Table B.4 gives such a table of critical values for χ^2 and the actual properties of this distribution are not of concern here. Note from the table that, like the t distribution, the chi-square distribution also has many different degrees of freedom. How are these degrees of freedom to be determined in the example? In the t test the degrees of freedom depended on the sample size; in the one-sample χ^2 test, however, the degrees of freedom depend on the number of categories in the variable being examined, and the appropriate degrees of freedom are given by one less than the number of categories. For the χ^2 test on tabular data, the degrees of freedom relate to the number of cells in the observed table that are free to vary, given the total sample size. The degrees of freedom thus increase with the number of $(O - E)$'s in the expression for χ^2, and the greater the number of these the higher the value of chi-square. A chi-square distribution with high degrees of freedom has higher critical values than a chi-square with lower degrees of freedom. Thus, since smoking had three categories the χ^2 test with 2 degrees of freedom is appropriate for the example.

A further point to note about the chi-square distribution is that the critical values are all positive; this is because χ^2 must itself be positive due to the squared term in Eqn. 6.9. The critical values given must then be exceeded for a significant result. For this one-sample test, only two-sided significance levels are appropriate, as the specification of differences in one particular direction has no real meaning. For a 5% two-sided test on 2 degrees of freedom, the critical χ^2 value is 5·991 from the table. The calculated χ^2 value of 9·127 is greater than this, so it can be concluded that there is a significant difference between the smoking habits of nurses and those of the general female population. ($\chi^2 = 9\cdot127$; d.f. $= 2$; $p < 0\cdot05$).

The one-sample χ^2 test as described above requires that theoretical population proportions are hypothesized without reference to the sample values. Such situations will often arise in genetic calculations for example. The one-sample χ^2 test can also be used in slightly different situations to test the goodness of fit of (grouped) data to a theoretical distribution like the normal. In these situations, the degrees of freedom are calculated differently however, and a more advanced text should be consulted.

The χ^2 test requires that the actual sample frequencies observed in the different categories of the variable be known — it is not sufficient to know only the percentages or proportions occurring in the sample. The test is limited in that it does not easily lead to confidence interval estimation, but with only two categories of a qualitative variable it is mathematically equivalent to the one-sample test for proportions discussed in the last section. (The chi-square distribution with one degree of freedom is the square of the standard normal distribution.) This test should only be used if not more than 20% of the expected frequencies are less than 5, and no single expected frequency is less than 1. If these assumptions are not met, combination of adjacent categories may increase the expected frequencies to the required levels. The one-sample χ^2 test is summarized in Section C.5 of Appendix C.

6.11 The one-sample z test for counts or rates

If the normal approximation to the Poisson distribution is valid then a significance test to check whether or not an observed count x (in a particular time period or spatial area) could have come from an underlying (population) with a true count of μ_0 is given by

$$z = \frac{x - \mu_0}{\sqrt{\mu_0}} \qquad (6.10)$$

where $\sqrt{\mu_0}$ is the standard error of the count and can be specified exactly under the null hypothesis. Note that, like the situation for a proportion, the standard error used for the confidence interval is based on the observed data (i.e. $\sqrt{x}$ — see Eqn. 4.14).

Suppose that 11 deaths from acute lymphatic leukaemia in children aged under 15 years occurred in a small geographical area over a 12-year period and also that, based on the population size and national figures, 5·45 cases would have been expected. Could the observed figure have been due to chance? Using Eqn. 6.10 the significance test is

$$z = (11 - 5 \cdot 45)/\sqrt{5 \cdot 45} = 2 \cdot 38.$$

The critical 5% two-sided z value is 1·96 and the result can be declared significant at $p < 0·05$. The one-sample significance test for a rate will be illustrated on the same data as above. If the average population age $0-14$ years in the geographical region were 28 560 the person-years at risk would be 12 times that figure or 342 720 (remember the observation period was 12 years). The average annual leukaemia rate in the region is then 11/342 720 or 32·10 per million. Suppose also that the average annual rate nationally were 15·90 per million. The null hypothesis states that the true population rate (θ) in the region is $\theta_0 = 15\cdot90$ while the observed rate is $32\cdot10$. The form of the significance test for a rate is

$$z = \frac{r - \theta_0}{\sqrt{(\theta_0/\text{PYRS})}} , \qquad (6.11)$$

where θ_0 is the hypothesized rate, r is the observed rate and PYRS is the person-years at risk — expressed in the same units as the rate. $\sqrt{(\theta_0/\text{PYRS})}$ is the expression for the standard error of the rate under the null hypothesis. Note that with this notation $\mu_0 = \theta_0$ (PYRS) or $5\cdot45 = 15\cdot90 \times 0\cdot3427$ (i.e. the null hypothesis count is obtained by multiplying the person-years at risk by the hypothesized rate).

In this example, PYRS must be expressed in millions since the rate is expressed per million. Thus

$$z = \frac{32\cdot10 - 15\cdot90}{\sqrt{(15\cdot90/0\cdot3427)}} = 2.38$$

which of course is identical to the value obtained when the same problem was analysed using counts. There is a significant difference between the rate of $32\cdot10$ per million found in the study region and the national rate of $15\cdot90$ based on a two-sided 5% significance level. The methods of this section are summarized in Section C.4 of Appendix C.

6.12 Small sample sizes and the validity of assumptions

A fundamental requirement for valid application of tests of significance is that the sampling distribution of the statistic of interest (sample mean, proportion or count for example) has a theoretical distribution whose properties are known.

Theoretically, the sampling distribution of the mean is normal only when the distribution of the variable in the population is itself normal. However, if the distribution of the variable in the population is not too skewed and the sample size is large enough, the central limit theorem assures us that the sampling distribution of the mean will closely approximate a normal distribution. For moderately skewed data sample sizes above 30 or so are sufficient. The same points apply for the t distribution which is used instead of the normal when the population standard deviation is not known. (The use of the t distribution instead of the normal has nothing to do with whether the parent population is normal or not; the choice depends totally on whether an exact or estimated standard error is used. With sample sizes above 60 or thereabouts the t distribution is closely approximated by the normal on the basis of examining the critical values but this is a separate question to that of dealing with skewed data.)

The distribution of the sample is the only guide to the population distribution, and if it is very skewed a transformation of the data (see Section 1.7) may be advisable prior to performing the z or t-test for a mean. The test is then performed on the transformed data. *Non-parametric tests* which make no assumptions about the distribution of the data are also available, and such tests for the two-sample situation will be discussed in the next chapter.

When the sampling distribution of proportions or counts is in question, slightly different problems arise. The sampling distribution of proportions and counts are binomial and Poisson respectively. The tests discussed in Sections 6.9 and 6.11 however made use of the normal approximation to these distributions. For small proportions or low counts the approximations given in this text may not be accurate enough. An acceptable alternative however is to perform the significance test using the confidence interval approach.

As discussed in Section 6.4 a two-sided 5% significance can be inferred if the null hypothesis value for the mean lies outside the 95% confidence interval for the mean. If the null hypothesis value is included in the confidence interval the result is equivalent to non-significance. The same result nearly holds when dealing with tests for proportions or counts. If the normal approximation is being used for both the significance test and the confidence interval, slight differences between the two approaches can arise however. This is because, for proportions and counts, the standard error is actually a function of the proportion or the count. Thus if the null hypothesis is true the exact standard error is known. There is no pre-specified population value for a confidence interval however and the standard error must be approximated by the sample value. (Complex confidence interval estimates are available when this approximation is not made, but are not considered in this text.) The fact that different expressions for the standard error are employed for hypothesis tests than for confidence intervals explains why the two procedures are not exactly equivalent. The discrepancies are small however, and differences in interpretation will only arise when a result just achieves or fails to achieve significance at whatever level is being considered, and the corresponding confidence interval just fails to include or just includes the null value.

In any case, for small sample sizes the normal approximation to the binomial or Poisson distribution as given in this text may not hold, and unless the result of the z test for a proportion or count (or rate) is very definitely significant an alternative approach is suggested. This is to use the tables for the exact binomial or Poisson confidence intervals as described in Sections 4.8 and 4.9 and to infer significance at the appropriate level if the (exact) confidence intervals exclude the null value of the hypothesis test. This is a perfectly acceptable procedure and is recommended for small sample sizes. Note however that one-sided tests cannot be performed with this method since the equivalence of the confidence interval is with a two-sided significance test.

6.13 Summary

In this chapter the development of the one-sample normal (z) test was described in detail to illustrate the underlying structure of hypothesis tests. The relationship of confidence intervals to hypothesis tests was discussed, as were the concepts of one- and two-sided tests and the principles of power and sample size calculations. Later sections in the chapter detailed calculations for the more widely applicable one-sample t test. The z test for a single proportion count or rate and the χ^2 test for many proportions were also described. Table 6.4 summarizes the one-sample tests discussed in this chapter, and the computational steps are repeated in Appendix C.

The following chapter details tests and confidence intervals for the comparison of two samples, which is a much more common situation in the medical area. The general principles discussed above however, in the context of the one-sample test, are applicable to all tests of hypotheses and are necessary for a full grasp of the remaining chapters.

Table 6.4. Summary of one-sample tests

Hypothesis test on	Test statistic	(Equation no.)
One mean:		
σ known	$z = \dfrac{\bar{x} - \mu_0}{\sigma/\sqrt{n}}$	(6.4)
σ unknown	$t_{n-1} = \dfrac{\bar{x} - \mu_0}{S/\sqrt{n}}$	(6.6)
One proportion	$z = \dfrac{p - \pi_0}{\sqrt{\dfrac{\pi_0 (1 - \pi_0)}{n}}}$	(6.8)
Many proportions	$\chi^2 = \sum \dfrac{(O - E)^2}{E}$	(6.9)
One count	$z = \dfrac{x - \mu_0}{\sqrt{\mu_0}}$	(6.10)
One rate	$z = \dfrac{r - \theta_0}{\sqrt{\theta_0/\text{PYRS}}}$	(6.11)

7

Confidence Intervals and Hypothesis Tests: Two-Group Comparisons

7.1 Introduction

In one sense medical research is all about examining associations between variables. If group membership is considered a qualitative variable, then comparing means in groups is the examination of an association between a quantitative and a qualitative variable, and comparing proportions in groups is the examination of the association between two qualitative variables. When the qualitative variable has only two categories the situation reduces to the comparison of two groups or samples. Two-group situations are exceptionally common in medical research, for example comparing cases and controls in a case-control study (see Chapter 10), or a treatment and a control group in a clinical trial (see Chapter 11), and it is often more convenient to reduce an analysis to a two-group comparison.

This chapter describes hypothesis tests and confidence intervals for the comparison of means, proportions, counts and rates in the two-group situation. It should be noted that, in the comparison of two groups, confidence intervals are preferably calculated for a single summary measure of the comparison (e.g. the difference between two means), rather than for each of the component statistics (e.g. the two separate means). This chapter only considers confidence intervals for difference measures however, while Chapter 10 describes confidence interval estimation for ratio measures such as the ratio of two proportions. The techniques considered here are among the most common in the medical literature and it is hoped that this 'cookbook' chapter will be of practical use to researchers who wish to analyse their own data.

Since all the methods described are based on the same underlying philosophy, detailed discussion is avoided and the formulae are not derived formally. Therefore a good grasp of the concepts of the confidence interval and significance test as described in the earlier chapters is necessary for the material that follows.

7.2 Independent and paired comparisons

One of the most common errors in statistical hypothesis testing is a failure to take cognizance of how the data were collected in the first place. Statistical analysis is not simply a tool applied to numbers, it is a methodology for examining real data which a researcher may have spent many months or years gathering together.

This chapter considers the comparison of two groups and is, therefore, in essence, concerned with the analysis of two samples taken from corresponding populations. Apart from issues relating to the accuracy of data collection, and whether or not the resulting numbers are truly a measure of what is being studied (see Chapter 15), the way in which samples are chosen from the populations is of vital importance.

Suppose that a sample has been taken from a population and it is of interest to compare blood pressures in alcohol drinkers and abstainers. Each of these groups can be considered to be a sample from one of the two populations defined by drinking and non-drinking. This is a common situation in medical research, where the comparison groups are defined by the value of some qualitative variable (such as drinking) in a single study group. Sometimes, however, the sampling from population groups is more explicit. Separate samples may, for instance, be taken of schoolchildren from rural and urban areas to compare IQs. The samples may be of equal size or may reflect the distribution of urban and rural children in the country as a whole (stratified samples).

Both of these examples have one important factor in common; the samples are *independent samples* from the populations being studied. By independent it is meant, in simple terms, that the actual selection of individuals for one sample group is not affected by the individuals already selected for the other group. It is vital to understand this notion of independence if the correct statistical test is to be chosen, and before undertaking any statistical analysis a researcher must be sure whether or not the comparison groups are independent.

At the other extreme from the comparison of independent samples is the comparison of *paired samples* or *individually matched* samples. A paired sample arises in two-group comparisons when every individual in one of the groups has a unique match or pair in the other group. A researcher, for instance, might be interested in comparing the smoking habits of a group of lung cancer patients with a control or comparison group of persons who do not have this cancer. Such a study is referred to as a *case-control study*, and is discussed in some detail in Chapter 10. The researcher, however, knows that smoking habits are related to both a person's age and sex, and wants to avoid a biased analysis which might arise if the age and sex distributions were different in the two groups being studied. (See a detailed discussion of *confounding variables* in Section 10.2 and Chapter 12). One solution to this problem would be to use paired samples. For every lung cancer case in the first group, the researcher would choose, from the general population, a control of the same age and sex who does not have lung cancer. In this way, each individual in one group is matched with an individual in the other group. This technique is sometimes called *artificial pairing*.

In animal experimentation, litter mates often provide the experimental material.

Two treatments may be compared in a group of rats by assigning one animal to one treatment and one of its litter mates to the other treatment. Thus, every animal in one group would have a litter mate in the other group. Such situations result in what is called *natural pairing*.

A third form of pairing is *self-pairing*, when the same individuals belong to both comparison groups. This can arise when, say, a new chemical is being tested for allergic reactions and compared with a non-allergic preparation. The chemical might be applied to a person's right arm, and the other preparation to the left arm. The arms of the people under study would be compared and for every right arm there is a left arm. A further example of a self-paired situation is when some variable is measured before and after a particular therapy. The measurements made before the therapy are matched with the measurements on the same individual after the therapy. The same situation arises when two different treatments are tested on the same individuals on two different occasions.

Although the examples of paired data above were for two-group comparisons, similar data may arise with more than two groups, although it is relatively uncommon in the medical literature. A point to note also is that in a paired situation the sample size in each of the groups must necessarily be the same, while this need not be so for independent comparisons.

Between the extremes of independent data and paired data lie what are called *frequency matched* data. These arise when the distribution of a variable, or variables, is forced to be the same in the two groups. For example, each group might end up with the same proportions of individuals in a number of age categories, without any matching of individuals. Studies giving rise to frequency matched data are described in Chapters 10 and 11, and the analysis of such data is considered in Chapter 12. The techniques of this present chapter are only applicable to independent or paired data.

If one fails to account for pairing or matching in an analysis the statistical test loses power and is more likely to miss a real difference if it exists. Thus, a test for independent data should not be used on paired groups. Occasionally, however, when suitable methods are not available, matching or pairing can be ignored with a consequent loss of power.

7.3 Parametric and non-parametric significance tests

Apart from how the data were collected, the measurement scale of the variable being studied can also determine the statistical hypothesis test to be used. In the discussion so far, it was sufficient to distinguish between quantitative and qualitative variables. In the medical literature, the vast majority of significance tests compare either proportions or means, operating on qualitative or quantitative data respectively.

It was noted in Chapter 1 that a qualitative variable can consist of ordered categories which will often take a numerical label or tag, although the concept of distance between these categories does not arise. Thus, while it can be said that a systolic blood pressure of 200 mmHg is twice as high as a systolic blood pressure of 100 mmHg, it cannot be said that an individual in social group I is twice as privileged as an individual in social group II. On this basis, a hierarchy of variables can be created: qualitative variables with no intrinsic order, qualitative variables with order; and quantitative variables based on measurement. For convenience, these three types of variables will from here on be referred to as nominal, ordinal and quantitative variables respectively. It is important to note that a quantitative variable, such as age, can be expressed in ordinal form (e.g. by ranking from youngest to oldest) or in nominal form (e.g. by categorizing into young, middle-aged or old and ignoring order). This means essentially that a significance test suitable for a low level of measurement can be applied to any higher level, if the scale of measurement is adjusted appropriately. Thus, tests suitable for nominal data can be applied to ordinal or quantitative data, and tests for ordinal data can also be applied to quantitative data.

One of the rules of good statistical analysis, all else being equal, is to use the highest level of test available for the data; but usually all is not equal, and in particular, many tests suitable for quantitative data make large assumptions about the distribution of variables in the populations being compared. It was seen in the last chapter, for instance, that an underlying assumption of normally distributed data was required for a valid application of the one-sample *t* test, but that with a large sample size violations of this assumption could be tolerated. Significance tests which make distributional assumptions about the variable being analysed are called *parametric tests*.

In some situations, it is not possible to check whether such assumptions are true, particularly when the sample size tends to be small, and there is often doubt about whether or not a particular test is valid for a set of quantitative data. As has been said however, quantitative data can be analysed as ordinal data, and most of the statistical tests of ordinal data are assumption-free. Such tests are called *non-parametric, distribution-free* or *rank tests* and provide a useful fallback in many situations.

A further point about many of the rank tests is that they test a null hypothesis relating to median values rather than mean values. The median however is probably much more appropriate for skewed data (see Section 2.2) and is close to the mean if the data have a nearly symmetrical distribution in the first place. It must be pointed out, however, that in general parametric tests are somewhat more powerful (in the sense of Section 6.7) in detecting differences between populations when the underlying assumptions hold, and many of the more complex parametric tests do not have a non-parametric equivalent. In general too, the non-parametric tests are not useful for estimation purposes, and confidence intervals for estimates are usually difficult to calculate.

In the two-sample situation however, non-parametric tests can be exceptionally useful in the analysis of quantitative data. With small sample sizes, many of the underlying assumptions of parametric tests may be invalid, and the non-parametric tests are probably the only valid ones to use. For this reason, such tests are sometimes called *small sample tests*, and, in fact, tables for the non-parametric tests in this text are only given for studies of up to moderate size. With fairly large sample sizes, on the other hand, many of the assumptions for the parametric tests may hold approximately, and they can be employed with a large degree of confidence. For large sample sizes too, the non-parametric tests are computationally more tedious.

The remainder of this chapter outlines the application of the more common parametric and non-parametric significance tests with confidence interval estimators for difference measures. Statistical tables are given in Appendix B, and Appendix C also summarizes the application of each test for easy reference.

7.4 Comparison of two independent means: confidence intervals and the *t* test

The parametric *t* test used for the comparison of means in two samples is one of the most commonly used tests in medical statistics. The test to be described in this section is for independent samples only and should not be used when the data are paired or matched (see Section 7.2). Failure to take note of this is an oft-repeated error and results in a loss of power in the comparison. In other words, an independent *t* test performed (incorrectly) on paired data will increase the chances of declaring a non-significant result when, in fact, the null hypothesis is false.

Suppose 20 regular users of oral contraceptives were studied to determine if cholesterol levels in such women are significantly different from those of women who do not use oral contraceptives. Because the cholesterol levels in the population were not known, a comparison or control group of 20 similarly aged women who were not on the 'pill' was also taken, without pairing or matching. The results of the study are shown in Table 7.1. The mean cholesterol levels in the contraceptive-users and controls were 5·20 and 4·81 mmol/l respectively with corresponding standard deviations of 0·53 and 0·48 mmol/l.

The null hypothesis is that the mean cholesterol levels in the populations of oral contraceptive-users and non-users are the same. The results of the samples suggest a difference of 0·39 mmol/l between the two groups. Could this be due to chance or does it reflect a real difference?

The statistical approach is similar to the situation with one sample only. If

Table 7.1. The independent *t* test comparing cholesterol levels in users and non-users of oral contraceptives

	Contraceptive-users	Controls
Sample size	20	20
Sample means	5·20	4·81
Sample standard deviations	0·53	0·48
Difference between means	0·39 mmol/l	

$t = 2\cdot439$; d.f. $= 38$; $p < 0\cdot05$

there really was no difference between the two groups, it would be expected that repeat samples, sized 20, from each group would generate a series of mean differences distributed around the value of 0. As in the one-sample case, a test statistic is calculated based on the difference obtained (0·39 mmol/l), divided by a factor which is the standard error of this difference. This test statistic has a known distribution from theoretical considerations, and tables can be used to see if the calculated value lies in the tails of the distribution. Moreover, since no prior knowledge is available concerning the direction of the difference in cholesterol levels, a two-sided test must be employed.

The actual test statistic to employ is defined

$$z = \frac{\bar{x}_1 - \bar{x}_2}{\text{SE}\,(\bar{x}_1 - \bar{x}_2)} \tag{7.1}$$

where $\bar{x}_1$ and $\bar{x}_2$ are the means in the groups being compared and $\text{SE}\,(\bar{x}_1 - \bar{x}_2)$ is the exact standard error of the difference between the means. In general the standard error of a difference between two statistics (if they are independent) is calculated as the square root of the sum of the squares of the individual standard errors:

$$\text{SE}\,(y_1 - y_2) = \sqrt{\text{SE}\,(y_1)^2 + \text{SE}\,(y_2)^2}$$

where y_1 and y_2 are any statistics. This result will be used throughout the chapter, and here

$$\text{SE}\,(\bar{x}_1 - \bar{x}_2) = \sqrt{\frac{\sigma_1^2}{n_1} + \frac{\sigma_2^2}{n_2}} \tag{7.2}$$

where σ_1 and σ_2 are the population standard deviations and n_1 and n_2 are the two sample sizes.

When, as is usual, the population standard deviations are not known, the sample values S_1 and S_2 must be used instead. How these sample values are employed depends on the assumptions which can be made. If it can be assumed that the two population standard deviations are equal, then what is called a *pooled variance* is calculated as the weighted average of the two sample variances:*

$$S_p^2 = \frac{(n_1 - 1)\,S_1^2 + (n_2 - 1)\,S_2^2}{n_1 + n_2 - 2}. \tag{7.3}$$

An appropriate test statistic for the comparison of two means is then obtained by substituting S_p^2 for each of the two population values in Eqn. 7.2

$$t = \frac{\bar{x}_1 - \bar{x}_2}{\sqrt{\dfrac{S_p^2}{n_1} + \dfrac{S_p^2}{n_2}}} \tag{7.4}$$

on $n_1 + n_2 - 2$ degrees of freedom. When the sample sizes are equal ($n_1 = n_2 = n$) this reduces to the simpler expression

$$t = \frac{\bar{x}_1 - \bar{x}_2}{\sqrt{\dfrac{S_1^2 + S_2^2}{n}}} \tag{7.5}$$

on $2n - 2$ degrees of freedom.

In the example, the two sample standard deviations are fairly close in value, and since the sample sizes are equal, Eqn. 7.5 is an appropriate test statistic. Substituting in the sample values

$$t = \frac{5{\cdot}20 - 4{\cdot}81}{\sqrt{\dfrac{(0{\cdot}53)^2 + (0{\cdot}48)^2}{20}}} = 2{\cdot}439.$$

This value must now be looked up in the tables of the t distribution for 38 degrees of freedom. Table B.3 does not give values for 38 degrees of freedom, but 40 is near enough for a valid approximation. The critical 5% (two-sided) level for t is $2{\cdot}021$ and the statistic exceeds this, so $p < 0{\cdot}05$. Note too, that the critical 1% value is $2{\cdot}704$, and that the result, although achieving a 5% level of significance, does not reach the 1% level. It can, therefore, be concluded that chance is not a likely explanation of the observed differences between the cholesterol levels of users and non-users of oral contraceptives at a 5% significance level.

A few words need to be said concerning the assumptions underlying this particular application of the t test. The first assumption is, of course, that the two samples are random and independent. The two-sample t test, like the one-sample test, also assumes that the populations from which the samples were taken are not too markedly skewed. The final assumption is that the standard deviations in the

---

* For technical reasons, a weighted average of the variances, rather than the standard deviations, is calculated.

two populations are the same (the technical term for this is *homoscedasticity*). If there is reason to doubt this assumption, it is not valid to pool the two sample variances into a single estimate, instead it is necessary to calculate

$$t' = \frac{\bar{x}_1 - \bar{x}_2}{\sqrt{\dfrac{S_1^2}{n_1} + \dfrac{S_2^2}{n_2}}} \tag{7.6}$$

using the separate sample values for the variances. This statistic does not have a Student's *t* distribution, and although some approximate solutions involving the *t* distribution with a complex formula for the appropriate degrees of freedom are available, they are not given here. If the sample sizes are large enough, it is suggested a normal approximation setting $t' = z$ be used. If the assumptions for the *t* test are not satisfied a transformation of the data might provide a solution. Skewness can be reduced using the suggestions of Section 1.7 and sometimes these transformations can also achieve equality of variances in the two groups. In particular the transformations for positively skewed distributions can be useful. Usually with heteroscedasticity the standard deviation tends to increase with the size of the mean. The easiest way to determine which transformation may be most appropriate is to examine the ratios of the standard deviation (S) to the square root of the mean ($\sqrt{\bar{x}}$), the mean itself ($\bar{x}$) and to the square of the mean ($\bar{x}^2$) in the two groups. Whichever set of ratios is closest in value in the two groups indicates whether the standard deviation is increasing in proportion to $\sqrt{\bar{x}}$, $\bar{x}$ or $\bar{x}^2$. The best transformation to use on each data observation (x) is then:

$S \propto \sqrt{\bar{x}}$: use $\sqrt{x}$ (square root)
$S \propto \bar{x}$: use log x (logarithmic)
$S \propto \bar{x}^2$: use $1/x$ (reciprocal)

where $\propto$ means 'is proportional to'. For small sample sizes however the non-parametric test outlined in the next section is likely to be far easier.

The confidence interval for the difference between two population means is given by

$$(\bar{x}_1 - \bar{x}_2) \pm t_c \text{ SE} (\bar{x}_1 - \bar{x}_2) \tag{7.7}$$

where t_c is the appropriate critical value of the *t* distribution, and the standard error term is given by the denominator of the appropriate *t* test. In the cholesterol example, the standard error is given by the denominator of Eqn. 7.5 and is 0·160. The critical *t* value for 40 (close enough to 38) degrees of freedom and a 95% confidence interval is 2·021, so that the confidence interval for the mean cholesterol difference between the contraceptive users and non-users is

$$0·39 \pm 2·021 \, (0·160)$$
or
$$0·39 \pm 0·32$$

Thus, it is 95% certain that the mean cholesterol level in contraceptive users is at least 0·07 mmol/l higher than in controls and could be as much as 0·71 mmol/l higher. Note that, as expected, the confidence interval for the cholesterol difference does not include the value specified by the null hypothesis which was a zero difference. Also note that when analysing a two-group comparison by means of a confidence interval one should calculate the confidence interval for a single summary measure of the association and not for the separate values (means) in the two groups. The difference between the means is the usual summary measure employed.

The independent *t* test is summarized in Section C.6 of Appendix C.

7.5 Comparison of two independent medians: the Wilcoxon rank sum test

In many situations, especially with small sample sizes, the assumptions underlying the parametric independent *t* test described in the last section may not hold. In such cases it may be wiser to employ a non-parametric alternative. Also, if the measurement scale of the data is ordinal, and not quantitative, the mean values are uninterpretable and the *t* tests cannot be used.

Suppose that systolic blood pressure has been measured on nine young adults with diabetes mellitus and on eight control patients of similar age (not matched) without this condition. The diabetes mellitus patients had systolic blood pressures of 114, 120, 120, 128, 130, 135, 138, 140 and 141 mmHg. The control patients had blood pressures of 110, 112, 112, 118, 120, 122, 125 and 130 mmHg. The purpose of the study is to see if there is a relationship between blood pressure and diabetes mellitus, and there is no prior conception about what the direction of this relationship may be. Also, since the sample size is small and the distribution of blood pressures may be quite skewed, it is decided that the two-sample *t* test is likely to be invalid. The most commonly used test in this situation is the *Wilcoxon two-sample rank sum test* or the entirely equivalent *Mann—Whitney U test* or *Kendall's S test*. The formulation which will be considered is that of Wilcoxon.

This test, like most non-parametric tests, is based on ranking or ordering the data. The data from the two groups are combined and ordered from lowest to highest, giving a rank of 1 to the lowest value and, in the example, 17 (the sum of the two sample sizes) to the highest observed value. The groups from which the different observations are taken must also be noted. If there are ties in the data (i.e. more than one individual has the same value for a measurement) the average of the ranks that would have been given to the observations are assigned instead.

In the example, the data would be laid out as in Table 7.2, underlining the observations from (say) the control group, and calling it group 1. The easiest way to assign the ranks correctly is to number the observations from lowest to highest.

If there are no ties, these numbers are the ranks. If there are ties as, for example, the two blood pressures of 112 mmHg, these are assigned a rank calculated as the average of the observation numbers. In this case the two measurements are given numbers 2 and 3, and are therefore assigned the average rank of $2\frac{1}{2}$ $[(2 + 3)/2]$. The three observations of 120 mmHg with numbers 6, 7 and 8 are all assigned rank 7 $[(6 + 7 + 8)/3 = 7]$.

The Wilcoxon test is based on examining the sum of the ranks in each group. If the two populations have similar distributions, then it would be expected that the sums of the ranks in each group would be close to each other. If the distributions are different, it would be expected that the group with the lower median would have a lower sum of ranks. In the example, the sum of the ranks of the observations in group 1 (the control group) is denoted

$$T_1 = 1 + 2 \cdot 5 + \ldots + 12 \cdot 5 = 49 \cdot 5$$

and the sum of the ranks in group 2 is

$$T_2 = 4 + 7 + \ldots + 17 = 103 \cdot 5.$$

Table 7.2. The Wilcoxon rank sum test comparing systolic blood pressures in nine diabetics (group 2) and eight controls (group 1)

Systolic blood pressures (mmHg)*	Ranks (observation numbers)	Ranks adjusted for ties*
110	1	1
112	2	$2\frac{1}{2}$
112	3	$2\frac{1}{2}$
114	4	4
118	5	5
120	6	7
120	7	7
120	8	7
122	9	9
125	10	10
128	11	11
130	12	$12\frac{1}{2}$
130	13	$12\frac{1}{2}$
135	14	14
138	15	15
140	16	16
141	17	17

* Control (group 1) values and ranks underlined.
T_1 = sum of ranks in group 1 = 49·5; T_2 = sum of ranks in group 2 = 103·5; $p < 0.05$

This immediately suggests that the median value in group 1 might be less than that in group 2.

The test statistic for the Wilcoxon rank sum test is the sum of the ranks in one of the groups — say group 1. As with all significance tests, this statistic is referred to tables of a particular distribution. The critical values for the Wilcoxon statistic are to be found in Table B.5 (Appendix B). Unfortunately the table is rather cumbersome and spread out over 12 pages of the appendix. The table allows for sample sizes of n_1 up to 25 and n_2 up to 35. The groups can be relabelled if one has more than 25 observations. For sample sizes outside this range a more detailed text should be consulted (see Appendix B).

Table B.5 is in three parts for values of n_1 of (a) 1−9, (b) 10−17, (c) 18−25. Firstly choose the appropriate part of the table depending on the value of n_1. For each range of values of n_1 there are four pages of tables, one for each of the two-sided (one-sided) significance levels of 0·10(0·05), 0·05(0·025), 0·02(0·01) and 0·01(0·005). Having chosen the required significance level the lower (T_l) and the upper (T_u) critical values for the sample sizes in group 1 (n_1) and in group 2 (n_2) can be read from the table. If the test statistic T_1 is greater than or equal to T_u or less than or equal to T_l a significant result can be claimed.

In the example the controls were labelled as group 1 and $T_1 = 49·5$. The lower and upper critical 5% two-sided values are, for $n_1 = 8$ and $n_2 = 9$, $T_l = 51$ and $T_u = 93$. The sum of ranks at 49·5 is less than T_l so there is a significant difference between the blood pressures of the two groups. Since T_1 is less than the lower critical value, it can be concluded that the blood pressure of controls is less than that of the diabetic patients ($p < 0·05$).

Unfortunately however, as with many non-parametric tests, a direct measure of the magnitude of the difference between the groups is not part of the test statistic, and it is necessary to rely on the examination of group medians to determine the importance of a given result. With the *t* test, on the other hand, the magnitude of the difference between the two groups, $\bar{x}_1 - \bar{x}_2$, is entered directly into the calculation of the *t*. Although possible, the calculation of confidence limits for the difference between medians is very tedious and is not considered here.

The main assumption for the Wilcoxon test is that there is an underlying continuous distribution of the variable of interest (even if the measurements are only on an ordinal scale). In essence, the test compares the two distributions in their entirety, so it is a valid test for the comparison of means or medians. It is nearly as powerful as the parametric *t* test, even when all the assumptions for that test are valid, and when the assumptions do not hold it is always to be preferred. There are some slight problems if there are many ties in the data, but the test as outlined should be adequate for most practical situations. The application of the test is summarized in Appendix C, Section C.7.

7.6 Comparison of paired means: confidence intervals and the paired *t* test

When data have been collected on pairs of individuals, and each member of one of the groups has a match or pair in the other group, the independent *t* test cannot be used. The statistical analysis must take account of how the data were collected. Suppose that a study on the effect of a particular drug on pulse rate is performed on eight volunteers; their pulses are measured before and after the administration of the drug, giving the data shown in Table 7.3. The mean pulse rate prior to drug administration is 67·0 beats per minute and afterwards it has increased to 70·375 beats per minute. One point to note is that in any paired situation such as this the sample sizes in the two groups must necessarily be the same.

The approach to hypothesis testing in a paired situation is to take advantage of the fact that observations in the groups come in pairs. If, under the null hypothesis, the means of the two populations (pulse rates before and after administration of the drug) are the same, then the mean of the differences calculated on a sample of pairs of individuals should be close to 0. Column 4 of Table 7.3 shows the differences in the pulse rates calculated by subtracting the 'before' reading from the 'after' reading. The mean of these differences denoted $\bar{d}$ is 3·375, which is the same as the difference between the means of the original two groups, 67·0 and 70·375 beats per minute. This is a general result, that the mean of the differences is the same as the difference of the means.

For the analysis of a paired experiment attention should be focused on the column of differences, essentially reducing the situation to a single sample of

Table 7.3. The paired *t* test. Pulse rates in eight subject before and after administration of a drug

Subject (pair)	Pulse rate (beats/min)		After minus before *d*
	Before drug	After drug	
1	58	66	8
2	65	69	4
3	68	75	7
4	70	68	−2
5	66	73	7
6	75	75	0
7	62	68	6
8	72	69	−3
Mean	67·0	70·375	3·375($\bar{d}$)

$t = 2 \cdot 167$; d.f. $= 7$; NS

differences. The null hypothesis states that the population mean difference should
be 0 and so, using an adaptation of the one-sample test (Eqn. 6.6), an appropriate
test statistic for the paired situation is

$$t = \frac{\bar{d} - 0}{S_d/\sqrt{n}} \tag{7.8}$$

on $n - 1$ degrees of freedom. $\bar{d}$ is the observed mean of the differences, and the 0
in the formula is the hypothesized value for the mean population difference. S_d
is nothing more than the standard deviation of the differences calculated in the
usual manner. Note though, that if any of the differences have a minus sign, this
must be taken into account, and also that zero differences should be included. n is
the number of pairs in the entire study, which, of course, is the number of
calculated differences. There are $n - 1$ degrees of freedom since, essentially, the
paired data have been reduced to a one-sample situation, with n observations of
differences.

The mean of the figures in column 4 of Table 7.3 is $\bar{d} = 3\cdot375$ and the standard
deviation can be calculated as $S_d = 4\cdot406$. With n equal to 8

$$t = \frac{3\cdot375}{4\cdot406/\sqrt{8}} = 2.167.$$

There are 7 degrees of freedom and it will be assumed that a two-sided test at
a 5% level of significance is to be performed. The critical 5% value for a two-
sided t test on 7 degrees of freedom is $2\cdot365$ (Table B.3) and since the calculated t
of $2\cdot167$ does not exceed this value a statistically significant result cannot be
claimed. Although the drug increased the mean pulse rate by over 3 beats per
minute in the subjects studied, this could be a spurious result due to sampling
variation.

A confidence interval for the mean difference between the pulse rates can be
calculated using

$$\bar{d} \pm t_c \, S_d/\sqrt{n} \tag{7.9}$$

where $S_d/\sqrt{n}$ is the standard error of the mean difference. In the example the
95% confidence interval turns out to be

$$3\cdot375 \pm 2\cdot365 \, (1\cdot558).$$

This gives confidence limits of $-0\cdot31$ and $7\cdot06$ beats per minute; thus the confidence
interval includes 0 as might have been expected from the result of the significance
test.

The approach to this analysis of paired quantitative data is to reduce the two
sets of observations to one set of differences, and the assumption underlying the
use of the paired t test is that the distribution of differences in the population is
not markedly skewed. The assumption required for the independent t test of

equal population standard deviations is not required, since there is now only one population of differences. Section C.8 (Appendix C) summarizes these calculations.

7.7 Comparison of paired medians: the sign test

An alternative to the parametric paired t test is the non-parametric *sign test*. Essentially, this examines the null hypothesis that the medians in the two populations are the same, and it is an exceptionally easy test to perform. As with the Wilcoxon rank sum test, the data may be quantitative or ordinal, but an underlying continuous distribution is assumed.

Suppose that the reactions of 10 patients to two different analgesics (A and B) have been studied, with the patients rating the effectiveness of each preparation on a scale from 0 to 9. On the basis of these scores, it is required to determine which analgesic might be judged more effective. The results of this study are laid out in Table 7.4. It can be seen immediately that analgesic A is superior to B according to eight of the persons studied. They are scored equally by one person, and another person judges B to be superior to A. If the median effects of the two analgesics were the same, it would be expected that, on average, half the persons would prefer A and the other half would prefer B; the sign test is, in fact, based on the number of preferences for one drug over the other, the superior drug being likely to have more preferences.

A preference (or superiority of one drug over the other) can be detected by the sign of the difference between the measured scores, a plus sign, say, representing a preference for A, and a minus sign a preference for B. Tied results

Table 7.4. The sign test (paired data). Scores assigned by 10 patients to two analgesics A and B

Patient (pair)	Analgesic A	Analgesic B	Sign of A−B
1	2	2	0
2	4	3	+
3	7	4	+
4	3	0	+
5	0	1	−
6	3	2	+
7	6	4	+
8	4	2	+
9	5	4	+
10	8	6	+

n_+ = number of '+' signs = 8; n = number of untied pairs = 9; $p < 0.05$

(e.g. subject number 1 who scored both drugs with a 2) must be ignored, and the number of preferences or 'pluses' denoted by n_+, should be recorded. In this case $n_+ = 8$, out of nine untied pairs. This number of preferences can be referred to critical values for the sign test, which depend on the number of untied pairs (n) and, as usual, on the significance level for the chosen one- or two-sided test. Table B.6 in Appendix B gives the lower (S_l) and upper (S_u) critical values. For $n = 9$, the two-sided 5% critical values are 1 and 8, and in this example n_+ at 8 is equal to the upper critical value. Thus, it can be concluded that there are more preferences for analgesic A in this study than could reasonably have arisen by chance, and a significant result can be claimed at the 5% level.

Note that this test does not, by its nature, take any account of the magnitude of the differences between the groups. The example shows, however, that small differences in a consistent direction, even with a small sample size, can lead to significant results. Section C.9 of Appendix C summarizes the applications of the sign test.

7.8 Comparison of paired medians: the Wilcoxon signed rank test

The non-parametric sign test for paired data described in the previous section took account only of the sign of the differences between the observations in the two groups, and took no cognizance of the magnitude of these differences. The test described below is more powerful than the sign test, in that the magnitude of the differences contributes to the test statistic.

The *Wilcoxon signed rank test* will be illustrated on the same data employed for the paired t test — the difference in pulse rates before and after administration of a drug (see Table 7.3). As with the paired t test (Section 7.6) the first step is to calculate the difference between the values for each pair ('after minus before' values). The next step is to rank these differences from smallest to largest ignoring the sign of the difference. This is done in Table 7.5. As usual, tied ranks are given the average of the ranks that would have been given if the values were not tied. Note that the zero difference on subject 6 is not included for the purpose of ranking. (In the paired t test, this zero difference did contribute to the test statistic.) Thus, the observed difference of -2 is given rank 1 and the difference of -3 is given rank 2. The difference 4 is the next largest, and is given the rank of 3. The remainder of the ranks are assigned similarly. Once the ranks have been calculated in this manner, the sign of the difference is given back to each rank, to form the signed ranks as shown in the last column of Table 7.5. The test statistic is then taken as the sum of the positive ranks, which is denoted T_+ and is in this example 25 ($3 + 4 + 5\cdot5 + 5\cdot5 + 7$).

Table 7.5. The Wilcoxon signed rank test (paired data). Differences between pulse rates before and after administration of a drug (see Table 7.3)

Subject (pair)	Difference* in pulse rates (after − before) beats/min d	Rank	Signed rank
6	0	—	—
4	−2	1	−1
8	−3	2	−2
2	4	3	3
7	6	4	4
3	7	5·5	5·5
5	7	5·5	5·5
1	8	7	7

* Ordered by magnitude.

T_+ = sum of positive ranks = 25; n = number of untied pairs = 7; NS

Again, this test statistic is intuitively reasonable. The null hypothesis states that the distribution from which the two sets of observations are sampled are identical and thus that the means, and/or medians, are the same. If this were the case, the differences (d) should be symmetrical about 0; that is, there should be as many negative differences as positive differences. Also, the sum of the positive ranks (T_+) should be close in value to the sum of the negative ranks, the sum of the ranks with the minus sign. If, however, the population mean (or median) of the 'after' group was greater than that of the 'before' group, there would be more positive differences, and thus T_+ would tend to be larger than expected under the null hypothesis. Similarly, if the differences were in the other direction T_+ would be smaller than expected. Table B.7 in Appendix B gives the lower (T_l) and upper (T_u) critical values of T_+ for different numbers of non-zero differences, since obviously these critical values will depend on the total number of differences that were ranked. In the example, there are 7 untied pairs, and T_+ is equal to 25. The critical values for a 5% two-sided test are, from the table, 2 and 26; thus T_+ does not lie in the critical region, and, as with the paired t test, it must be concluded that the difference between the pulse rates before and after treatment with this particular drug is non-significant, and could be ascribed to chance.

As with many of the non-parametric tests considered so far, it is necessary to assume an underlying continuous distribution for the variable, and there should not be too many ties among the differences. The calculation of confidence limits is again not considered. Section C.10 in Appendix C summarizes the use of the sign test.

7.9 Comparison of two independent proportions: confidence intervals and the z test

In many medical investigations, the variable of interest is binary and takes on two values only. Thus, one might want to compare the proportions or percentages alive or dead in two groups. In this and the following sections techniques for the comparison of proportions in two groups are described. This section deals with the comparison of proportions in two independent samples. As with the one-sample situation, the analysis here is in terms of proportions, and if working with percentages is preferred, translation back to this measure at the end of the analysis is suggested.

As an example, take the clinical trial discussed in Chapter 5, where the 5-year survival expressed as a proportion of the two treated groups, each of 25 subjects, was found to be 0·68 in those on drug A and 0·48 in those on drug B. Table 7.6 presents these data in a 2 × 2 table, often called a 2 × 2 *contingency table*. The test to be described for use in this type of situation is approximate, insofar as the normal distribution is being used to approximate the binomial distribution (see Section 6.9). For this reason, the applicability of the test is in doubt with small sample sizes. The test, however, is non-parametric in that it makes no assumptions in relation to the distribution of the variables being examined.

As with the two-sample test for means, the test statistic for the comparison of the two proportions is in the form

$$\frac{\text{Difference between the proportions}}{\text{SE (difference)}}.$$

The standard error of the difference between the two proportions depends on the value for the proportions specified by the null hypothesis. The null hypothesis specifies that the proportions in the two populations from which the samples were taken are the same. If, in the example quoted, survival is being analysed, then

Table 7.6. Results of a clinical trial comparing survival in two drug-treated groups (proportions given in parentheses)

	5-year outcome		
	Alive	Dead	Total
Drug A	17 (0·68)	8 (0·32)	25 (1·0)
Drug B	12 (0·48)	13 (0·52)	25 (1·0)
Totals	29 (0·58)	21 (0·42)	50 (1·0)

$z = 1·433$; NS

letting π_1 and π_2 represent the population proportion of survivors in the drug A- and drug B-treated groups respectively,

$$H_0: \pi_1 - \pi_2 = 0$$

or

$$H_0: \pi_1 = \pi_2.$$

If this common value for the proportion of survivors as specified by the null hypothesis is denoted π then it can be shown that

$$SE(p_1 - p_2) = \sqrt{\pi(1 - \pi)\left(\frac{1}{n_1} + \frac{1}{n_2}\right)} \tag{7.10}$$

where p_1 and p_2 are the observed proportions of survivors in samples size n_1 and n_2 taken from the two populations of interest, and $SE(p_1 - p_2)$ is the standard error of the difference between these two proportions. In practice, of course, this common value of π in the populations is not known and the best estimate of the quantity is the proportion of survivors observed in the two treated groups combined. In the example, there were 29 survivors in the two groups out of a total of 50 patients studied (see Table 7.6), so that the overall proportion of survivors is 29/50 or 0·58. This pooled estimate of the proportion of survivors can also be obtained as a weighted average of p_1 and p_2:

$$p = \frac{n_1 p_1 + n_2 p_2}{n_1 + n_2} \tag{7.11}$$

where the weights are the respective sample sizes, and p denotes the pooled value. Substituting this into Eqn. 7.10,

$$SE(p_1 - p_2) = \sqrt{pq\left(\frac{1}{n_1} + \frac{1}{n_2}\right)} \tag{7.12}$$

where q is defined as $1 - p$.

Combining these results, the following test statistic is appropriate for testing the difference between proportions in independent samples.

$$z = \frac{p_1 - p_2}{\sqrt{pq\left(\frac{1}{n_1} + \frac{1}{n_2}\right)}}. \tag{7.13}$$

This should be referred to tables of the standard normal distribution (Table B.2)

Substituting in the results in the clinical trial example, this equation becomes

$$z = \frac{0·68 - 0·48}{\sqrt{0·58(0·42)\left(\frac{1}{25} + \frac{1}{25}\right)}} = 1·433.$$

For a two-sided test at a 5% level of significance, the critical z value is 1·96 and, since the calculated value of 1·433 is not greater than this, it must be concluded that the difference between the drug effects is not statistically significant. In fact, examining the table of the standard normal distribution, it can be seen that the *p* value is just greater than 10%.

In some texts, the estimate of the standard error of the difference between two proportions may be given as

$$\text{SE}(p_1 - p_2) = \sqrt{\frac{p_1 q_1}{n_1} + \frac{p_2 q_2}{n_2}}. \tag{7.14}$$

This is an acceptable approximation so long as n_1 and n_2 are nearly equal and p_1 and p_2 do not differ substantially. This formula for the standard error results in a figure of 0·137 for the example, as opposed to a value of 0·140 obtained with the more exact expression given by Eqn. 7.12. The standard error formula given by Eqn. 7.14 should, however, be used for estimating confidence intervals for the difference between two proportions, and 95% or 99% confidence intervals are given by

$$(p_1 - p_2) \pm z_c \sqrt{\frac{p_1 q_1}{n_1} + \frac{p_2 q_2}{n_2}} \tag{7.15}$$

where z_c is the 5% or 1% critical value for the normal distribution. For example, the 95% confidence interval for the difference between the proportions alive on drug A and drug B is

$$0·2 \pm 1·96 \,(0·137)$$

or from −0·069 to 0·469.

The summary measure used here (the difference between the proportions) is not the only measure possible when a proportion is being compared between two groups. In Chapter 10 the *odds ratio* and *relative risk* will be introduced, which are alternative measures of association.

The conditions under which the normal distribution can be used as an approximation to the binomial are that the total sample size be greater than 20, and that $n_1 p$, $n_2 p$, $n_1 q$ and $n_2 q$ are all greater than 5 for sample sizes between 20 and 40. The approximation should be quite valid for a total sample size, that is in the two groups, above 40. These criteria are satisfied in the example. If the criteria do not hold, then an exact test for the comparison of proportions based on the binomial distribution is available (see Section 7.11). The *z* test for independent proportions is summarized in Section C.11 of Appendix C.

7.10 Comparison of two independent proportions: the χ^2 test

A more common alternative to the *z* test discussed in the last section is to employ a χ^2 test to compare differences between two independent proportions. This test is easier to apply, but the computational approach, though mathematically equivalent, is quite different.

The data are laid out in a 2 × 2 table, and the test statistic is based on the observed and expected (under the null hypothesis) frequencies in each of the four cells of the table. It is essential, however, that the actual numbers in the cells are used rather than the percentages or proportions. Table 7.7 shows the results obtained when cigarette smoking in a group of 150 patients with an upper respiratory tract infection (URTI) is compared with that of a control group of 140 patients without URTI. The aim is to determine if smoking is associated with URTI or, equivalently, if there is a difference in the proportion of smokers amongst the population of URTI patients and the comparison population. As in previous examples, it will be assumed that the comparison is valid, and that the design of the study has been adequate. It is important, however, that the two

Table 7.7. The χ^2 test. Smoking status in 150 patients with upper respiratory tract infection (URTI) compared to 140 controls

(a) Observed numbers

	URTI	Controls	Total
Smokers	95 (63·3%)	70 (50·0%)	165 (56·9%)
Non-smokers	55 (36·7%)	70 (50·0%)	125 (43·1%)
Totals	150 (100·0%)	140 (100·0%)	290 (100·0%)

(b) Expected numbers

	URTI	Controls	Total
Smokers	85·345	79·655	165
Non-smokers	64·655	60·345	125
Totals	150	140	290

(c) Calculation

Observed (O)	Expected (E)	O − E	(O − E)²	(O − E)²/E
95	85·345	9·655	93·219	1·092
55	64·655	−9·655	93·219	1·442
70	79·655	9·655	93·219	1·170
70	60·345	−9·655	93·219	1·545
				5·249

$\chi^2 = 5\cdot249$; d.f. = 1; $p < 0\cdot05$

samples should have been independently chosen. The null hypothesis then states that the proportion of smokers in each group is the same.

The first step in applying the test being considered is to calculate the numbers of people expected to be observed in the four cells of the table if, in fact, the null hypothesis were true. If there really is no difference between the groups, it would be expected that the proportion of smokers observed in the total sample, 165/290 = 0·5690, would be seen in each of the groups, thus out of 150 cases of URTI it would be expected that 0·5690 × 150 = 85·345 individuals would be smokers. Similarly, for the controls, 0·5690 × 140 = 79·655 persons would be expected to be smokers. Now, the overall proportion of non-smokers in the two groups combined is 125/290 = 0·4310, so that in 150 cases of URTI 0·4310 × 150 = 64·655 non-smokers are expected and a similar calculation leads to 60·345 expected non-smokers in the comparison group.

The middle of Table 7.7 shows these expected numbers filled into the corresponding cells of a 2 × 2 table. Note that when these expected numbers are added up across the rows and columns, the same total numbers of cases and controls and smokers and non-smokers as were in the original table are obtained. This is an important property of the expected numbers, and it can be seen that, in fact, for such a table only one of the expected numbers need be calculated and that all the others may be obtained by subtracting from the totals at the edge of the table (the marginal totals). In practice, it is advisable to calculate all the expected values, and to check the calculation by ensuring that they do add up to the original totals. It is usually sufficient to keep to three decimal places in the calculation.

Once the expected numbers have been calculated in this way, the significance test is fairly straightforward. Obviously, the greater the difference between the observed and the expected figures, the more evidence there is to reject the null hypothesis. The test statistic is based on this observation, and also includes a factor to allow for the relative magnitude of these differences (e.g. a difference of 10 is much more striking if it arises from values of 30 and 20 than from values of 310 and 300). The test statistic used is

$$\chi^2 = \sum \frac{(O - E)^2}{E} \tag{7.16}$$

where the Os are the four observed numbers in the body of the table and the Es are the four expected numbers. Summation is over the four cells of the table. The bottom of Table 7.7 illustrates the calculation of this sum which turns out to be 5·249. Note that the magnitude of the $O - E$ quantities is the same for each cell of the table in the 2 × 2 case but this is not so for larger tables. (The sum of the $O - E$ quantities is always 0 however.)

The sum 5·249 is then referred to tables of the χ^2 distribution on one degree of freedom (Table B.4). (For a 2 × 2 table there is only one degree of freedom. If the marginal totals are fixed, the number of observations in only one of the four cells of the table is free to vary.) Note that the chi-square test statistic as calculated must always have a positive sign, and unlike the other tests considered so far, it does not indicate which of the groups has the larger proportion. The critical values given in the χ^2 table must be *exceeded* for a significant result.* The two-sided critical value for χ^2 with one degree of freedom is 3·841 for a 5% level of significance, and since the calculated value of 5·249 is greater than this, it can be concluded that there is a significant difference in the proportion of smokers among the URTI cases and controls. The exact same result would have been obtained if the methods of the last section, using the z test, had been employed. Which test to use is quite arbitrary, though the χ^2 test is by far the most popular. Although it does not enable confidence intervals to be calculated, it has the great advantage, as will be seen later, that the method extends to tables larger than 2 × 2.

The applicability of the χ^2 test for 2 × 2 tables depends on the same criteria as used in the z test, which can be restated in terms of the expected values. For total sample sizes less than 20, the usual wisdom is that a more exact test should be used (see next section). For sample sizes between 20 and 40, the test is quite valid as long as none of the expected frequencies falls below 5. For sample sizes greater that 40, there should be no problem with the use of the χ^2 test. Recent work however, suggests that the 2 × 2 table χ^2 should be used even if the sample size is smaller than noted above, as Fisher's test (in the next section) may be too conservative (D'Agostino *et al.* 1988). The application of the χ^2 test is summarized in Appendix C, Section C.12.

7.11 Comparison of two independent proportions: Fisher's exact test

As has been pointed out, the χ^2 test may not be valid whenever the expected frequency in any of the cells in a 2 × 2 table falls below 5. In this case, an exact test is available called *Fisher's exact test*. Unlike all the other significance tests so far described, this test involves the calculation of the p value directly, without the use of a particular test statistic. Of all the tests encountered, Fisher's exact test is, without any doubt, the most difficult to calculate but, nonetheless, is useful in

---

* The χ^2 table gives both one- and two-sided critical values for various significance levels. The one-sided critical values, however, do not refer to areas in one tail of the χ^2 distribution, but the interpretation of a one-sided test is as described before. The one-sided test is really only valid for the 2 × 2 tables being considered in this section.

many situations, and the computational method is outlined below. (Many statistical computer packages will also perform the test for you.)

The χ^2 test for a 2 × 2 table has been described as a test for the comparison of proportions in two independent samples. In such a situation, the numbers of individuals in each sample are determined by the investigator, and thus, depending on the layout of the table, the column totals are fixed while the row totals are free to vary according to the results of the study.

The χ^2 test, however, may also be used where one sample is classified by two binary variables; thus, the numbers of smokers and non-smokers in males and females in a single sample from a population might be examined. This is still a two-group comparison though based on a single sample. In this case, both the row totals and the column totals are free to vary; they are determined by the sex and smoking distributions in the sample, and are not fixed in advance of the study. The only quantity fixed is the total sample size. The χ^2 test is also appropriate for 2 × 2 tables arising in this manner. It is also possible that in a 2 × 2 table both the row and column totals are fixed beforehand by the investigator. This type of situation rarely arises in medical applications, but again the χ^2 test is appropriate.

Now Fisher's exact test is in fact based on fixed row and column totals, and so, theoretically, is not applicable to 2 × 2 tables arising from either the two-sample or one-sample situations described above. However, the test is often used in these cases also, with the proviso that it is conditional on (i.e. assumes) fixed row and column totals (fixed marginals), thus the test is not 'exact' in the situations in which it is often applied.

Underlying the approach to all hypothesis tests is the distribution of a specific test statistic, and the calculation of the area (areas) — corresponding to probabilities — in the tail(s) of the distribution cut off by the test statistic actually calculated on the basis of the observed results. In Fisher's exact test, the distribution of all possible 2 × 2 tables with the same fixed column and row totals as the one observed in the study are examined. The probability of obtaining each of these tables, if there is no relationship between the two factors being studied, can be calculated. For a general 2 × 2 table laid out as shown in Table 7.8, this probability is

$$P = \frac{r_1! \; r_2! \; s_1! \; s_2!}{n! \; a! \; b! \; c! \; d!} \tag{7.17}$$

The letters r and s with the subscripts refer to the row and column totals, and a, b, c and d are the numbers in each of the cells; n is the total sample size. The exclamation mark denotes 'factorial' and means successive multiplication of the integers in descending order, thus $5! = 5 \times 4 \times 3 \times 2 \times 1 = 120$. $0!$ is defined as equal to 1.

Now, to calculate a p value for Fisher's exact test, it is necessary to add up the

Table 7.8. Fisher's exact test: general layout for a 2×2 table and its exact probability (p)

a	b	r_1
c	d	r_2
s_1	s_2	n

$$p = \frac{r_1!\, r_2!\, s_1!\, s_2!}{n!\, a!\, b!\, c!\, d!}$$

probabilities of the observed table, and any even more unlikely ones, in the tail of the distribution of all possible tables. This will give a one-sided test if only tables showing a more extreme result than that actually obtained are included, which at the same time also suggest the same direction of difference in the result. A two-sided test is obtained by doubling the one-sided p value.

Suppose that 16 elderly insulin-dependent patients with diabetes mellitus were studied and that six of these were classified as having had poor diabetic control during their illness. The patients were also examined to determine if they suffered any of the long-term complications of diabetes, such as deteriorating eyesight or circulatory problems. Table 7.9a displays these results in a 2×2 table. The aim is to determine if good control of diabetes is associated with a lower rate of complications. Among the seven patients with complications, four or 57·1% had poor control, while among the nine patients without complications, only two or 22·2% could be so classified. Thus, on the basis of the sample results, there seems to be an association between the two factors, but is it statistically significant? From the usual viewpoint, since the sample size is less than 20, the χ^2 test would not be valid, and Fisher's test should be used instead.

The easiest way to apply Fisher's exact test is firstly to rearrange the observed 2×2 table so that the number in the top left cell is the smallest of the observed cell frequencies. In this example the smallest cell frequency is 2, and the rearranged table is shown in Table 7.9b. Labelling the table by the number in the top left cell, this is called set 2. The tables with more extreme results are then obtained by successively reducing the top left figure by 1 with the remainder of the table determined by the fact that the row and column totals are fixed. This process is repeated until a table with a top left cell having a 0 entry is obtained. In the example, set 1, with a 1 in the top left cell, has 5, 8 and 2 in the other three cells determined by the fixed rows and columns (Table 7.9c). This table has more extreme results in the same direction as the original, in that only 1/9 (11·1%) of those with no complications had poor diabetic control compared to 22·2% in the original table. The final set in the example, set 0 with a zero in the top left, has again even more extreme results.

The one-sided p value for the test is now obtained by summing the probabilities of these three sets or tables. In general, the number of such tables will be one more

Table 7.9. Fisher's exact test: diabetic control and complications in 16 patients

(a) Original table

	Diabetic complications		
Diabetic control	Present	Absent	Total
Good	3(42·9%)	7(77·8%)	10(62·5%)
Poor	4(57·1%)	2(22·2%)	6(37·5%)
Totals	7(100·0%)	9(100·0%)	16(100·0%)

(b) Rearranged table (set 2)

	Diabetic complications		
Diabetic control	Absent	Present	Total
Poor	2	4	6
Good	7	3	10
Totals	9	7	16

(c) Set 1

1	5	6
8	2	10
9	7	16

(d) Set 0

0	6	6
9	1	10
9	7	16

than the smallest frequency observed in any cell of the original. The probability of set 0 is calculated first. Using Eqn. 7.17,

$$P = \frac{6! \; 10! \; 9! \; 7!}{16! \; 0! \; 6! \; 9! \; 1!}$$

and cancelling this reduces to (using the subscript 0 to denote the set)

$$P_0 = \frac{10! \; 7!}{16! \; 1!}.$$

This probability can be computed directly by cancelling a little more, noting that $10!/16! = 1/(16 \times 15 \times 14 \times 13 \times 12 \times 11)$. Calculated in this manner, $P_0 = 0·0008741.$* If some of the numbers are fairly large, tables of log factorials may be employed. Table B.8 gives the logarithms of all the factorials from 0 to 99. From this table, $\log P_0 = \log 10! + \log 7! - \log 16! - \log 1! = 6·55976 + 3·70243 -$

---

* Many small calculators now have a factorial key, which can make this calculation even easier.

$13 \cdot 32062 - 0 \cdot 0 = -3 \cdot 05843$. The decimal part of this log value must be positive to get the antilog from a table, so that $\log P_0 = \overline{4} \cdot 94157 \ (- \ 4 \cdot 0 + 0 \cdot 94157)$. The $0 \cdot 94157$ must now be looked up in an antilog table* (Table B.9) where its antilog is found to be $8 \cdot 742$. Thus, the antilog of $\overline{4} \cdot 94157$ is $0 \cdot 0008742$ which is almost identical to the value previously obtained for P_0.

Once P_0 (the probability of set 0) is calculated, the probabilities for the remaining sets (if any) are easily obtained. If the four entries in the body of set i, where i is any number, are denoted as a_i, b_i, c_i and d_i then

$$P_{i+1} = P_i \times \frac{b_i \times c_i}{a_{i+1} \times d_{i+1}}. \tag{7.18}$$

That is, to obtain the probability of a set it is necessary to multiply the probability of the previous set by b and c from that set and divide by a and d from the new set. Thus

$$P_1 = P_0 \times \frac{6 \times 9}{1 \times 2} = 0 \cdot 0236007$$

$$P_2 = P_1 \times \frac{8 \times 5}{2 \times 3} = 0 \cdot 157338.$$

In this case, $P_0 + P_1 + P_2 = 0 \cdot 1818$. Under the assumption of fixed rows and columns, and independence of the two factors being studied, this is the probability that the result, or one even more extreme, is spurious. This, of course, defines the one-sided p value and the two-sided value is obtained by doubling this figure $(0 \cdot 3636)$. Thus, in this example, diabetic complications are not significantly associated with poor control (Fisher's exact test; two-sided; $p = 0 \cdot 36$).

As can be seen, this test is quite complex to perform, but a little practice does help. Section C.13 in Appendix C summarizes the steps involved.

7.12 Comparison of two independent sets of proportions: the χ^2 test

In Section 7.10 the use of the χ^2 test for analysing independent data laid out in a 2×2 table was described. In many cases, however, data will be laid out in a larger table than a 2×2. Either a qualitative variable with perhaps more than two categories is to be compared in two (or more) independent samples, or the relationship between two qualitative variables is being examined in one sample. (The discussion in the previous section on Fisher's exact test drew attention to

---

* Looking up $0 \cdot 9416$.

such situations in a 2 × 2 context.) The χ^2 test is the appropriate test to employ for such tables larger than 2 × 2 also.

The use of the χ^2 test for a 3 × 2 table with three rows and two columns will be illustrated. Chapter 1, Table 1.1, gave the smoking status of males and females in a study of 2724 persons, and is reproduced in Table 7.10. The null hypothesis in this case would be that the distribution of smoking category is the same in males and females. The data can be equivalently interpreted as a comparison of the proportion of males (or females) between the three smoking categories, in which case the null hypothesis is that the proportion of males (females) is the same in each category.

The figures in the table suggest a definite difference between males and females and with such a large sample size it could be presumed that the observed result actually does reflect a population difference between males and females. For illustrative purposes however, a χ^2 test will be performed on these data. The approach is identical to that used in the 2 × 2 table. Firstly, the expected numbers (E) under the null hypothesis are calculated. For instance, since there were *in toto* 1168 current smokers from a total of 2724 persons (42·9%) this percentage of males would be expected to be current smokers; 42·9% of 1353 males is 580·14 which is the expected number of male smokers. All the other expected numbers may be calculated in a similar manner, and are also given in Table 7.10. In general, to calculate the expected number in any cell, multiply the corresponding row total by the corresponding column total and divide by the total sample size. Thus, the expected number of male smokers can be obtained from 1168 × 1353/2724 = 580·14. Note that in this example, once two of the expected numbers in a particular column are calculated, the remainder follow by subtraction from the row and column totals which remain fixed as usual.* It is suggested however that each expected number be calculated directly as above, and that a check on the calculations be made by confirming that they do add up to the correct row and column totals.

Once the expected numbers are calculated, the quantities $(O - E)^2/E$ are determined as before for each cell of the table, where O represents the observed numbers in the cells. (Note again that the $O - E$ quantities should sum to zero, apart from rounding errors.) The test statistic is then

$$\chi^2 = \sum \frac{(O - E)^2}{E} \tag{7.16}$$

as in the 2 × 2 table, but with two degrees of freedom in this example. In general, for a table with I rows and J columns there are $(I - 1)(J - 1)$ degrees of freedom

---

* In the light of the discussion of the 2 × 2 table in Section 7.10 it can be said that a 2 × 3 table has two degrees of freedom.

Table 7.10. The χ^2 test. Smoking status by sex in 2724 persons (see Table 1.1). O'Connor & Daly (1983) with permission

(a) Observed numbers

	Male	Female	Total
Current smokers	669 (49·5%)	499 (36·4%)	1168 (42·9%)
Ex-smokers	328 (24·2%)	215 (15·7%)	543 (19·9%)
Non-smokers	356 (26·3%)	657 (47·9%)	1013 (37·2%)
	1353 (100·0%)	1371 (100·0%)	2724 (100·0%)

(b) Expected numbers

	Male	Female	Total
Current smokers	580·14	587·86	1168
Ex-smokers	269·71	273·29	543
Non-smokers	503·15	509·85	1013
	1353	1371	2724

(c) Calculation

Observed (O)	Expected (E)	$O - E$	$(O - E)^2$	$(O - E)^2/E$
669	580·14	88·86	7896·100	13·611
328	269·71	58·29	3397·724	12·598
356	503·15	−147·15	21653·123	43·035
499	587·86	−88·86	7896·100	13·432
215	273·29	−58·29	3397·724	12·433
657	509·85	147·15	21653·123	42·470
				137·579

$\chi^2 = 137·579$; d.f. = 2; $p < 0·001$

which, with $I = 3$ and $J = 2$, is two degrees of freedom here, and of course one degree of freedom for a 2×2 table. In the smoking example, an extremely large value for χ^2 of 137·579 is obtained which, when referred to Table B.4 on two degrees of freedom, is seen to be highly significant. Unless the sample size is very large, χ^2 values of this magnitude are most unusual. Note that for tables larger than the 2×2 a one-sided χ^2 test is not applicable, since it is impossible to specify beforehand, or indeed interpret, a one-sided alternative hypothesis.

The χ^2 test can be employed so long as not more than 20% of the expected numbers in the cells are less than 5, with no cell having an expected frequency of less than 1. In the 2×2 situation, of course, this requires that all the expected numbers are greater than 5, which was the condition given already for this case.

As has been said, this example could be interpreted as a three-group comparison of the proportion of males, without any change of interpretation. As will be discussed in Section 8.7, the χ^2 test easily extends to any size table (3×3, 4×3, etc.) and has applicability in many situations. It is the most widely used test in medical research and one of the most useful tests to know. Its application is summarized in Section C.14 of Appendix C.

7.13 Comparison of paired proportions: confidence intervals and the McNemar test

The tests for proportions in the previous sections assume that the groups being compared are independent. In this section, a simple test for use with paired samples, where the variable under examination is binary, is described. The test is sometimes called a test for correlated proportions.

Suppose that 18 patients on two different antihypertensive drugs were studied. Each patient was given either drug A or drug B for a 1-month period, and a drop in systolic blood pressure of more than 15 mmHg was considered a success, and a lesser drop or rise, a treatment failure. After a washout period the treatments were switched around so that those previously on drug A were now given drug B and *vice versa*. The same criteria were again used to assess the effectiveness of the treatment. Essentially then, there exists a paired sample with each of the 18 patients on each of the two treatments, with the effectiveness of the drugs determined on a qualitative binary scale as either a success or failure.

Paired data like these are often incorrectly analysed. The tendency is to create a 2×2 table for the results as shown in Table 7.11a and perform the usual chi-square test on it. Unfortunately however, this is incorrect; the two groups (drug A and drug B) are not independent and the analysis must take this into account. The table, although suitable for the presentation of results, cannot be used for significance testing since the 18 persons on each treatment are the same. The analysis must be performed in terms of the 18 pairs of observations — the result on drug A and the result on drug B for each individual. This requires more information than is contained in Table 7.11a and a table must be formed for analysis purposes as shown in Table 7.11b. The entry in the top left cell of 1 means that one person (one of the pairs) had a success with both treatments. The entry of 3 means that three persons were treated successfully with drug B but unsuccessfully with drug A. Nine persons, on the other hand, had a successful outcome on drug A and not on drug B. In five persons, neither drug worked. When analysing correlated or paired proportions, the data must be laid out in this way. Table 7.12 shows this general layout. The plus and minus signs can refer to whatever the binary outcome is in the particular data being analysed. McNemar's test for this type of data is truly

Table 7.11. The McNemar test. Outcome of a paired experiment on 18 patients

(a) Summary of results

	Drug A	Drug B	Total
Success	10 (55·6%)	4 (22·2%)	14
Failure	8 (44·4%)	14 (77·8%)	22
Totals	18 (100·0%)	18 (100·0%)	36

(b) Layout for test

		Drug A		Total
		Success	Failure	
Drug B	Success	1	3	4
	Failure	9	5	14
	Totals	10	8	18

$$\text{McNemar's } \chi^2 \text{ on 1 d.f.} = \frac{(9-3)^2}{9+3} = 3\cdot0; \text{ NS}$$

one of the few tests that can be done in one's head. A χ^2 on one degree of freedom is calculated as

$$\chi^2 = \frac{(c-b)^2}{b+c}. \tag{7.19}$$

In the example, $\chi^2 = 6^2/12 = 3\cdot0$. For a two-sided, 5% significance level, the critical χ^2 value is 3·841 (Table B.4) so that no significant difference can be claimed between the effects of the drugs.

Note that only the untied observations contribute to this test statistic. The persons (pairs) on whom the effects of the two drugs were the same (two successes or two failures) do not enter into the calculation. These are called tied pairs; only the untied pairs are used. An alternative analytical procedure for such data (*sequential analysis*) is discussed in Chapter 11.

Table 7.12. The McNemar test: general layout

		Group 1	
		+	−
Group 2	+	a	b
	−	c	d

$$\text{McNemar's } \chi^2 \text{ on 1 d.f.;} \quad \frac{(c-b)^2}{b+c}$$

For small sample sizes, an exact test statistic can be used. The number of pairs with a preference for one drug rather than the other one can be referred to the table for the sign test (Table B.6) entered at n equal to the *total number of untied pairs*. Thus, in the example, the test statistic could be 9 (the number of pairs denoting a preference for drug A). For a 5% two-sided significance test for 12 untied pairs, the lower and upper critical values are 2 and 10. The test statistic falls within the acceptance region, and therefore the results are non-significant. The use of this exact test is advisable when the sample sizes in the statistical table are adequate, even though the χ^2 approach is much easier to perform.

It may seem strange that the significance test only uses the untied pairs, a and b, and takes no account of the total sample size. This is because it is only the untied pairs that contribute information relating to the existence of a difference. However in estimating the magnitude of the difference between the paired proportions all the data is used.

The difference between the success rate on drug A and drug B is (from Table 7.11) $0.566 - 0.222 = 0.334$ (expressed as a proportion). Denoting these proportions by p_1 and p_2 it can be shown that

$$\text{SE}\,(p_1 - p_2) = \frac{1}{N}\sqrt{c + b - \frac{(c-b)^2}{N}}, \tag{7.20}$$

where c and b are the untied pairs in Table 7.12, and N in this case is the *total number of pairs*.* The 95% confidence interval for the difference between paired proportions is then given by the usual formula

$$(p_1 - p_2) \pm 1.96\,\text{SE}\,(p_1 - p_2). \tag{7.21}$$

In the example this is

$$(0.556 - 0.222) \pm 1.96\,\sqrt{12 - (36/18)}/18$$

which is 0.334 ± 0.344 or from -0.010 to 0.678. Thus at a 95% level of confidence drug A could be from 1.0% worse than drug B or up to 67.8% better. Section C.15 in Appendix C summarizes the analysis of paired proportions.

7.14 Comparison of two counts or rates: confidence intervals and the z test

If two counts are to be compared directly then the counts must be based on the same time period or same underlying distribution in space or time. If this is not the case then the counts must be converted to rates to correct for the different

---

* Some texts give the standard error formula as $(1/N)\sqrt{(b+c)}$. Equation 7.20 however is more correct.

periods of observation and it is the rates that must be compared. For the methods described in this section the two counts should be greater than 10.

Suppose that two cultures of bacteria were prepared in equal volumes and incubated on nutrient media. The number of colonies eventually growing on the two plates is 11 and 27. Is there evidence of different bacterial concentrations? The significance test for this is rather simple. If x_1 and x_2 are the observed counts then a test using the normal approximation to the Poisson is

$$z = \frac{x_1 - x_2}{\sqrt{(x_1 + x_2)}} \tag{7.22}$$

where

$$SE(x_1 - x_2) = \sqrt{(x_1 + x_2)} \tag{7.23}$$

is the standard error of the difference between the counts. For this example the z statistic is $(27 - 11)/\sqrt{(27 + 11)}$ which is 2·60, showing a significant difference between the counts and thus between the bacterial concentrations (5% two-sided test). A 95% confidence interval for the difference between the two counts is given by

$$(x_1 - x_2) \pm 1·96 \sqrt{(x_1 + x_2)}. \tag{7.24}$$

Note that the same standard error estimator is employed for both the confidence interval and the hypothesis test. In this case the confidence interval for the difference between the counts is $16 \pm 1·96 \sqrt{(38)}$ or from 3·9 to 28·1; the difference measure is not directly interpretable in the example however, whereas the ratio of the counts would estimate the ratio of the concentrations. A confidence interval for the ratio of two Poisson variables will be considered in Section 10·11 when the more general ratio of two rates will be discussed.

When two rates are being compared account must be taken of the possibly different person-years at risk in the two groups. Suppose that the 32·10 per million population annual death rate from acute lymphatic leukaemia, discussed in Section 6.11, was to be compared to a rate of 22·41 per million in a second region. The first figure arose from 11 deaths in 0·3427 million person-years and suppose the second figure is based on 17 deaths in 0·7586 million person-years. (Remember that the person-years at risk must be expressed in the same units as the rates themselves.) Table 7.13 illustrates the data.

Table 7.13. Childhood deaths from acute lymphatic leukaemia in two regions

Group i	Region 1	Region 2
No. deaths (x_i)	11	17
Person-years at risk ($\times 10^6$) (PYRS$_i$)	0·3427	0·7586
Annual rate per 10^6 (r_i)	32·10	22·41

Using similar arguments to those in Section 7.9 for the comparison of two proportions, letting θ be the common rate in the two regions under the null hypothesis,

$$\text{SE}\,(r_1 - r_2) = \sqrt{\frac{\theta}{\text{PYRS}_1} + \frac{\theta}{\text{PYRS}_2}}. \tag{7.25}$$

The best estimate of this common rate θ is the total number of deaths divided by the total person-years at risk. This is equivalent to a weighted average of the two observed rates weighted by the person-years. The pooled estimate of θ is

$$r = \frac{\text{PYRS}_1\,(r_1) + \text{PYRS}_2\,(r_2)}{\text{PYRS}_1 + \text{PYRS}_2} \tag{7.26}$$

giving as an estimate of the standard error under the null hypothesis

$$\text{SE}\,(r_1 - r_2) = \sqrt{\frac{r}{\text{PYRS}_1} + \frac{r}{\text{PYRS}_2}}, \tag{7.27}$$

where r, the pooled rate, is given by Eqn. 7.26. The significance test for comparing two rates is then formulated as

$$z = \frac{r_1 - r_2}{\sqrt{\dfrac{r}{\text{PYRS}_1} + \dfrac{r}{\text{PYRS}_2}}}. \tag{7.28}$$

This is referred to tables of the normal distribution. In the example the pooled value of the rate (r) is 25·42 and

$$z = \frac{32\cdot10 - 22\cdot41}{\sqrt{\dfrac{25\cdot42}{0\cdot3427} + \dfrac{25\cdot42}{0\cdot7586}}} = \frac{9\cdot69}{10\cdot38} = 0\cdot93.$$

This does not reach the two-sided critical value of 1·96 so that a significant difference between the regions is not demonstrated at a 5% two-sided level.

For confidence intervals the standard error of the difference between two rates is not based on a pooled estimate of the rates but rather on

$$\text{SE}\,(r_1 - r_2) = \sqrt{\frac{r_1}{\text{PYRS}_1} + \frac{r_2}{\text{PYRS}_2}} \tag{7.29}$$

which for the example is 11·10, compared to 10·38 based on Eqn. 7.27. The formula for the confidence interval is then

$$(r_1 - r_2) \pm z_c\,\text{SE}\,(r_1 - r_2) \tag{7.30}$$

where as usual z_c is the appropriate value from the normal distribution. The 95% confidence interval for the rate difference in the example is

$$9.69 \pm 1.96 \ (11.10)$$

which is from -12.07 to $+31.45$. At a 95% level of confidence Region 1 could have an annual childhood mortality rate from leukaemia ranging from a figure of 12.07 per million lower than Region 2 to 31.45 per million higher. The significance tests and confidence interval formulae for comparing two counts or rates are summarized in Section C.16, Appendix C.

7.15 Significance testing versus confidence intervals

It is worth while commenting at this stage on the two different approaches to statistical inference — significance testing and confidence intervals. This chapter has illustrated how each of the methods can be used in the comparison of two groups. Up to recently most statistical analyses in medical research were via significance tests, but many medical journals are now calling for a reduced emphasis on p-values and an increased use of confidence intervals.

It goes without saying that the results are the most important part of any research endeavour. As much effort should go into examination of the data as into its collection. As discussed in later chapters this should include evaluation of possible biases related to study design and execution, and to the influence of confounding factors such as age and sex. This teasing out of the results is vital to determine the medical importance or relevance of a particular finding and is in one sense far more important than a formal statistical analysis. The purpose of a statistical analysis is purely to determine the extent to which sampling variation could explain the observed results and whether they can be validly extended to the population(s) from which the study sample(s) were drawn.

Too often however, results have been sacrificed to the gods of significance tests and p-values. A statistically significant difference between two groups does not guarantee medical importance, it just indicates that the result is unlikely to be due to chance or more formally that one can reject the null hypothesis of no group difference. With a large enough sample size even the smallest and most unimportant difference can be made statistically significant.

At the other end of the scale a non-significant difference between two groups is not synonymous with no difference. A non-significant difference means that there is not enough evidence to reject the null hypothesis. Chance may be an explanation of the observed result but the possibility of a real difference cannot be excluded either. In many situations medically important results can be statistically non-significant due to an inadequate sample size. Again it is the magnitude of the result that is critical to its interpretation rather than its statistical significance.

The confidence interval approach to statistical analysis, on the other hand, rather than concentrating on the decision reject/do not reject, draws attention to the results actually obtained. It gives a range of values which, at a given probability level, are likely to contain the true population value for the measure of association employed. The confidence interval at the same time presents the result and conveys the inherent variability in the estimate of that result. In addition, as discussed, statistical significance can generally be inferred by observing whether the null value of the hypothesis test falls inside or outside the confidence interval. Confidence intervals however do not require the prespecification of a null value, which explains why the two approaches are not completely equivalent.

The confidence interval can be particularly illuminating for the presentation of non-significant results. If the sample size is too small the width of the confidence interval shows clearly the large range of values compatible with the observed result and thus allows one to see the possibly important effects that would be glossed over by giving only the negative result of the significance test. If the sample size is adequate for non-significant results the range covered by the confidence interval should be narrow enough to exclude the possibility of medically important effects.

The advantages of using confidence intervals in statistical analysis are many, and there is no doubt that their use will expand. Hypothesis testing however has served medical research well in the past, and a mixture of both approaches will no doubt be present for some time to come.

7.16 Summary

In this chapter an overview was given of the confidence interval and hypothesis-testing approaches for the comparison of two groups. It was shown how the sampling procedure, in terms of whether or not the groups were matched, and the level of measurement of the data both determine the specific method to employ. A point that must be made is that one cannot apply all possible valid tests to a given set of data and then choose, for presentation purposes, the one that gives a significant result. The most appropriate test must be chosen beforehand and its results accepted.

Computational details were given for the common two-group parametric and non-parametric tests and confidence interval estimates were explained. Tables 7.14 and 7.15 summarize the methods discussed, giving formulae, though the text will have to be consulted for the notation used.

It is hoped that this chapter will prove useful to researchers who wish to analyse their own data. Appendix C outlines, in step-by-step form, the computational details for all the procedures described, and Appendix B provides a

Table 7.14. Summary of hypothesis tests for the comparison of two groups

Comparison of:	Hypothesis test		Eqn. no.
Independent means	(*t* test)	$$t = \frac{\bar{x}_1 - \bar{x}_2}{\sqrt{\dfrac{S_p^2}{n_1} + \dfrac{S_p^2}{n_2}}}$$	(7.4)
		$$S_p^2 = \frac{(n_1 - 1) S_1^2 + (n_2 - 1) S_2^2}{n_1 + n_2 - 2}$$	(7.3)
		d.f. $= n_1 + n_2 - 2$	
Paired means	(paired *t* test)	$$t = \frac{\bar{d}}{S_d/\sqrt{n}}$$	(7.8)
		d.f. $= n - 1$	
Independent proportions	(*z* test)	$$z = \frac{p_1 - p_2}{\sqrt{\dfrac{pq}{n_1} + \dfrac{pq}{n_2}}}$$	(7.13)
		$$p = \frac{n_1 p_1 + n_2 p_2}{n_1 + n_2}$$	(7.11)
	(χ^2 test)	$$\chi^2 = \sum \frac{(O - E)^2}{E}$$	(7.16)
	(Fisher's exact test)	—	
Paired proportions	(McNemar test)	$$\chi^2 = \frac{(c - b)^2}{b + c}$$	(7.19)
Independent counts	(*z* test)	$$z = \frac{x_1 - x_2}{\sqrt{x_1 + x_2}}$$	(7.22)
Independent rates	(*z* test)	$$z = \frac{r_1 - r_2}{\sqrt{\dfrac{r}{PYRS_1} + \dfrac{r}{PYRS_2}}}$$	(7.28)
		$$r = \frac{PYRS_1 (r_1) + PYRS_2 (r_2)}{PYRS_1 + PYRS_2}$$	(7.26)
Independent medians	(Wilcoxon rank sum test)		
Paired medians	(Sign test) (Wilcoxon signed rank test)		

Table 7.15. Summary of confidence intervals for two-group difference measures

Difference between two:	Confidence interval	Eqn. no.
Independent means	$(\bar{x}_1 - \bar{x}_2) \pm t_c \sqrt{\dfrac{S_p^2}{n_1} + \dfrac{S_p^2}{n_2}}$ S_p^2 as in Table 7.14 d.f. $= n_1 + n_2 - 2$	(7.7)
Paired means	$\bar{d} \pm t_c\, S_d/\sqrt{n}$ d.f. $= n - 1$	(7.9)
Independent proportions	$(p_1 - p_2) \pm z_c \sqrt{\dfrac{p_1 q_1}{n_1} + \dfrac{p_2 q_2}{n_2}}$	(7.15)
Paired proportions	$(p_1 - p_2) \pm z_c \dfrac{1}{N} \sqrt{c + b - \dfrac{(c - b)^2}{N}}$	(7.20/7.21)
Independent counts	$(x_1 - x_2) \pm z_c \sqrt{x_1 + x_2}$	(7.24)
Independent rates	$(r_1 - r_2) \pm z_c \sqrt{\dfrac{r_1}{\text{PYRS}_1} + \dfrac{r_2}{\text{PYRS}_2}}$	(7.29/7.30)

useful set of statistical tables. Beware, however, that different texts may give the statistical tables in a different format, and that the actual test statistics for a given test, particularly for one of the non-parametric ones, although equivalent, can differ from book to book. For this reason, it is advisable to become familiar with one particular set of tables and the associated test statistics.

The next chapter moves on to consider the comparison of means and proportions in more than two groups.

8

Comparisons of More than Two Groups: Analysis of Variance and the Chi-square Test

8.1 Introduction

The previous chapter considered in detail the comparison of two groups using hypothesis tests and confidence intervals. Here the analysis of more than two groups is considered. The major part of what follows deals with the so-called analysis of variance, which despite its name is actually a technique for the comparison of means. The logic behind the approach is explained together with computational details in simple examples. It is hoped that this will provide the reader with enough detail to appreciate the very general applications of this methodology. The comparison of proportions in more than two groups using a simple extension of the chi-square test is examined, and a test for a trend in proportions is introduced.

There is a vast body of analytical techniques for multigroup analysis and the material in this chapter can only be considered a brief foray into this area. As has been pointed out previously however, two-group comparisons are much more common in medical applications, and in many cases problems may be reduced to the two-group case by appropriate grouping of categories. The contents of this chapter are somewhat difficult and require the reader to be conversant with much of the material covered so far in this text.

8.2 Comparison of independent means in more than two equal-sized groups: introduction to analysis of variance and the *F* test

When analysing means in more than two groups, which are not paired or matched, it would seem tempting to employ the usual independent *t* test and compare the groups in pairs. Thus for three groups, A, B and C, one might compare A with B, A with C and finally B with C. With more than three groups the number of comparisons increases quite quickly. Such a procedure is not to be recommended however for two basic reasons. The first is that *in the one analysis* many *t* tests would be used and, overall, the chances are greater than 5% that any single one of them might give a statistically significant result, even if the groups being compared had the same population means. The second reason is that the correct approach uses the data from all groups to estimate standard errors, and this can increase the power of the analysis considerably.

The correct technique to compare means in three or more groups is called *analysis of variance* or ANOVA for short. When there is only one qualitative variable which defines the groups a *one-way* ANOVA is performed. ANOVA is a very powerful method and can be extended to quite complex data structures. (A two-way ANOVA is used when groups are defined by two qualitative variables. See Chapter 12 for a fuller discussion.) Despite its misleading name the analysis of variance is a technique for the comparison of means, which happens to use estimates of variability in the data to achieve this.

The logic behind an analysis of variance is quite different from anything encountered so far in this text. Supposing blood pressures in three groups are being compared. Figure 8.1 shows the distribution of the blood pressures in two possible situations. In Fig. 8.1a the blood pressures in the three groups are fairly tightly spread about their respective means and it is easy enough to see that there is a difference between the means in the three groups. In Fig. 8.1b the three groups have the same means as previously but the individual blood-pressure

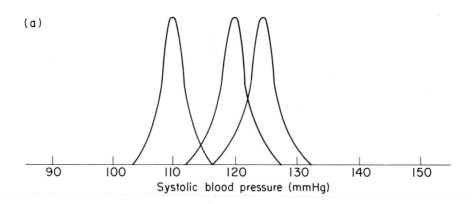

(a)

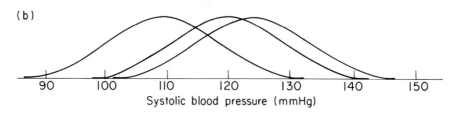

(b)

Fig. 8.1. Distribution of blood pressure in three groups: (a) with low variance, (b) with high variance.

distributions are much more spread out and it is quite difficult to see that the means are in fact different.

On this basis one could say more formally that to distinguish between the groups, the variability *between* or among the groups must be greater than the variability of, or *within*, the groups. If the within-group variability is large compared to the between-group variability any differences between the groups are difficult to detect. Thus, the determination of whether or not group means are significantly different can be achieved by a comparison of between- and within-group variability, which is measured by the variance. (Remember the variance is the square of the standard deviation and is a measure of variability or spread in the data.)

A simple example comparing three groups should suffice to explain the basic concepts involved. In general the number of groups will be denoted by k, and here $k = 3$. Suppose that systolic blood pressure is to be compared among current, ex- and non-cigarette smokers, and that there are four persons in each group. (The sample size in each group will be denoted n for the equal sample-size situation considered in this section.) The null hypothesis for this example is that the mean (population) systolic blood pressure is the same in the three smoking categories. Table 8.1 shows the data, with the means and variances in the three groups separately. ($\bar{x}_i$ and S_i^2 represent the mean and variance in the ith group. $\bar{x}$ without a subscript represents the mean of all the observations, called the grand mean, and N is the total sample size $-$ $3n$ or 12 in this example.)

One of the assumptions of the analysis of variance is that the (population) variances in the groups being compared are all equal. From an examination of the data in the table, this seems to be a reasonable assumption and is the same as that made for the independent t test also (see Section 7.4). Under this assumption the three sample variances within current, ex- and non-cigarette smokers all estimate this common value, which will be denoted σ^2. In this case of equal sample sizes the best estimate of the common population variance from the within sample values is the average of the three of them. This estimate is called the *within-group*

Table 8.1. Data for one-way analysis of variance in three equal sized groups

Group (i)	Smokers (1)	Ex-smokers (2)	Non-smokers (3)	$k = 3$
Systolic	125	110	95	
blood	135	125	100	
pressure	145	125	105	
	155	140	120	
n	4	4	4	$N = 12$
$\bar{x}_i$	140·00	125·00	105·00	$\bar{x} = 123·33$
S_i^2	166·67	150·00	116·67	

variance or, more commonly, the *within-group mean square* or the *error mean square*, and is denoted S_W^2 (the use of the latter two terms will be explained later):

$$S_W^2 = \Sigma S_i^2 / k \qquad \text{(equal sample sizes)} \qquad (8.1)$$

which in this case is

$$S_W^2 = (166 \cdot 67 + 150 \cdot 00 + 116 \cdot 67)/3 = 144 \cdot 45.$$

Note that the summation is over the k ($i = 1, 2, 3 \ldots k$) values of S_i^2. Since equal population variances have been assumed this estimate of the population variance, derived from the separate within-groups estimates, is valid whether the null hypothesis holds or not.

If the null hypothesis were true, the three groups could be considered three random samples, each of size n, from the same population, and the three sample means would be three observations from the sampling distribution of the mean. Now the sampling distribution of the mean has variance σ^2/n (the square of the standard error, where n the sample size is in this case equal to 4 and σ^2 is the population variance) and this gives a method for obtaining a further estimate of the population variance. The variance of the sample means is obtained directly from the usual formula for a variance (cf. Eqn. 2.3) where in this case the three sample means ($\bar{x}_i$) replace the observations and the grand mean ($\bar{x}$) is the figure subtracted from each value. In general the summation is over the k groups and the divisor is $k - 1$:

$$\frac{\Sigma(\bar{x}_i - \bar{x})^2}{k - 1}.$$

If this is equated with σ^2/n then the between-groups estimate of the population variance, denoted S_B^2 is

$$S_B^2 = \frac{n \, \Sigma(\bar{x}_i - \bar{x})^2}{k - 1} \qquad \text{(equal sample sizes).} \qquad (8.2)$$

This quantity, which is calculated from the between-group variance is called the *between-groups mean square*. If the null hypothesis is true then it is an estimate of the population variance. However, if the population means of the groups are not all equal, S_B^2 should be greater than the population variance. On this basis, a comparison of S_B^2 and S_W^2 (which always estimates the population variance), should indicate if the null hypothesis is likely to be true. If S_B^2 is much greater than S_W^2 there is more variability between the groups than would be expected given the variability within the groups, and the null hypothesis might be suspect. In the example the between-groups mean square is

$$S_B^2 = \frac{4 \, [(140 - 123 \cdot 33)^2 + (125 - 123 \cdot 33)^2 + (105 - 123 \cdot 33)^2]}{3 - 1}$$

which is equal to 1233·33. Now this is considerably larger than S_W^2 which was calculated as 144·45 so that one might doubt the null hypothesis in this case.

The question is, of course, how much larger than S_W^2 must S_B^2 be before the null hypothesis can be rejected formally at a particular level of significance. Now there is a significance test available which will test the hypothesis that two variances are equal. It is based on the ratio of the two variances and is called the *F* test.

$$F = S_B^2/S_W^2. \tag{8.3}$$

In the example, $F = 1233·33/144·45 = 8·54$. If *F* is sufficiently larger than unity one can reject the hypothesis that the two variances are equal, which in the situation considered here translates to a rejection of the null hypothesis that the means of the groups being compared are equal. This is how an analysis of variance allows for a comparison of group means. As for the *z*, *t* and χ^2 distributions, tables of the *F* distribution are available. The validity of the *F* test is based on a requirement that the populations from which the variances were taken are normal, but as usual approximate normality will suffice.

Note that the critical value, F_c, for the *F* distribution must be equalled or exceeded for a significant result and, in the analysis of variance a one-sided *F* test must be employed. This is because no interpretation can be attached to the ratio $F = S_B^2/S_W^2$ if it is less than one. An *F* value of less than one must be a chance occurrence and it is only when *F* exceeds one that the null hypothesis can be rejected.

An unusual property of the *F* distribution is that, unlike the *t* and χ^2 distributions, it has a *pair* of degrees of freedom. These are based on the degrees of freedom for the two variances in the *F* ratio. Looking at Eqn. 8.1, S_W^2 is based on the sum of *k* variances each with $n - 1$ degrees of freedom, so that its degrees of freedom are $k (n - 1)$. Now since *k* (the number of groups) multiplied by *n* (the sample size in each group) is equal to *N* (the total sample size), this gives a total of $N - k$ degrees of freedom for S_W^2. From Eqn. 8.2, S_B^2 obviously has $k - 1$ degrees of freedom. For a one-way analysis of variance $F = S_B^2/S_W^2$ has then $k - 1$ and $N - k$ degrees of freedom, the first member of the pair taken from the numerator of the *F* ratio and the second from the denominator.

Table B.13 in the Appendix gives tables of the *F* distribution. Separate pages are provided for *one-sided p* values of 0·05 and 0·01. (As stated above, two-sided tests are inappropriate for the analysis of variance.) Degrees of freedom for the numerator run from 1 to 10 along the top of the table, allowing for comparison of up to 11 groups. The degrees of freedom for the denominator are given down in the table from 1 to 20 with all values, up to 100 in jumps of 10 and up to 500 in jumps of 100. If the value of the degrees of freedom for a particular analysis is not given then the next lowest should be taken and used.

In the example the F ratio was 8·54 on 2 and 9 degrees of freedom. From the table the critical 5% (one-sided) value is 4·26 and the 1% value is 8·02. Thus the F value is sufficiently large to enable rejection of the null hypothesis at a 1% level of significance. The mean blood pressures are not the same in the three smoking categories ($F = 8·54$; d.f. $= 2,9$; $p < 0·01$). The question of which mean is significantly different from which will be discussed below.

8.3 One-way analysis of variance with unequal sample sizes

The discussion above and the formulae for the two estimates of the population variance were for equal sample sizes in the three groups. Although it is somewhat easier to understand the logic with equal sample sizes, extension to unequal sample sizes is not difficult. Table 8.2 shows almost identical data relating to blood pressure by cigarette smoking status, but this time rather than four persons in each group, there are five smokers, three ex-smokers and four non-smokers. The sample size in group i will be denoted n_i.

Table 8.2. Data for one-way analysis of variance in three unequal sized groups

Group (i)	Smokers (1)	Ex-smokers (2)	Non-smokers (3)	$k = 3$
Systolic	125	115	95	
blood	135	125	100	
pressure	140	135	105	
	145		120	
	155			
n_i	5	3	4	$N = 12$
$\bar{x}_i$	140·00	125·00	105·00	$\bar{x} = 124·58$
S_i^2	125·00	100·00	116·67	

As before, there are three separate estimates of the population variance within the three groups, but they are based on different sample sizes. With equal sample sizes the average of the three was taken, but now a weighted average is required. Remember that in the independent t test a weighted average of the two variances was taken to get what was called the pooled variance (see Eqn. 7.3 in Section 7.4). A similar procedure is followed here and each variance is weighted by its degrees of freedom ($n_i - 1$):

$$S_W^2 = \frac{(n_1 - 1)S_1^2 + (n_2 - 1)S_2^2 + (n_3 - 1)S_3^2}{(n_1 - 1) + (n_2 - 1) + (n_3 - 1)}.$$

This of course reduces to an unweighted average when the sample sizes are all equal. For the smoking example

$$S_W^2 = \frac{4\ (125) + 2\ (100) + 3\ (116\cdot67)}{4 + 2 + 3} = \frac{1050}{9} = 116\cdot67.$$

This generalizes to

$$S_W^2 = \frac{\Sigma\ (n_i - 1)S_i^2}{N - k} \qquad \text{(unequal sample sizes).} \qquad (8.4)$$

The extension of the formula for S_B^2 is slightly more difficult to justify. The usual result for the sampling distribution of the mean under the null hypothesis cannot be invoked because the sample size is not the same in each group. However, it can be taken on faith that instead of Eqn. 8.2

$$S_B^2 = \frac{n\ \Sigma\ (\bar{x}_i - \bar{x})^2}{k - 1} \qquad \text{(equal sample sizes),} \qquad (8.2)$$

the correct expression with unequal sample sizes is

$$S_B^2 = \frac{\Sigma\ n_i\ (\bar{x}_i - \bar{x})^2}{k - 1} \qquad \text{(unequal sample sizes).} \qquad (8.5)$$

This is, in the example

$$S_B^2 = \frac{5\ (140 - 124\cdot58)^2 + 3\ (125 - 124\cdot58)^2 + 4\ (105 - 124\cdot58)^2}{3 - 1}$$

$$= 2722\cdot9/2 = 1361\cdot45.$$

Again the significance test is performed by calculating the F ratio $F = S_B^2/S_W^2 = 1361\cdot45/116\cdot67 = 11\cdot67$, with 2 and 9 degrees of freedom as before. The 1% critical value is $8\cdot02$ and again in this example the null hypothesis of no group differences in means is rejected at this level of significance.

It should be noted that if the one-way ANOVA is used for the comparison of two groups only, the analysis is exactly and mathematically equivalent to the use of the independent t test of Section 7.4. The one-way ANOVA, like the independent t test, requires that the groups under comparison are independent. Adaptations of the method must be employed for paired or frequency matched data. It is important also to remember the assumptions underlying an analysis of variance. In the situation of a straightforward comparison between groups the distribution of the variable must be near normal in each group, with the same underlying variance. If, on examination of the data, these assumptions appear suspect a transformation of the variable may alleviate the problem (see Sections 7.4 and 1.7). Section C.17 of Appendix C summarizes calculations for the one-way ANOVA.

8.4 Sums of squares, mean squares and degrees of freedom

It is hoped that the above description of the analysis of variance is sufficient to allow an understanding of the basic ideas behind the technique. Usually, however, the approach is explained and carried out from a slightly different perspective. This section can be omitted without any loss of understanding of the technique.

So far in this text the sigma sign (Σ) has been used in a fairly straightforward manner to denote summation and it has been obvious what exactly is being summed up. For this section a slight extension of the use of Σ and the general notation must be made. Instead of using x on its own to denote one of the observations in a group, x_{ij} will explicitly refer to the jth observation in the ith group. j can thus have values ranging from one up to n_i (the sample size in the ith group). The summation sign will also have an explicit subscript to indicate what is being summed. Σ_i will mean summation over the k groups, Σ_j will mean summation over the observations in a group, and $\Sigma_i\Sigma_j$ will mean summation over all observations. To give an example, the mean and variance in the ith group would be expressed as

$$\bar{x}_i = \frac{\Sigma_j x_{ij}}{n_i} \tag{8.6}$$

$$S_i^2 = \frac{\Sigma_j(x_{ij} - \bar{x}_i)^2}{n_i - 1} \tag{8.7}$$

where the summations are over the n_i observations in the ith group.

Now the deviation of any individual observation (x_{ij}) from the grand mean ($\bar{x}$) can be expressed

$$(x_{ij} - \bar{x}) = (x_{ij} - \bar{x}_i) + (\bar{x}_i - \bar{x}). \tag{8.8}$$

This states simply that the deviation of any observation from the grand mean can be split into two components, a deviation of the observation from *its own* group mean, and the deviation of the group mean from the grand mean. It can be shown that if each of these deviations is squared and summed over all observations, that the following equality also holds

$$\Sigma_i\Sigma_j(x_{ij} - \bar{x})^2 = \Sigma_i\Sigma_j(x_{ij} - \bar{x}_i)^2 + \Sigma_i\Sigma_j(\bar{x}_i - \bar{x})^2. \tag{8.9}$$

Each of these is referred to as a *sum of squares*. The expression on the left is called the total sum of squares, and the two components, on the right, are called the within-group and between-group sums of squares respectively. Letting 'SSq' denote sum of squares

$$\text{Total SSq} = \text{Within-group SSq} + \text{Between-group SSq.} \tag{8.10}$$

In some sense the sums of squares are measures of the variability observed in the data. The total SSq measures the total variability independently of group membership, the within-group SSq measures the variability within the groups only (irrespective of how the group means differ), and finally the between-group SSq measures the variability between the groups with no contribution from the variability within.

As well as partitioning the total sum of squares into components within and between groups, the total degrees of freedom can be similarly partitioned. Remember that degrees of freedom refer to how many of the components of an expression are free to vary. Using the same arguments of Section 2.4, the total SSq has $N - 1$ degrees of freedom because there is a total of N observations and the grand mean is included in the SSq. The within-group SSq has $N - k$ degrees of freedom because all observations are included in its calculation in addition to the k group means. Note that the between-group SSq can be expressed as

$$\Sigma_i\Sigma_j(\bar{x}_i - \bar{x})^2 = \Sigma_i n_i(\bar{x}_i - \bar{x})^2 \tag{8.11}$$

since the Σ_j just repeats the summation n_i times in each group. With this formulation it is clear that the between-group SSq has $k - 1$ degrees of freedom.

$$\text{Total d.f.} = \text{Within-group d.f.} + \text{Between-group d.f.} \tag{8.12}$$
$$N - 1 = N - k + k - 1$$

When a sum of squares is divided by its degrees of freedom the result is called a mean square (MSq for short). Comparing Eqns. 8.11 and 8.5 it is obvious that

$$S_B^2 = \text{Between-group MSq.}$$

Also, by substituting the value for S_i^2 from Eqn. 8.7 into Eqn. 8.4 for S_W^2, and comparing with Eqn. 8.9

$$S_W^2 = \text{Within-group MSq.}$$

The analysis of variance F test can thus be expressed as

$$F = \text{Between-group MSq/Within-group MSq} \tag{8.13}$$

on $k - 1$ and $N - k$ degrees of freedom.

Note that the total mean square (total SSq/total d.f.) is nothing more than an estimate of the variance of all the observations taking no account of group membership. It is often given the symbol S_T^2.

$$S_T^2 = \frac{\Sigma_i\Sigma_j(x_{ij} - \bar{x})^2}{N - 1}.$$

The actual magnitude of this quantity is not very important in an analysis of variance however.

For the unequal sample size example in the last section, the total SSq can be calculated as 3772·9. From earlier calculations in the same example the values for the other two sums of squares are seen to be

$$\text{Within-group SSq} \quad = 1050\cdot0$$
$$\text{Between-group SSq} = 2722\cdot9$$

which add to the total SSq. Most computer printouts and presentations of the analysis of variance are in terms of the sums of squares, giving rise to what is called an ANOVA table, and analyses of variance for more complex situations (see Chapter 12) are all based on an appropriate partitioning of both the total SSq and degrees of freedom. Short-cut formulae for calculating sums of squares are given in Appendix A. The ANOVA table for the second example with unequal sample sizes is given in Table 8.3 below.

Table 8.3. ANOVA table for the study of blood pressure and smoking (unequal sample size example)

Source of variation	d.f.	SSq	MSq	*F* ratio
Between groups	2	2722·9	1361·45	11.67
Within groups	9	1050·0	116·67	($p < 0\cdot01$)
Total	11	3772·9		

The between-group SSq is sometimes referred to as the *model sum of squares* and the within-group figure is often called the *residual sum of squares* (what is left over when the between-group variation is taken out) or the *error sum of squares* (the variation that cannot be explained by anything else).

8.5 Multiple comparisons and the interpretation of a significant *F* test

It was already pointed out that when means in more than two groups are being compared, use of many independent *t* tests on pairs of groups is not valid because of the possibility of misinterpretation of a significant result. For *k* groups there are $k(k-1)/2$ pairs of means which could be compared, and for seven groups there would be 21 *t* tests. One of these is likely to be significant at a 5% level (1/20), even if the null hypothesis were true and there were no real differences between the groups.

When an *F* test is significant, the correct conclusion is that the population means in the groups are not all the same. There is a difference among the means somewhere but it is not clear where. Perhaps the most straightforward solution is to just examine the data and note which means are different from which, without further formal statistical analysis. If however the design of the study was specifically to compare certain *prespecified* means, then the approach below is quite acceptable as long as the comparisons were chosen before examination of the data. If the data are examined just to see what significant comparisons turn up, more complex *multiple comparison* techniques must be used. These essentially correct for the large number of comparisons that must be made and allow an appropriately interpretable significance test to be performed. Multiple comparison tests are not considered in this text.

If certain specific comparisons were chosen beforehand then the equivalent of an independent t test can be used on the relevant means. The general wisdom is, however, that this should only be done if the overall F test is itself significant. Essentially an independent t test (Eqn. 7.4) is used

$$t = \frac{\bar{x}_1 - \bar{x}_2}{\text{SE}\,(\bar{x}_1 - \bar{x}_2)} \tag{8.14}$$

where, without loss of generality, the comparison is assumed to be between groups 1 and 2. However for the standard error term, the estimate of the population variance based on all groups in the analysis (S_W^2) replaces the usual pooled estimate based on the specific two groups being compared (cf. Eqn. 7.3)

$$\text{SE}\,(\bar{x}_1 - \bar{x}_2) = \sqrt{\frac{S_W^2}{n_1} + \frac{S_W^2}{n_2}}. \tag{8.15}$$

Note that the divisors in the standard error term are n_1 and n_2, but the degrees of freedom for the test are $N - k$ (rather than $n_1 + n_2 - 2$ for the usual t test). These are the degrees of freedom that the variance estimate is based on. Remember that one of the assumptions of the analysis of variance was that the variances in the groups were the same so that S_W^2 estimates the variance of each of the groups. This is a far more accurate estimate than that based on two groups but it is the increase in the number of degrees of freedom for the t test that increases the efficiency of the analysis. For small sample sizes this is quite important since the increased degrees of freedom mean that the critical t value for the test will be smaller and more easily exceeded.

Assume that in the smoking/blood pressure (unequal sample size) example that prior interest had been on the comparison of blood pressures between current cigarette smokers and the other two groups. For the comparison of smokers and non-smokers the t test gives

$$t = \frac{140 - 105}{\sqrt{\dfrac{116{\cdot}67}{5} + \dfrac{116{\cdot}67}{4}}} = 35/7{\cdot}25 = 4{\cdot}83$$

on 9 degrees of freedom. The critical 1% (two-sided) t value is 3·25 so there is a highly significant difference between the blood pressures of current cigarette smokers and non-smokers. For the comparison between cigarette smokers and ex-smokers the t can be calculated:

$$t = \frac{140 - 125}{\sqrt{\dfrac{116{\cdot}67}{5} + \dfrac{116{\cdot}67}{3}}} = 15/7{\cdot}89 = 1{\cdot}90$$

again on 9 degrees of freedom. The critical two-sided 5% value is $2{\cdot}262$ so that the smokers and ex-smokers do not have significantly different blood pressures. The significant differences between the groups determined by the omnibus F test seems to be due to differences between smokers and non-smokers.

8.6 Confidence intervals in the analysis of variance

Confidence intervals for individual means or for the difference between two means are based on the usual approaches described in Sections 4.7 and 7.4 except that the within-group mean square S_W^2 is used as the estimate for the population variance in the standard errors, and the degrees of freedom are $N - k$ (total sample size in all groups less the number of groups). The confidence interval for the mean in a single group (group i) is given by

$$\bar{x}_i \pm t_c \frac{S_W}{\sqrt{n_i}} \tag{8.16}$$

where S_W is the square root of S_W^2, and there are $N - k$ rather than n_i degrees of freedom for the t statistic (cf. Eqn. 4.7). The 95% confidence interval for the mean systolic blood pressure in current smokers (unequal sample-size example) is therefore

$$140 \pm 2{\cdot}262 \sqrt{(116{\cdot}67/5)} \quad \text{or} \quad 140 \pm 10{\cdot}93$$

which is from $129{\cdot}07$ to $150{\cdot}93$ mmHg. Note that the critical value of the t distribution for 9 degrees of freedom ($2{\cdot}262$) was used rather than the value for 4 degrees.

Similarly the confidence interval for the difference between the means in groups 1 and 2 is given by

$$(\bar{x}_1 - \bar{x}_2) \pm t_c \sqrt{\frac{S_W^2}{n_1} + \frac{S_W^2}{n_2}}. \tag{8.17}$$

Again there are $N - k$ degrees of freedom (cf. Eqns. 7.4 and 7.7). For the difference between the blood pressures of smokers and non-smokers the 95% confidence interval is

$$(140 - 105) \pm 2\cdot262 \sqrt{\frac{116\cdot67}{5} + \frac{116\cdot67}{4}}$$

which is $35 \pm 16\cdot40$. Confidence interval calculations for ANOVA are summarized in Section C.17 of Appendix C.

8.7 Comparison of independent proportions in more than two groups: the χ^2 test

Section 7.12 considered the Chi-square (χ^2) test for comparing many proportions in two groups, using an example of the association of smoking status (current, ex- and non-smokers) in males and females. Equivalently this example could have been considered a comparison of the proportion of males in the three groups defined by smoking status. Thus the usual chi-square test is appropriate for multigroup comparisons. In fact the test is applicable to tables of any dimension (3×3 for instance) as long as the groups in the table are independent. The expected numbers in each cell (E) are calculated in the usual manner and the observed (O) and expected (E) numbers are entered into the standard formula

$$\chi^2 = \Sigma \frac{(O - E)^2}{E}. \tag{7.16}$$

As mentioned in Section 7.12 the degrees of freedom for the test are $(I - 1)(J - 1)$ where I and J are the numbers of rows and columns. It is usually suggested that for valid application of the test not more than 20% of the cells should have expected numbers less than 5 and no cell should have an expected frequency less than 1. If these conditions are not met then adjacent categories should be combined and the chi-square recalculated.

When comparing proportions in say k groups, the analysis is that of a $2 \times k$ contingency table. As an example, Table 8.4 examines in-hospital mortality after coronary artery bypass surgery in groups defined by increasing severity of angina using the New York Heart Association classification.

The proportions being compared are denoted p_i in the table, and the usual chi-square can be calculated from Eqn. 7.16. In the special case of a $2 \times k$ table, however, there is a short cut computational formula which is entirely equivalent. Firstly, the deaths (or whatever the proportion is being calculated on) in each group are squared and divided by the total number in the group. This quantity is then summed over all k groups and denoted $\mathcal{A}$. The chi-square, on $k - 1$ degrees of freedom is then

$$\chi^2 = \frac{N(N\mathcal{A} - D^2)}{D(N - D)} \tag{8.18}$$

Table 8.4. In-hospital mortality after coronary artery bypass surgery by severity of angina

Classification of angina:		I	II	III	IV	
Group:	i	1	2	3	4	Row totals
Dead	d_i	2	12	11	22	$D = 47$
Alive	$n_i - d_i$	160	545	403	559	$N - D = 1667$
Total	n_i	162	557	414	581	$N = 1714$
Proportion dead	$p_i = d_i/n_i$	0·0123	0·0215	0·0266	0·0379	
For χ^2 calculation:	d_i^2	4	144	121	484	
	d_i^2/n_i	0·0247	0·2585	0·2923	0·8330	$\mathcal{A} = 1·4085$

where N is the total sample size, D is the total number of deaths and

$$\mathcal{A} = \Sigma(d_i^2/n_i).$$

In the example

$$\chi^2 = \frac{1714\,[1714\,(1·4085) - (47)^2]}{47\,(1714 - 47)} = 4·49.$$

The reader should verify that this is exactly the same answer that would have been obtained if Eqn. 7.16 had been employed instead. The critical 5% chi-square on 3 $(k - 1)$ degrees of freedom is 7·815 so that on the basis of the usual chi-square test the differences between the proportions of deaths in the four anginal categories is non-significant.

If a chi-square test comparing more than two groups is significant, the question is often asked, as with the comparison of means, which groups are significantly different from which. Formal, more advanced, methods are available to help answer this, but it is often sufficient just to examine the data and draw conclusions from a visual inspection of the table.

Without doubt the chi-square test is the most commonly used test in medical statistics. The fact that it is as equally applicable to multigroup comparisons as to the comparison of two groups explains this in part. The popularity of the chi-square test, however, is mainly due to the fact that it can be used to analyse quantitative data also. All one has to do is categorize the quantitative variable (working with, for example, age groups rather than exact age) and apply the chi-square test in the usual way. The loss of information by categorizing into four or five groups is not great and often a table with a grouped variable can be more informative than working with the mean of the (ungrouped) variable. The categories however must be chosen before examination of the data and should not be selected to maximize group differences. This application of the chi-square test is summarized in Section C.14 of Appendix C.

8.8 The χ^2 test for a trend in proportions

When analysing proportions in more than two groups it is often of interest to know if the proportions increase or decrease as one moves along the groups. Such a question can only be asked of course if the groups have some intrinsic order.

If *prior to the analysis* a trend in the proportions had been considered likely, then a more powerful statistical test than the usual chi-square for a $2 \times k$ table is available. Note that this test should be applied only if the trend is hypothesized prior to examination of the data. Essentially the test is based on a null hypothesis of no group differences against an alternative hypothesis of a linear trend in proportions. If there is a real linear trend (in the population) then the test is more likely to give a significant result than the usual chi-square. On the other hand, if there are real group differences without a clear trend, the test is less powerful than the usual test.

The exact formulation of the chi-square test for trend is somewhat difficult to justify so the formula will be given here without explanation. The method is illustrated on the data for mortality after coronary bypass related to anginal status already examined in Table 8.4, and it is assumed that the researchers involved wished to examine whether mortality increased with increasing severity of angina. For examination of a trend a score must be assigned to each of the groups being compared. The choice of this score is arbitrary and usually it is quite adequate to assign scores of 1, 2, 3, etc. to each category. If the categories represent a grouping of a continuous variable (e.g. age groups) then the mid-point of the group could be used instead. In the example scores of 1 to 4 will be assigned to the four anginal groups. The data for the example, together with the quantities required for calculation of the chi-square for trend, are given in Table 8.5.

The chi-square for trend χ^2_{TR}, on 1 degree of freedom, is calculated as

$$\chi^2_{TR} = \frac{N(N\mathscr{C} - D\mathscr{B})^2}{D(N-D)(N\mathscr{D} - \mathscr{B}^2)} \tag{8.19}$$

where N is the total sample size, D is the total number of deaths,

$$\mathscr{B} = \Sigma n_i x_i$$
$$\mathscr{C} = \Sigma d_i x_i$$
$$\mathscr{D} = \Sigma n_i x_i^2$$

Table 8.5. In-hospital mortality after coronary artery bypass surgery by severity of angina (chi-square test for trend)

Classification of angina:		I	II	III	IV	
Group:	i	1	2	3	4	Row totals
Dead	d_i	2	12	11	22	$D = 47$
Total	n_i	162	557	414	581	$N = 1714$
For χ^2 calculation:	Score x_i	1	2	3	4	
	$n_i x_i$	162	1114	1242	2324	$\mathcal{B} = 4842$
	$d_i x_i$	2	24	33	88	$\mathcal{C} = 147$
	x_i^2	1	4	9	16	
	$n_i x_i^2$	162	2228	3726	9296	$\mathcal{D} = 15412$

and x_i is the assigned score. From the table

$$\chi_{TR}^2 = \frac{1714\,[1714\,(147) - 47\,(4842)]^2}{47\,(1714 - 47)\,[1714\,(15412) - (4842)^2]} = 4\cdot38.$$

This value exceeds the critical 5% value for chi-square on 1 degree of freedom so that one can conclude that there is a significant tendency for increased mortality rates to be associated with an increased severity of angina. Note that in the last section the ordinary chi-square (on 3 degrees of freedom) did not achieve significance for the same data, illustrating clearly the increased power of this test to detect a trend if it exists. No matter how many groups are involved, χ_{TR}^2 has 1 degree of freedom, and if significant the null hypothesis of no group difference is rejected in favour of a trend of increasing (or decreasing) proportions with group membership.

One can also test if there is a significant departure from a linear trend. (A linear trend holds if the proportions increase at a constant rate in proportion to the score assigned to the groups.) The chi-square for this test is obtained by subtracting the trend chi-square from the total (usual) chi-square and has $k - 2$ degrees of freedom where k is the number of groups.

$$\chi_{DEP}^2 = \chi^2 - \chi_{TR}^2. \tag{8.20}$$

In the example $\chi_{DEP}^2 = 4\cdot49 - 4\cdot38 = 0\cdot11$ which on 2 degrees of freedom is obviously non-significant. Thus, there is no evidence that the trend is not linear in this case. A significant departure from trend can arise together with a significant trend if there is an increase (decrease) in proportions that is not linear. A significant departure from trend in the absence of a significant trend is interpreted to mean that group differences exist but that there is no trend in the data.

Different formulae for the chi-square test for trend are to be found in different texts. Mostly these are equivalent formulations of the version given above (Eqn. 8.19) but sometimes there is a factor of $N - 1$ rather than N. This makes no difference in practice. As with the ordinary chi-square test, the test for trend should not be used if more than 20% of the expected numbers in the cells of the table fall below 5, or if any fall below 1. The chi-square test for trend is summarized in Section C.18, Appendix C.

8.9 Summary

In this chapter the comparison of independent proportions and means in more than two groups has been discussed. The analysis of variance (ANOVA) was introduced as the appropriate technique for the comparison of means, and it was indicated that this is a very powerful method that can extend to very complex data structures. The comparison of means in individually matched data was not

Table 8.6. Summary of formulae for comparison of means in more than two groups (one-way ANOVA) (see Appendix A for computational formulae)

Application	Formulae	Eqn. nos.
Overall comparison between means (F test)	$F = S_B^2 / S_W^2$ d.f. $= k - 1$ and $N - k$	(8.3)
	$S_B^2 = \dfrac{\Sigma n_i (\bar{x}_i - \bar{x})^2}{k - 1}$	(8.5)
	$S_W^2 = \dfrac{\Sigma (n_i - 1) S_i^2}{N - k}$	(8.4)
Comparison between two means (t test)	$t = \dfrac{\bar{x}_1 - \bar{x}_2}{\sqrt{\dfrac{S_W^2}{n_1} + \dfrac{S_W^2}{n_2}}}$ d.f. $= N - k$	(8.14/8.15)
Confidence interval for a single mean	$\bar{x}_i \pm t_c \dfrac{S_W}{\sqrt{n_i}}$ d.f. $= N - k$	(8.16)
Confidence interval for difference between two means	$(\bar{x}_1 - \bar{x}_2) \pm t_c \sqrt{\dfrac{S_W^2}{n_1} + \dfrac{S_W^2}{n_2}}$ d.f. $= N - k$	(8.17)

Table 8.7. Summary of formulae for comparison of proportions in more than two groups ($2 \times k$ table)

Hypothesis test	Formulae	Eqn. nos.
Overall test	$$\chi^2 = \sum \frac{(O - E)^2}{E}$$	(7.16)
	$$= \frac{N(N\mathscr{A} - D^2)}{D(N - D)}$$	(8.18)
	d.f. $= k - 1$	
Test for linear trend	$$\chi^2_{\text{TR}} = \frac{N(N\mathscr{C} - D\mathscr{B})^2}{D(N - D)(N\mathscr{D} - \mathscr{B}^2)}$$	(8.19)
	d.f. $= 1$	
Test for departure from linear trend	$\chi^2_{\text{DEP}} = \chi^2 - \chi^2_{\text{TR}}$	(8.20)
	d.f. $= k - 2$	

$$\mathscr{A} = \sum (d_i^2/n_i)$$
$$\mathscr{B} = \sum n_i\, x_i$$
$$\mathscr{C} = \sum d_i\, x_i$$
$$\mathscr{D} = \sum n_i\, x_i^2$$
$$N = \sum n_i$$
$$D = \sum d_i$$

x_i is the assigned sine

considered but the analysis of variance (two-way ANOVA) can be adapted for this situation. Though not discussed either, some non-parametric techniques are available for the comparison of medians in more than two groups. It was also shown how the chi-square test for the comparison of two groups extends to multigroup comparisons, and the chi-square test for a trend in proportions was described.

Tables 8.6 and 8.7 briefly summarize the formulae discussed in this chapter, and Sections C.14, C.17 and C.18 in Appendix C review the approach.

9

Regression and Correlation

9.1 Introduction

The previous two chapters of this book showed how one could statistically analyse differences between groups as regards quantitative variables (comparing mean values) and qualitative variables (comparing percentages or proportions). As already mentioned such a comparison of two or more groups can be viewed as an examination of the association or relationship between two variables, one of which is qualitative and defined by group membership. If, for instance, the proportions of smokers in groups of individuals with and without lung cancer are being compared, essentially the relationship between two qualitative variables is being examined. These are the variable 'lung cancer' (present or absent) and the variable 'smoking category'. If blood pressure is being compared in males and females the relationship between a quantitative variable (blood pressure) and a qualitative variable (sex) is being examined.

The third possible combination of two variables is that both are quantitative and this chapter examines associations between two such variables. For instance, for a group of children, an association would be expected between height and weight. *On average*, taller children would weigh more. Similarly, an association might be expected between coronary heart disease mortality and increasing age. Although details of some of the simpler calculations are included, these can be omitted at first reading.

9.2 Regression lines and regression equations

In Chapter 2 it was indicated that a scattergram could be used to display the relationship between two quantitative variables. Figure 9.1 shows, for instance, the relationship between systolic blood pressure (SBP) in mmHg and weight (W) in kilograms in 40 10-year-old schoolchildren.* The points on the scattergram

---

* Adapted from Pollock *et al.* (1981) with permission. Although the regression equation and correlation coefficient (to be discussed later) are taken from this article which is actually based on a study of 675 children, the scattergram presented here is not based on the actual data and is used for illustrative purposes only.

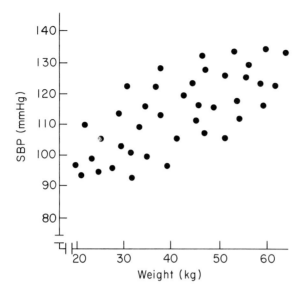

Fig. 9.1. A scattergram of systolic blood pressure (SBP) and weight in 40 10-year-olds.

show a trend upwards and to the right; this indicates a direct or positive relationship between the two sets of readings. High (low) values of one variable, blood pressure, are associated with high (low) values of the other (weight).

Having identified an apparent relationship between two quantitative variables, it might be asked — 'Is it possible to describe or summarize the relationship in some compact way?' For instance, is it possible to obtain an equation that would express the relationship or association in numerical terms? Equations are often used to describe relationships; for instance, $y = 2{\cdot}54x$ describes the exact relationship between inches and centimetres, where y represents centimetres, and x represents inches. Such a relationship could also be represented graphically by a straight line, with centimetres on the y-axis and inches on the x-axis, as in Fig. 9.2. A 'straight line' relationship such as this is called *linear*. In a linear relationship, the change in one variable associated with a given change in the other variable is not dependent on the absolute magnitude of the values concerned. Thus, in the example, an increase in length from 10 inches to 12 inches means an increase of $5{\cdot}08$ cm, from $25{\cdot}40$ to $30{\cdot}48$ cm. An increase from 25 inches to 27 inches is, of course, also associated with a length increase of $5{\cdot}08$ cm.

More generally, the equation of a straight line can be expressed as $y = a + bx$, where 'a' is the intercept of the line on the y-axis and 'b' is the slope of the line. In the special case in which the line passes through the origin (0) of the two axes, as in Fig. 9.2, $a = 0$, and the equation of the line reduces to $y = bx$. The coefficient b may take any value. In the equation $y = 2{\cdot}54x$ for example, $b = 2{\cdot}54$. An equation always implies an exact relationship, which in the case of two variables x and y means that given a value for x a value for y can be precisely

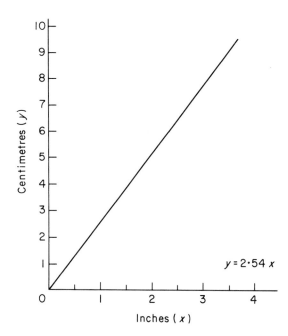

Fig. 9.2. A direct linear relationship.

determined. A linear relationship is said to be *direct* if the two variables involved increase together, in which case the coefficient *b* has a positive sign. Linear relationships can also be *indirect* or *inverse*, as illustrated in Fig. 9.3. In this case, the coefficient *b* will be negative ($y = a - bx$) and as one variable increases the other will decrease. In Fig. 9.4 a curvilinear (non-linear) exact relationship is

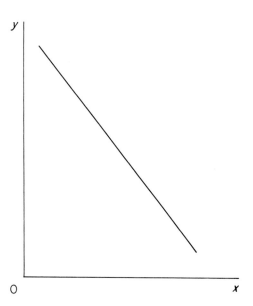

Fig. 9.3. An indirect or inverse linear relationship.

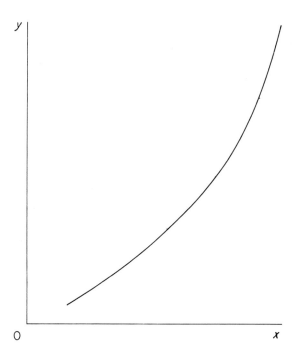

Fig. 9.4. An exact curvilinear relationship.

shown, but the equation for such a relationship is more complex than for a linear one. $y = bx^2$ is an example of such an equation.

Now return to the example of the relationship between weight and blood pressure for which the scattergram was given in Fig. 9.1. It is obvious that there is some form of relationship between the two variables but, obviously, this relationship cannot be described exactly by means of an equation. No line (straight or smoothly curved) could pass through all the points on the scattergram. However, some sort of 'average' equation could summarize the relationship, and might be obtained by drawing a smooth line through the middle of the data points. In Fig. 9.1 a straight line would seem to be the best choice, and although such a line could be fitted by using a ruler there would be a subjective element about this and different people would fit different lines. There is, however, a mathematical technique for fitting such a line to a set of data points, and the line so fitted to the data is called a *regression line*, and its corresponding equation is called a *regression equation*. This text deals, for the most part, with linear regression, which means the relationship as seen in the scattergram should at least appear to be linear in the first place. For the moment also, only relationships between two variables, or what is technically referred to as *bivariate regression*, will be considered. The regression equation then, in some sense, measures the average relationship between two variables. It could be expressed in the form

$$\hat{y} = a + bx \tag{9.1}$$

where $\hat{y}$ is the 'computed' or 'expected' value of y given any value of x. 'a' and 'b' are constants, to be determined on the basis of the data, as described later, by the *method of least squares*. In many situations, the '$\hat{}$' above the y variable will be omitted although it should always be remembered that in a regression equation it is an expected value which is being calculated. In the blood pressure study, the actual regression equation calculated turns out to be

$$\text{SBP} = 79\cdot7 + 0\cdot8\text{W} \tag{9.2}$$

where SBP represents systolic blood pressure in mmHg, W represents weight in kilograms, and the coefficients 79·7 and 0·8 are calculated from the data. This regression line is drawn in on the scattergram in Fig. 9.5. The line passes through the middle of the scatter points, and the regression line might reasonably be claimed to represent, approximately, the relationship between the two variables. On the basis of the regression line, it would be expected that a child weighing 40 kg, for instance, would have a systolic blood pressure of

$$\text{SBP} = 79\cdot7 + 0\cdot8(40) = 111\cdot7\,\text{mmHg}.$$

This result could also have been read off Fig. 9.5 using the regression line. Note, however, that there may not have been anyone in the study who actually weighed 40 kg, and even if there was, he or she need not necessarily have had a blood pressure of 111·7. The figure of 111·7 mmHg is interpreted as the average blood pressure that would be expected among a large number of children, all of whom weighed 40 kg, or in other words, the average blood pressure associated with this weight.

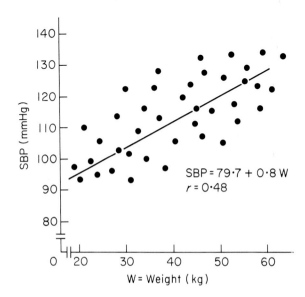

Fig. 9.5. Scattergram of systolic blood pressure (SBP) and weight with the regression line drawn in.

The regression equation also implies that systolic blood pressure will increase by 0·8 mmHg with every 1 kg increase in weight. The coefficient 0·8 in the equation is called the *regression coefficient* and, in general, means the change in *y* per unit change in *x*. It is, in fact, the slope of the regression line. One further point may be noted; if a value of zero is substituted for weight in Eqn. 9.2, an expected systolic blood pressure of 79·7 would be calculated. It is plainly nonsensical to estimate a blood pressure for a child weighing nothing. The regression equation is derived from the observed values of the two variables, and it is only valid within the ranges actually observed for the variables. Extrapolation beyond this range may be misleading, and often totally invalid.

Another example of a regression analysis relates to indicators of prognosis after a myocardial infarction (heart attack). The left ventricular ejection fraction (LVEF) is one such indicator, but, unfortunately, is difficult to measure, and also expensive. On the other hand, the taking of an electrocardiograph (ECG) is much faster and cheaper, and a particular index called the QRS score is easily derived from an ECG tracing. Twenty-eight patients had their LVEF measured three weeks after their heart attack. This was then compared with the patients' QRS score to evaluate the usefulness of this score in determining LVEF. Figure 9.6 shows the scattergram and regression line for the relationship between these two variables. From inspection of the plot points on the diagram, it is clear that the relationship is linear but inverse. The regression equation can be calculated as

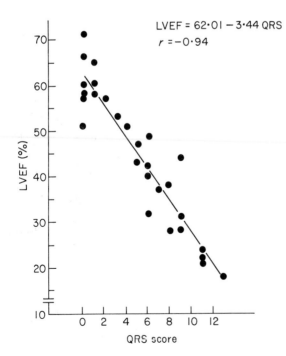

Fig. 9.6. Scattergram showing relationship between the left ventricular ejection fraction (LVEF) and the QRS score in 28 patients after a myocardial infarction. Palmeri *et al.* (1982) with permission.

$$\text{LVEF} = 62 \cdot 01 - 3 \cdot 44 \text{QRS} \qquad (9.3)$$

where the LVEF is measured as a percentage. In this case, the regression coefficient is $-3 \cdot 44$, which means that for every increase of 1 unit in the QRS score the value of the LVEF decreases by $3 \cdot 44\%$. An inverse relationship will always give rise to a negative regression coefficient.

In both of these examples, it was meaningful to consider how one variable depended on the other. In the first case, the aim was to determine how blood pressure depended on weight, and in the second case, how the LVEF could be determined by the QRS score. Blood pressure and the LVEF are both called *dependent* variables, while weight and the QRS score are considered the *independent* variables. (Note that this use of the word independent is different from that in Chapter 3, where the question of independent events was considered.) The question of which variable in a regression analysis is independent and which is dependent is decided on the basis of logic (a child's weight is hardly dependent on blood pressure) or on the precise question the researcher is trying to answer. (In the heart attack example, the purpose was to predict a patient's LVEF on the basis of the QRS score.) It is important to note however that a regression equation expresses a numerical association between two variables, but it does not establish a causal link between the two, or prove that one variable is causally dependent on the other.

In a regression equation, the dependent variable is written on the left-hand side of the equation, and the independent variable is written on the right-hand side; it is usual to talk about the regression of the dependent variable on the independent one. Thus, the first example is of the regression of blood pressure on weight. In the scattergram, the dependent variable is put on the y-axis. It is important in calculating regression equations that one is clear which variable is to be considered independent. Without going into detail, the regression of a variable y on a variable x does not give the same mathematical relationship as the regression of x on y, although unless there is a large scatter of points around the regression line the relationships are usually very close.

9.3 Correlation analysis

Consider the regression Eqn. 9.2. For a given value of W (body weight) a corresponding value of SBP (systolic blood pressure) can be calculated. This calculated value can be written SB̂P. SB̂P can be interpreted as the expected or average value of systolic blood pressure associated with the given value of weight. Now, if all the points in the scattergram lay on the regression line, for any given value of W the expected and observed values of SBP would be identical. The regression equation would describe the relationship between systolic blood pressure and weight exactly. The variation in systolic blood pressure would be completely explained by, or be dependent upon, the variation in weight.

In practice, this is not the case. Systolic blood pressure can vary independently of variation in weight, so that two children of the same weight may have different blood pressures. Weight is not the only factor affecting systolic blood pressure. Given any particular value for weight, the expected blood pressure can be calculated. However, since blood pressures do vary independently of weight, the blood pressure associated with any particular weight cannot be predicted exactly. In this sense, the regression equation can be described as measuring the average relationship between the two variables. It does not measure the *strength* or *goodness of fit* of the relationship.

In the blood pressure and weight example (Fig. 9.5) there is a fairly large dispersion of the plot points around the regression line. This suggests a fairly weak relationship between the two variables. Given a weight of 40 kg a child's systolic blood pressure could be estimated as 111·7 mmHg, but the child's actual blood pressure could vary quite appreciably around this. A considerable amount of the variation in the dependent variable is unexplained by the variation in the independent variable. Although, on average, systolic blood pressure increases with weight, there are obviously many other factors that influence this variable.

In Fig. 9.6, which shows the relationship between the LVEF and QRS score, the plot points lie close to the regression line, which suggests a strong relationship between the two variables. The observed values for LVEF do not differ markedly from the expected values represented by the regression line. This implies that most of the variation in LVEF can be 'explained' by the variation in the QRS score. Given a particular QRS score, the estimated left ventricular ejection fraction could be predicted, and it would be fairly certain that the actual value would be quite close to this predicted one.

A measure of the strength of the relationship between two variables is provided by the coefficient of correlation, denoted by 'r'. If the relationship between the two variables is of linear form, r is called *the coefficient of linear correlation*. r is also called *Pearson's product moment correlation*.

Values of r vary between $+1$ and -1, the sign of r depending on whether or not there is a direct relationship between the two variables, as in Fig. 9.5, or an inverse relationship, as in Fig. 9.6. If the relationship between the two variables is perfect or exact, that is if all the points on the scattergram lie on the regression line, r will be equal to $+1$ or -1. A positive sign indicates a direct relationship; a negative sign indicates an inverse one. If there is no relationship at all between the two variables, r will be 0. The greater the numerical value of r, the stronger the relationship between the two variables.

Methods for calculating the coefficient of correlation (or, as it is often called, the correlation coefficient) are given in the next section, but for the moment only the results for the two examples are given. The correlation coefficient for the relationship between blood pressure and weight in 10-year-old children is $r = 0.48$ which is not very high. On the other hand, $r = -0.94$ for the relationship between LVEF and the QRS score, which confirms the strength of that relationship as determined visually. (Note that r is negative for this inverse relationship.)

It has been said that r ranges from -1 to $+1$, but it is not immediately clear how to interpret different values of this coefficient. It happens however that the value of r^2 has a readily understandable interpretation in terms of the strength of a relationship. Take the example of blood pressure in 10-year-old children. Blood pressures will show a fair degree of variation from child to child due to the many factors, one of which is body weight, that affect blood pressure. This can be referred to as the total variation in the variable. Prediction of the systolic blood pressure of a 10-year-old without reference to these factors would be subject to quite a degree of uncertainty. If, however, only children of a particular weight were examined, the variation in their blood pressures would be considerably less. (See Fig. 9.5 where the scatter of blood pressures for a given weight is far less than the total scatter of blood pressure in all the children studied.) Some of the total variation in blood pressure measurements can be explained by the variation in children's weights (the 'explained' variation), while the remainder of the variation must be due to other factors which were not considered explicitly or are unknown (the 'unexplained' variation). The larger the first component is, relative to the second, the stronger is the relationship between the two variables.

It can be shown that r^2 (the square of the correlation coefficient — sometimes called the *coefficient of determination*) is equal to the proportion of the total variation in the dependent variable (SBP) that is explained by the regression line. If the relationship between the two variables is perfect, all the variation in the dependent variable is explained by the regression line, and thus r^2 equals 1 so that r equals ± 1. r is written plus or minus, according to whether the relationship is direct or inverse. The more closely the points in the scattergram are dispersed around the regression line, the higher will be the proportion of variation explained by the regression line, and hence the greater the value of r^2 and r. In the blood pressure example, it was said that r equals 0.48, so that r^2 equals 0.2304. Thus, the variation in the weights of the children explains just over 23% of the total variation in blood pressure. The other 77% of the variation is unexplained and must be due to many other factors not considered in this analysis. In the left ventricular ejection fraction example, $r^2 = (0.94)^2 = 0.8836$, which means that over 88% of the variation in LVEF is explained by the variation in the QRS score.

In most cases involving the use of regression analysis, it is advisable to include the value of the correlation coefficient or its square. There are situations, however, where determination of the exact form of a linear relationship is not relevant, or

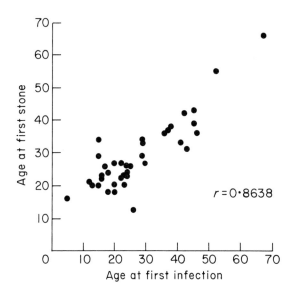

Fig. 9.7. Relation between age at first stone and age at first infection in 38 females with two or more stone-associated urinary tract infections (see Fig. 1.12). Parks *et al.* (1982) with permission.

where identification of which of the variables being examined is dependent and which independent is not obvious. In these cases a correlation analysis examining only the strength of a relationship may be all that is required, and the actual regression equation(s) may be irrelevant. A regression analysis is not symmetrical, in that one variable must be taken as dependent and the other as independent. Correlation, however, results in a measure of association that does not imply any dependence of one variable on the other.

Figure 9.7 is a case in point. This shows a scattergram for the relationship between the age at which 38 females with frequent urinary tract infections (UTI) developed their first kidney stone, and the age at which they first developed UTI. Rather than one age determining the other age, it is much more likely that another factor or factors determined the timing of each event. A regression analysis would not seem to be appropriate, but a correlation analysis examining the strength of the relationship would be. For this example, r turns out to be equal to 0·86 ($r^2 = 0.74$), showing a reasonably strong association between the age at first infection and the age at first stone. The interpretation of this association in terms of a causal hypothesis is much more difficult, however.

9.4 Calculation of regression and correlation coefficients

In Section 9.2 it was pointed out that a regression line could be fitted by hand by drawing a line through the middle of the points on the scattergram. Obviously, as was said, this is rather a haphazard way of fitting the line, and a more systematic procedure is required. A number of different methods may be used, the best-known of which is the *method of least squares*. Assume that the scatter of points is such that a straight line would be appropriate to describe the relationship. From the infinite number of straight lines which could be drawn it is desirable to select that line to which the points on the scattergram are, in some sense, closest. That is, the line should be drawn in such a way as to minimize the distance between the scatter points and the line. In Fig. 9.8 a line has been fitted to minimize the sum of vertical distances between the four plot points and the line. Actually, since some of these distances will be positive (points above the line) and some will be negative (points below the line) the line is fitted to minimize the sum of squares of the vertical distance between the plot points and the line. This is why it is called the method of least squares.

When the line is fitted in this way, the overall difference between the plot points and the line is minimized. This is the line of 'best fit'. The mathematical derivation of the regression coefficients a and b in the regression line

$$\hat{y} = a + bx \tag{9.1}$$

are not given here, but they can be calculated from the following formulae

$$b = \frac{\Sigma(x - \bar{x})(y - \bar{y})}{\Sigma(x - \bar{x})^2} \tag{9.4}$$

$$= \frac{\Sigma(x - \bar{x})(y - \bar{y})}{(n - 1)S_x^2} \tag{9.5}$$

$$a = \bar{y} - b\bar{x}. \tag{9.6}$$

These are the slope and intercept of the regression line as determined by the method of least squares. The numerator in the expression for b, $\Sigma(x - \bar{x})(y - \bar{y})$, looks formidable, and as it stands requires subtraction of the mean of the x variable from each x value, the mean of the y variable from each corresponding y value, multiplication of the two results together, and summing over all the pairs of xy values. Appendix A, however, outlines an easier computational approach. The

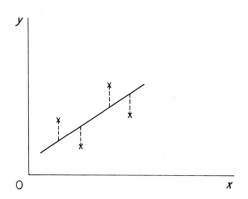

Fig. 9.8. Illustration of the 'method of least squares'.

denominator of the expression for b is identical to $(n - 1)S_x^2$ where S_x^2 is the variance (square of the standard deviation) of the x values (see Eqn. 2.3). The equation for a requires only the means of both x and y, together with the calculated value of b.

Once the regression equation has been estimated, it can easily be drawn in on the scattergram. Choose two representative values for x; calculate the predicted or expected $\hat{y}$ values; plot in these points and connect with a straight line.

The formula for the correlation coefficient r is also fairly cumbersome.

$$r = \frac{\Sigma(x - \bar{x})(y - \bar{y})}{\sqrt{\Sigma(x - \bar{x})^2\ \Sigma(y - \bar{y})^2}} \tag{9.7}$$

$$= \frac{\Sigma(x - \bar{x})(y - \bar{y})}{(n - 1)S_x S_y} \tag{9.8}$$

where S_x and S_y are the standard deviations of the x and y variables respectively. Appendix A outlines in detail the calculation of these quantities for the left ventricular ejection fraction data of Fig. 9.6.

9.5 Statistical inference in regression and correlation

In the examples used so far, and in general, analysis is based on a sample of the pairs of variables of interest. Thus, the data in Fig. 9.1 are based on a sample of 10-year-old children. Now, in the same way that the mean and standard deviation of a random sample are estimates of the mean and standard deviation of the population from which it is drawn, so the regression coefficient and correlation coefficient of a sample of pairs of two variables are estimates of the regression coefficient and correlation coefficient for the population of pairs of these values. Let the regression coefficient for the sample be denoted by b and the correlation coefficient by r; similarly, denote the regression coefficient for the whole population by β (beta) and the correlation coefficient by ρ (rho — the Greek letter 'r'). Then, the sample statistics b and r are estimates of the unknown population parameters β and ρ. The regression equation in the population may thus be written

$$y = \alpha + \beta x \tag{9.9}$$

where α and β are the regression coefficients in the population. (a and α are also called regression coefficients although the term is more usually employed for b and β.)

An interesting possibility now arises: suppose, for the whole population of pairs of values, that $\beta = 0$ and $\rho = 0$. This would occur in cases where there was no relationship between the two variables.* The two variables are said to be independent of one another. An example would be pairs of values that arise in throwing two dice simultaneously. There is no relationship (or should not be!) between the number that turns up on one die and the number turning up on the other. A regression analysis between pairs of values should yield $\beta = 0$ and $\rho = 0$.

However, if a sample of pairs of values is analysed, it is quite possible that, just by chance, non-zero values will be obtained for b and r. In the same way that the mean ($\bar{x}$) of a single sample is unlikely to be exactly equal to a population mean (μ), the values of a regression coefficient b and a correlation coefficient r derived from a sample are unlikely to be exactly equal to the population values β and ρ. Hence, it is likely that even if β and ρ equal 0, b and r will be non-zero. This means that the results of a regression analysis may suggest a relationship between two variables that is quite spurious. To guard against this possibility, some method is needed to make inferences about the population values of b and r (β and ρ respectively) on the basis of the sample results. In Chapters 4, 6 and 7 it was explained how confidence intervals for, and significance tests on, unknown population parameters could be based on the sample statistics and their standard errors. Similarly, confidence intervals and significance tests are available for the regression and correlation coefficients (β and ρ) based on the standard errors of their sample values. Tests for the value of α (the y-intercept) are also available, although less commonly employed.

As before however, some assumptions concerning the underlying distribution of the data must be made for valid use of these inferential approaches. For inferences relating to a regression analysis, it must be assumed that the distribution of y for each fixed value of x is normal (or nearly so), that the standard deviation of this normal distribution of y is the same for each x, and that the mean values of the y distribution are linearly related to x. These assumptions are explained below in the specific example of the regression of blood pressure on weight in 10-year-old children, considered earlier. The assumptions state that for children of a given weight (40 kg say) the distribution of systolic blood pressure is normal, with a standard deviation (σ), and that no matter which weight is chosen children of that weight will have a normally distributed blood pressure with this standard deviation. This assumption, which is often stated in terms of variances rather than standard

---

* β is a measure of the average change in one variable (y) per unit change in the other (x). If there is no relationship between x and y, an increase of 1 unit in x is equally likely to be associated with a decrease or increase in y. Hence the average change in y per unit change in x will be 0. Similarly, if no relationship can be postulated between x and y, $\rho = 0$.

deviations, is called the assumption of homoscedasticity. The final assumption is that the population mean systolic blood pressure for each different weight is a linear function of weight. Given these assumptions it can be shown that the standard error of b is

$$\text{SE}(b) = \frac{\sigma}{\sqrt{\Sigma(x - \bar{x})^2}} \qquad (9.10)$$

$$= \frac{\sigma}{\sqrt{(n - 1)}\, S_x} \qquad (9.11)$$

where σ is the (unknown) standard deviation of the y variable at each x value. The assumption of homoscedasticity is important, and more advanced techniques may have to be used if the assumption is not tenable, or perhaps a transformation of the data (see Section 9.6) may suffice. Note, of course, that σ is unknown, and must be estimated from the data. Again, without deriving the result, it can be shown that an estimate of σ is given by

$$S_{y.x} = \sqrt{\frac{\Sigma(y - \hat{y})^2}{n - 2}} \qquad (9.12)$$

where y represents the observed y values obtained, and $\hat{y}$ is the predicted or expected y calculated from the regression equation on the corresponding x (Eqn. 9.1). The similarity of this formula to that of the usual standard deviation should be noted. The quantity is some sort of average of the deviations of each point from its predicted value but, as for the standard deviation, it is the squared deviations that are averaged. It can be seen however, that $S_{y.x}$ is a reasonable estimator for σ. (An easier computational form is given in Appendix A.) $S_{y.x}$ is variously referred to as *the standard deviation from regression* or *the standard error of the estimate* or when squared as *the residual mean square*. $n - 2$ is sometimes called the residual degrees of freedom. The subscript $y.x$ on S means that we are talking about the regression of y on x.

The standard error of b is estimated as (see Eqn. 9.11)

$$\text{SE}(b) = \frac{S_{y.x}}{\sqrt{(n - 1)}\, S_x}. \qquad (9.13)$$

This standard error of b has $n - 2$ degrees of freedom so that

$$b \pm t_\text{c}\, \text{SE}(b)$$

gives a confidence interval for b where t_c is the critical value of the t distribution on $n - 2$ degrees of freedom for the required confidence level. In the LVEF example, it can be shown that (see Appendix A) $S_{y.x}$ equals 5·102 on 26 degrees of freedom, and S_x equals 4·118. It has already been seen that b equals $-3·438$ (to three decimal places) so that a 95% confidence interval for β is given by

$$-3·438 \pm 2·056 \ (0·238)$$

where $SE(b) = 0·238$ from Eqn. 9.13, and $t_c = 2·056$ is the critical t value on 26 degrees of freedom, corresponding to 5% of the area in both tails. The lower and upper confidence limits are thus $-3·927$ and $-2·949$.

To recap — usually, a calculated regression equation is determined on a sample of values so that, in particular, the regression coefficient b is a sample estimate of the regression coefficient (β) in the population. As with sample means and proportions, it is possible (given certain assumptions) to calculate the standard error of the regression coefficient and thus give a confidence interval estimate for the unknown value of β. A hypothesis test for β is also easily derived. If the null hypothesis specifies a particular value β_0 for the regression coefficient in the population, the test statistic is

$$t = \frac{b - \beta_0}{SE(b)} \tag{9.14}$$

where b is the sample value of the regression coefficient, β_0 is the hypothesized value and $SE(b)$ is given by Eqn. 9.13. This provides a t test on $n - 2$ degrees of freedom. The usual null hypothesis specifies a value of $\beta = 0$ so that the test is of the existence of any relationship in the first place, and Eqn. 9.14 becomes, when Eqn. 9.13 is used for $SE(b)$,

$$t = \frac{bS_x\sqrt{n - 1}}{S_{y.x}} \cdot \tag{9.15}$$

If t is greater than the appropriate (usually two-sided) critical value then the existence of a real relationship in the population can be accepted. For the LVEF data, $t = -14·42$, d.f. $= 26$, $p < 0·01$. Thus, the value of b is significantly different from zero. This, of course, is consistent with the confidence interval for β calculated above which did not include zero as a possible value.

Although formulae are not given in this text, it is also possible to derive standard errors for a predicted $\hat{y}$ value, given a particular value for x, or for the population mean y value for that x. Confidence intervals can then be obtained.

The null hypothesis of zero population correlation $(\rho = 0)$ uses the test statistic

$$t = r\sqrt{\frac{n - 2}{1 - r^2}} \tag{9.16}$$

on $n - 2$ degrees of freedom. For the LVEF data, $t = -14·42$ on 26 degrees of freedom. This is numerically the same as that obtained using the *t* test of zero regression coefficient mentioned above (Eqn. 9.15). This is not an accident; it can be shown that the two tests are mathematically equivalent. Confidence intervals for ρ and tests of hypotheses for population values other than $\rho = 0$ are more complex and require additional assumptions relating to the distribution of the variables in the population. They are not considered here.

It is important to distinguish between the strength of a relationship as measured by the correlation coefficient, or its square, and its statistical significance for a null hypothesis of zero population correlation. A significant correlation does not mean a strong relationship, thus an *r* of 0·12 explaining only 1·4% $[(0·12)^2 = 0·0144]$ of the variation in the dependent variable could be highly significant from the statistical point of view, but would probably be of little consequence. On the other hand, a high value for *r* may be non-significant if based on a very small sample size. Correlation coefficients can only be interpreted if both their magnitude and significance are reported.

Section C.19 of Appendix C summarizes the statistical calculations of this section.

9.6 Non-linear regression and data transformations

The assumptions underlying the regression techniques discussed in this chapter are important. These are essentially, a linear relationship, homoscedasticity (equality of variances) and normality of the data. In previous sections it was shown how suitable transformation of the data may reduce skewness (Section 1.7) or decrease differences between group variances (Section 7.4). Data transformations may also linearize a curved relationship. Figure 9.9 shows some curvilinear relationships and the transformations that could be applied to either the *y* or the *x* variable to linearize the relationship. Essentially non-linearity is caused by a skew in the distribution of one or both of the variables and the transformations to reduce skewness are used. If a transformation succeeds then a linear regression analysis can be carried out on the transformed data. An example of the logarithmic transformation that linearized a relationship is given in Chapter 1, Fig. 1.13. In practice you may have to experiment with different transformations of either the *x* or *y* variable to produce the best result.

Another approach to curvilinear regression is to run a *polynomial regression* on the data, where without transformations a dependent variable *y* might be related to an independent variable *x* with a polynomial equation of the following form

$$y = a + bx + cx^2 \tag{9.17}$$

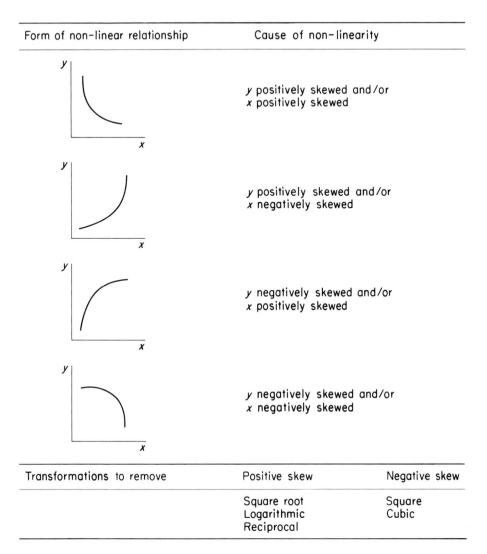

Form of non-linear relationship	Cause of non-linearity	
	y positively skewed and/or *x* positively skewed	
	y positively skewed and/or *x* negatively skewed	
	y negatively skewed and/or *x* positively skewed	
	y negatively skewed and/or *x* negatively skewed	
Transformations to remove	Positive skew	Negative skew
	Square root Logarithmic Reciprocal	Square Cubic

Fig. 9.9. Data transformations to linearize relationships.

with terms in x^3 and x^4, etc., if necessary. With such an approach more than one regression coefficient must be estimated (e.g. *b* and *c* above). Often curvilinear relationships can be expressed in such a polynomial form and the analysis is very similar to that of *multiple regression* to be discussed in Section 12.2.

One method of checking on the assumptions underlying linear regression is to perform what is called an analysis of residuals. The residual is the difference between the observed value *y* and the predicted value $\hat{y}$ obtained by applying the regression equation to the corresponding *x* value for the dependent variable. Plots of the residuals against x or $\hat{y}$ can provide insights into how well the assumptions hold and can aid greatly in choosing the correct approach. A more advanced text should be consulted for details on this topic.

When other assumptions underlying linear regression do not hold, non-parametric alternatives are available and are discussed in the next section.

9.7 Rank correlation

Rank correlation is a non-parametric procedure for calculating a correlation coefficient. As such, it does not require the assumptions made for the usual approach when Pearson's product moment correlation coefficient is employed. There are two common rank procedures which will be encountered in the medical literature. The first is called *Kendall's rank correlation coefficient* or *Kendall's tau* (tau is the Greek letter 't'). The calculations can be complex and are not given in this text. An alternative rank correlation method due to Spearman is given instead, which results in the calculation of *Spearman's rank correlation coefficient*. When in doubt about the underlying assumptions required for an ordinary correlation analysis, when a transformation of the data will not work or when perhaps only a ranking of the data is available, recourse to this method should be made. The first step is to rank the observations on each variable. Suppose 10 children are subjected to a form of an intelligence test by two independent assessors. The ranks assigned to the children by each investigator are shown in Table 9.1.

The ranking order given by the two assessors, although similar, is different. If the ranking orders were exactly the same, a coefficient of correlation of $+1$ would be expected. On the other hand, if the ranking order of assessor B were exactly the *reverse* of assessor A, the coefficient of correlation would be expected to be -1. If there is no relationship at all between the two rankings, the coefficient of correlation would be expected to be almost 0.

Table 9.1. Spearman's rank correlation coefficient. Rank assigned to 10 children by two assessors

Child	1	2	3	4	5	6	7	8	9	10
Assessor A	7	6	1	2	3	8·5	8·5	10	4	5
Assessor B	6	7	3	2	1	4	9	8	10	5
d	1	−1	−2	0	2	4·5	−0·5	2	−6	0
d^2	1	1	4	0	4	20·25	0·25	4	36	0

$$\Sigma d^2 = 70\cdot5; \quad r_s = 1 - \frac{6(70\cdot5)}{10(99)} = 0\cdot5727; \text{ NS.}$$

For each student, one calculates the differences between the ranks given by the two assessors: d = 'the rank for assessor A' minus 'the rank for assessor B'. These differences are shown in Table 9.1. They are squared and summed up to

$$\Sigma d^2 = 70.5. \tag{9.18}$$

Spearman's rank correlation coefficient is then simply calculated as

$$r_s = 1 - \frac{6\Sigma d^2}{n(n^2 - 1)} \tag{9.19}$$

where n is the number of pairs (10 in this case). r_s in the example turns out to be 0.5727. This correlation coefficient can be interpreted in a similar manner to the parametric correlation coefficient discussed earlier. The formula given is not quite exact if there are a lot of tied ranks in the data.

A significance test can also be performed on Spearman's rank correlation coefficient. The test statistic is actually r_s itself, and Table B.10 gives the critical values for a given number of pairs. If the calculated correlation coefficient is equal to or outside the limits defined by $\pm r_c$ given in the table, a significant result can be declared. For 10 pairs and a two-sided significance level of 5%, r_s would have to lie outside ± 0.6485. The calculated r_s in the example is not outside these limits, and so it can be concluded that there is no significant difference between the ranks assigned by these two assessors. Section C.20 of Appendix C summarizes the steps required to do these calculations.

9.8 Regression to the mean

The term 'regression' for the type of analysis that has been considered seems a bit strange and was first used by Sir Francis Galton in describing his 'law of universal regression' in 1889. 'Each peculiarity in a man is shared by his kinsman, but *on the average* in a less degree'. Thus, intelligent fathers will tend to have intelligent sons, but the sons will, on average, be less intelligent than their fathers. There is a regression, or 'going back', of the sons' intelligence towards the average intelligence of all men. Sons of intelligent fathers will, of course, be more intelligent than the average in the population. Galton's 'law' can be shown graphically, as in Fig. 9.10. For any parental IQ, the son's IQ is closer to the mean IQ (about 100) than his father's was. The word 'regression' is now applied to the analysis of any such relationship, as has been discussed in this chapter.

Regression to the mean, as this phenomenon is called, is not confined to genetic stituations, and its existence can cause confusion in the interpretation of certain results. Take a simple example. Suppose the mid-year examination results of 100 first-year medical students in statistics have been obtained and the group of 25 who obtained the highest marks have been identified. The average mark for

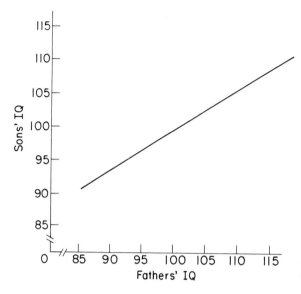

Fig. 9.10. Regression to the mean of sons' IQ

these 25 is 62% and, of all the students, is 50%. It can be predicted that when these 100 students sit their end-year examination the average mark of the 25 identified on the basis of the first examination will be less than 62%. This will occur even if the average mark for the whole group remains at 50%, with an overall similar spread of marks. Why this happens is not very hard to see. Some of the 25 students will have got very high marks in the mid-year examination that they are most unlikely to improve on. On the other hand, some of the 25 could drop their marks appreciably in the second examination; this could be due to luck on the first examination or a bad day on the second. As a consequence, the *average* mark of the group is likely to fall, or regress downward, to the mean of the full group. If instead the 25 worst students on the first examination had been taken, their average mark would have been likely to increase or regress upward to the mean.

Regression to the mean occurs when a variable is measured on two separate occasions, when that variable can change its value in the individual on whom it is measured and when a subgroup of a larger study group is defined on the basis of high (or low) values of the variable at the first measurement. Any subgroup so defined will have an average value for the variable that is lower (or higher) the second time it is measured. If, for instance, a group of patients was selected on the basis of systolic blood pressure being above 180 mmHg at a particular examination, the average blood pressure of this group would be lower on a repeat examination. Such a decrease could be mistakenly interpreted as the effect of a particular treatment, whereas it would occur without any intervention whatsoever.

Regression to the mean relates to the experience of the whole group, and not to any defined individuals. Allowing for regression to the mean mathematically is not usually an easy procedure. The problem is probably best solved by ignoring the first measurement on the basis of which the individuals were categorized and to take, as a baseline, measurements taken at a subsequent examination when spuriously high (or low) levels have 'settled down'.

9.9 Summary

In this chapter, it has been explained how the relationship between two quantitative variables may be described by means of regression equations, and how the strength of the relationship between the variables may be measured. It has been shown, also, how the significance of statistics such as the regression coefficient and the correlation coefficient may be tested. The calculations are summarized in Sections C.18 and C.19 in Appendix C, and Table 9.2 outlines the relevant formulae.

Table 9.2. Summary of formulae for regression (see Appendix A for computational formulae)

Application	Formulae	Eqn. nos.
Regression equation	$\hat{y} = a + bx$	(9.1)
	$b = \dfrac{\Sigma(x - \bar{x})(y - \bar{y})}{(n - 1) S_x^2}$	(9.5)
	$a = \bar{y} - b\bar{x}$	(9.6)
Correlation coefficient	$r = \dfrac{\Sigma(x - \bar{x})(y - \bar{y})}{(n - 1) S_x S_y}$	(9.8)
Hypothesis test ($\beta = 0$)	$t = \dfrac{bS_x\sqrt{n - 1}}{S_{y.x}}$	(9.15)
	d.f. $= n - 2$	
Confidence interval for β	$b \pm t_c \dfrac{S_{y.x}}{\sqrt{n - 1}\, S_x}$	(9.13)
	d.f. $= n - 2$	
Hypothesis test ($\rho = 0$)	$t = r\sqrt{\dfrac{n - 2}{1 - r^2}}$	(9.16)
	d.f. $= n - 2$	
Spearman's rank correlation coefficient	$r_s = 1 - \dfrac{6\Sigma d^2}{n (n^2 - 1)}$	(9.19)

It is appropriate to complete this chapter with a word of caution concerning the interpretation of measures of regression and correlation, and indeed any statistical analysis. The establishment of a functional relationship in the form of a regression equation between one variable and another, or others, does not establish a *causal* link between the variables concerned. It is possible to establish a positive relationship between the growth of private vehicle registrations and the average number of telephone calls in Ireland. Both may reflect a more affluent society, but it is not suggested that there is a causal link between the two. Both may depend on a third factor, such as income, but be independent of one another. Many variables move in the same direction, or in opposite directions, over time without being in any way causally related. In practice, measures of regression and correlation are used to support hypotheses of causality, but cannot of themselves provide *proof* of causal relationships.

10

Medical Studies and Epidemiological Statistics

10.1 Introduction

So far in this book, the emphasis has been on the statistical analysis of medical data. One point that has been particularly stressed is that data are not only numerical values but also information collected in a particular way for a particular purpose. The method of data collection and the design of a medical study are intimately related to the purposes for which the data are collected, and if the study design is inappropriate to, or inadequate for, the purposes of the study, no amount of statistical manipulation or analysis can rescue it.

The sampling techniques that can be used in population surveys were discussed in Chapter 3, and it was pointed out that in many situations random sampling is not employed as a basis for studies in medicine. This chapter examines some standard designs employed in observational studies, and looks at some of the methods used for the analysis and presentation of results.

10.2 Observational and experimental studies

Studies in medicine may be divided into two distinct categories: *experimental studies* in which the investigator manipulates the allocation of individuals to different groups (discussed in the next chapter), and *observational studies* or *medical surveys* where the investigator merely makes observations on individuals, without experimental manipulation. In an observational study, different groups are compared without group membership being determined by the investigator, or alternatively relationships between different factors are examined in a single study group. Observational studies are often concerned with identifying factors that could be regarded as causal in the development of a disease or condition (risk factors), or with determining predictors of outcome or prognosis (without experimental manipulation) in patients who already have a specific condition. Observational studies may be classified into three broad groups: the *cross-sectional study*, the *prospective (cohort follow-up or longitudinal) study* and the *retrospective (case-control) study*. This terminology is by no means ideal, but is fairly commonly employed. These three study designs are discussed individually below. In essence, the cross-sectional study takes no account of time; the prospective study goes forward in time from a risk factor to the disease; the case-control study goes backward in time from the disease to the risk factor.

Although case reports and clinical observations do not fall into the framework of statistical studies in medicine, they of course form the basis and foundation-stone for most medical research. Clinical observations and 'hunches' often provide the initial ideas which may eventually lead to a formal study, and to new knowledge being scientifically tested. Perhaps one of the best-known examples of this process started with the observation of Gregg (1941), an ophthalmologist, who noted an unusual number of congenital cataracts appearing in Australia. He suggested that this might be related to the exposure of the pregnant mother to German measles, of which there had been a severe epidemic in the previous year. This clinical observation led eventually to the implication of rubella virus in congenital malformations. Clues provided by studies in vital statistics may also lead to new and important findings, and such studies are discussed in Chapter 13.

As has been said, most studies in medicine eventually involve the comparison of two or more groups, and the determination of differences between the groups as regards a single factor of interest. Statistical analysis of a study is performed on the results as obtained, with the assumptions that the groups were randomly sampled from defined populations, and that measurements taken on the sample were true reflections on what one was actually trying to measure. In practice, of course, there are many biases in both the selection of study subjects and the measurements actually taken. Such biases may distort or completely invalidate the conclusions drawn from any study. Statistical analysis however cannot correct for such biases, and they must be avoided by careful study design and implementation. In the sections that follow, the design and analysis of observational studies and a few of the biases that can occur and may be preventable are discussed. Chapter 15 of this book considers the subject of bias in medical research in more detail, and to some extent the rest of this chapter assumes that such problems have been overcome, and do not affect the validity of presented results and analyses.

The problem of confounding in the examination of associations between variables must also be addressed. Essentially, a confounding variable is one that distorts an existing real relationship. It might be found, for example, that the mortality rate in one community was substantially higher than in another. Such an association, however, could be due to the fact that the first community was much older, and the observed effect could be explained totally by age rather than by any other adverse influences on mortality. Age would be said to act as a con-founder of the association of mortality with community membership. A con-founder can make it appear that there is a relationship present when there is none, or, at the other extreme, hide a real relationship. Chapter 12 will consider statistical techniques for the control of confounding in the analysis of medical studies and Chapter 13 will discuss the problem in the context of vital statistics (see also Section 7.2).

The alternative to the control of confounding at the analysis stage of a study is to use an appropriate study design to eliminate the effect of confounding variables. This is an important aspect of the setting up of medical studies and will be considered in this and in the next chapter.

10.3 Association and causality

It has been indicated at various stages in the book that a statistical association or relationship between two factors does not imply a causal connection. Even if the effects of confounders are eliminated the identification of causal factors requires investigations that go far beyond mere statistical calculation. Criteria for evaluating the causal significance of an association between some factor and the occurrence of a disease have been suggested (*Smoking and Health*, 1964) and these are outlined below in the context of the causal link between cigarette smoking and lung cancer. These criteria include the *consistency, strength, specificity, temporality* and *coherence* of the association. An association between a risk factor and a disease which satisfies these criteria can be taken as a strong, if not absolute, indication of causality.

The consistency of an association requires that different methods of study design, and studies in different populations all lead to similar conclusions. With few exceptions, all the studies of the association of cigarette smoking and lung cancer show a positive result.

The strength of an association means that the effect of the risk factor is large, and it is seen below how this might be quantified in studies of disease aetiology. A dose response effect is also related to the strength of an association and means that, in the example being considered, lung cancer risk increases with the amount smoked.

In simple terms, the specificity of the association between cigarette smoking and lung cancer demands that most persons with lung cancer are, in fact, cigarette smokers. Of course, lung cancer can arise in non-smokers, due to the multifactorial causation of the disease, but the specificity of this association is fairly clear. Note, however, that this does not mean that most cigarette smokers get lung cancer.

Before a risk factor for a particular disease can be judged causal, it must be certain that in fact the risk factor was present before the disease occurred. Although fairly easy to show for cigarette smoking and lung cancer, this temporality requirement can cause difficulties for other diseases and other risk factors.

For an association to be coherent, the association should not be at odds with known facts concerning the natural history and biology of a disease, and there should be a reasonable explanation for the association in this light. The dose–response relationship in the development of lung cancer and the numbers of cigarettes smoked, and the known carcinogenic effects of tobacco smoke, all contribute to the coherence of the association.

These five criteria are fairly stringent, and it must be admitted that many statistical associations between risk factors and disease do not meet them all. The criteria do however provide a reference by which to judge the likely causal significance of an association, and act as a reminder that statistical association on its own does not necessarily imply causality. With this caveat in mind, different study designs to detect associations in medicine are examined.

10.4 The cross-sectional study

Essentially, a cross-sectional study takes no account of the temporal relationship between the factors studied, and usually involves the examination of a cross-section of a particular population at one point in time. It gives a 'snapshot' view. Cross-sectional studies may be based on a random sample from a defined population, or on a presenting sample of patients with a particular condition. The sampling techniques discussed in Section 3.6 are relevant in this context. If a study is hospital-based, one must be careful not to over-generalize results, and be wary of the selection biases which lead to hospital admission (see discussion in Chapter 15 also).

Cross-sectional studies may be employed to study associations between different diseases, but they cannot often determine which disease might have occurred first. In terms of explaining disease aetiology (cause of disease), they provide only limited information. The *prevalence* of a disease can be broadly defined as the proportion of persons in a population who have the disease in question at a particular point in time (point prevalence), or over a short time period (period prevalence). Cross-sectional studies are ideally suited to study prevalence. Such studies also have a use in estimating health needs or health attitudes and behaviour in a community, and the results of such studies may be a help in planning services or appropriate health education programmes. Screening programmes also fit into this category. (These programmes, however, are not designed for research purposes, but are set up to identify persons in the community who may have early evidence of a particular disease. The object of these studies is to commence early treatment of such persons.)

Although cross-sectional surveys are not as common in medical research as prospective or retrospective studies, they are widely used in many areas of social research including government surveys of household budgets and unemployment. The opinion poll itself is also of course a cross-sectional survey.

10.5 The prospective study

The *prospective* or, as it is often called, the *cohort, longitudinal or follow-up study* requires that individuals be followed up over a, sometimes quite long, period of time. This follow-up may require periodic examination of the individuals studied, or may just be based on the notification of the date of death for each individual as he or she dies. Prospective studies have two main areas of application.

In studies of disease aetiology, a group of individuals without the disease in question may be followed forward in time until the particular disease develops, or until they die. The purpose of such studies is to identify which factors are related to the particular end-point being studied and typically will start with a cross-sectional survey. In studies of prognosis, patients with a specific disease are followed up to determine which factors relate to further morbidity (illness) and/or mortality. Studies of prognosis are usually based on a presenting sample of patients with a disease, and thus patients do not enter into observation at the same point in calendar time, but often over an extended period. Prognosis studies should, however, start at some fixed point in the natural history of the disease, usually at its first manifestation. As with all prospective studies, complete follow-up of all patients is essential, and this will often necessitate much work on the part of the investigator. When the end-point of the study is not death a regular follow-up is also required to ensure that, say, in a study of cancer recurrence no events are missed.

Two famous and long-running prospective studies to determine risk factors for specific diseases deserve mention. The Doll and Hill smoking study, as it is generally called, surveyed in 1951 all the 59 600 doctors on the medical register who were resident in the United Kingdom. Postal questionnaires were used, and nearly 41 000 usable replies were received. The questionnaire elicited very simple information regarding the respondents' cigarette smoking habits; each person was asked to classify himself/herself as a current smoker, a person who had smoked but had given up, or a person who had never smoked at all. Current and ex-smokers were asked the age at which they started to smoke, and how much they smoked. Ex-smokers were asked the age at which they ceased, and all respondents were requested to give their age at the time of the survey. Subsequent to the receipt of these questionnaires, all deaths among the doctors were notified to the study team through medical associations and the Registrar General (who is in charge of death certification). The study still continues, and a 20-year report was published in 1976 (Doll and Peto). This study has shown, very conclusively, that the death rates (number of deaths per 1000 in a defined population over a specified period) from lung cancer, and indeed all causes, among the smokers were very much higher than among the non-smokers, with the ex-smokers in an intermediate position. Death rates also increased with increasing use of tobacco.

A large sample size was required for this study, since the death rate from lung cancer was low, and a sufficient number of deaths had to be obtained. In England and Wales in 1951, eight out of every 10 000 males aged over 25 would have been expected to die from lung cancer. Note, however, that the study was not based on a random population sample and the generalization of the results requires that the relationship between lung cancer and smoking be judged the same in the general population as in doctors. The very long duration of this study is also noteworthy, although initial results were available a few years after the study commenced. As has been said, the important point about any prospective study is that the presence or absence of the end-point (death or development of disease) be determined in all subjects. The Doll and Hill study employed routinely available records, in that the basic source of information was the death certificate. Stringent confirmation of cause of death was sought, however, and error checks on the time of death were also made.

A second famous prospective study is the Framingham Heart Study (Dawber, 1980). This study also commenced in the early 1950s, with a random sample of nearly 5000 male and female residents, aged 30 − 59 years, in the town of Framingham, Massachusetts (USA). The purpose of this study was to determine the many risk factors for coronary heart disease (CHD). Subjects underwent an initial comprehensive medical examination, which concentrated on the suspected risk factors for CHD. Subjects were then, and still are, examined every two years to determine the change of risk factors with time, and also the occurrence of the many manifestations of CHD. This study has provided much of what is now known about the aetiology of this condition.

10.6 Comparative measures of risks in prospective studies

At this stage, it is necessary to consider the analysis and presentation of the results of a prospective study. Central to this is the notion of *risk*. There are three terms in epidemiology, which are, for most practical purposes, synonymous. These are rates, risks and probabilities. For a disease, it is usual to talk about its *incidence rate* — the number of *new* cases of the disease over a particular period of time (usually a year) per 1000 (usually) of the population. (Compare this with the definition of the point prevalence rate which is the number of cases per 1000 of the population *existing* at a point in time.) A mortality rate is similarly defined as the incidence rate for the end-point of death. The *risk* of a disease or of death is the number of events occurring in a specific period of time divided by the total number of persons alive at the start of the period. Thus, a risk and a probability are measuring exactly the same thing. In this text, the subtle distinctions between rates and risks* are not of concern. Thus, if out of 200 individuals 15 developed

---

* The distinction between a rate and a risk is that the denominator of the former is usually the average population over the study period, while for a risk it is the number of persons at the start of the study period. The terms rate and risk are often used interchangeably, however.

CHD in one year, the risk of CHD among similar persons is 15/200 or 7·5%. Note that the estimation of an incidence rate or risk requires a prospective study design, and that the definitions only allow for one event per person to occur — usually the first occurrence of an illness; death can of course occur only once.

There are many descriptive measures that can compare two risks, and they will be illustrated on the results of a study of survivors of a first heart attack (Daly *et al.* 1983). A total of 368 male cigarette smokers aged less than 60 years, who survived their first heart attack by at least 2 years*, were categorized by whether or not they had ceased cigarette smoking at this time. The patients were then followed up to determine if cessation of cigarette smoking was related to subsequent mortality. The data presented in Table 10.1 relate to the mortality experience of these patients in the two years following their categorization into continued and stopped smokers (i.e. 4 years after the initial heart attack). The data are laid out in a 2 × 2 table and, as was seen previously, an appropriate significance test for the mortality difference would be the χ^2 test. These 2-year mortality results are non-significant at a 5% two-sided level ($\chi^2 = 3\cdot03$; d.f. = 1), although over a

Table 10.1. Risk comparisons in a prospective study. Subsequent 2-year mortality related to cessation of cigarette smoking in 368 survivors of a first heart attack

| | Survival at 2 years | | |
	Dead	Alive	Total
Continued smokers	19 (12·3%)	135 (87·7%)	154 (100·0%)
Stopped smokers	15 (7·0%)	199 (93·0%)	214 (100·0%)
	34 (9·2%)	334 (90·8%)	368 (100·0%)

$\chi^2 = 3\cdot03$; d.f. = 1; NS

Absolute risks of death:
  continued smokers: 19/154 = 12·3%
  stopped smokers: 15/214 = 7·0%
  total: 34/368 = 9·2%

Comparing continued and stopped smokers:
  relative risk: 12·3%/7·0% = 1·76
  attributable risk: 12·3% − 7·0% = 5·3%
  attributable risk per cent: 5·3%/12·3% = 43·1%

---

* Six patients who were not followed for this 2-year period are excluded from this illustrative analysis. See Section 10.7 where the complete results on 374 patients are presented.

longer period of follow-up (see Section 10.7) a significant difference was obtained.

To distinguish it from other measures, the risk of an event is often termed the *absolute risk*. The absolute risk of a continued smoker dying within the 2 years of the study period is given by the number of deaths in this group divided by the total number in the group: $19/154 = 12·3\%$. The absolute risk for a stopped smoker is, similarly, $7·0\%$, and for the group as a whole it is $9·2\%$ (see Table 10.1). The risks of $12·3\%$ and $7·0\%$ in continued and stopped smokers may be compared in two basic ways. Their ratio can be taken and the *relative risk* (RR) of death for continued smokers relative to stopped smokers can be derived as $12·3\%/7·0\% = 1·76$. This means that a continued smoker has $1·76$ times the risk of death of a stopped smoker. This relative risk measure is the most commonly employed comparative measure of risk.

The relative risk, however, does not take account of the magnitude of its two component risks. For instance, a relative risk of $2·0$ could be obtained from the two absolute risks of 90% and 45%, or from the two absolute risks of 2% and 1%. For this reason, an alternative comparative measure between two risks is also used. This is the *attributable* or *excess risk*. It is calculated by subtracting the two risks in question; thus, continued smokers have an excess risk of death of $12·3\% - 7·0\% = 5·3\%$ relative to stopped smokers. The term attributable risk is used because, all else being equal, continued smokers, had they not continued, would have experienced a risk of $7·0\%$ so that (assuming a significant result) the $5·3\%$ excess can be attributed to their smoking. Both these comparative measures of risk display different aspects of the data.

Another comparative measure which is sometimes used is the attributable risk per cent. This is the attributable risk as a percentage of the absolute risk in the group exposed to the risk factor (in this case exposed to continued smoking). The attributable risk per cent is then $5·3\%/12·3\% = 0·431 = 43·1\%$. This can be interpreted to mean that, again all else being equal, $43·1\%$ of the total risk of death in a continued smoker is attributable to smoking. Which of these or any of the many other comparative risk measures to employ depends on the purpose of a particular analysis. The relative risk is generally accepted as the best measure of the strength of an association between a risk factor and disease, because it is less likely to be influenced by unmeasured confounding or nuisance variables. The attributable risk on the other hand, or the attributable risk per cent, is a more useful indicator of the impact of prevention. For instance, on the basis of the above study, just over 40% of the risk of death in two years among the continued smokers could be eradicated if they had been persuaded to stop smoking; or in other words, 40% of the deaths among continued smokers were, in theory, preventable.

Although many comparative risk measures are available, the appropriate test of significance remains the same — the χ^2 test (see Section 7.10). Section 10.10 explains how confidence intervals can be calculated for comparative measures of

Table 10.2. Risks (per 100 000) of developing a disease X in groups defined by drinking and smoking habits

	Non-drinkers	Drinkers
Non-smokers	24	36
Smokers	32	50

risk in 2 × 2 tables. This illustrative analysis has assumed that comparison between the continued and stopped smokers was valid and that there are no confounding variables. In fact the excess of mortality in the continued smokers cannot be explained by confounding factors and age, for example, was similar in the two groups. Chapter 13 discusses the analysis of such data when confounding is present.

In a prospective study, one might often be interested in the joint effect of two or more risk factors on the end-point being considered. Table 10.2 shows the (hypothetical) risk of developing a disease X in groups defined by drinking and smoking habits. An important question in relation to such data is whether or not the combined effect of both factors is greater than that expected on the basis of their individual effects in isolation. A *synergistic* effect is said to be present if the observed effect is greater than expected, and an *antagonistic* effect obtains if the effect is less than expected. Variables that interact in this way are called *effect modifiers* and are discussed further in Chapter 12.

In the example, the observed effect of drinking and smoking is given by an absolute risk per 100 000 of 50, and the main question is how to calculate the expected effect. There are at least two methods of doing this, and they are best illustrated on a more concrete example. Table 10.3 shows the same numerical data, but this time relating the price of a cup of tea or coffee to whether it is drunk on the premises, or bought to take away. The price of a cup of coffee to drink at a table is not given, however. What would it be expected to be, on the basis of the prices displayed? It could be argued that since it costs 8p extra

Table 10.3. Costs in pence of buying tea and coffee either to take away or to drink at a table in the premises (1984 prices)

	Tea	Coffee
To take away	24	36
To drink at a table	32	?

Cost to drink coffee at a table. Additive model: $36 + 8 = 44$; multiplicative model: $36 \times 1\frac{1}{3} = 48$.

(32p − 24p) to drink tea at a table it should also cost 8p extra to drink coffee at a table; thus, the cost of this should be 36p + 8p = 44p. The same result could be obtained by noting that coffee costs 12p more than tea (to take away), so that coffee at a table should be 12p dearer than tea at a table, i.e. 44p. For obvious reasons this is considered an *additive* model for the expected price of coffee at a table.

An alternative method of calculating the expected price of drinking coffee at a table is to note that drinking tea at a table costs one-third extra, so that the expected price of drinking coffee at a table would also be one-third extra or 36p × $1\frac{1}{3}$ = 48p. This is the expected price under a *multiplicative* model. Going back to the same data as representing risks, the expected risk of disease X in smoking drinkers can be calculated at 44 per 100 000 on an additive model, or 48 per 100 000 on a multiplicative model. It can be seen that the expected risk in the additive model is based on equality of attributable or excess risks, for one variable at each level of the other, and in the multiplicative model on equality of relative risks. There is no definite answer as to which of the two models is more appropriate, although many favour the additive one. In the example, the observed risk of 50/100 000 is greater than that expected on either model, so that a synergistic effect of tobacco and alcohol consumption can be claimed unambiguously. In other situations, model choice may affect the interpretation of results on the combined effect of two risk factors.

10.7 Estimation of risk with variable follow-up: person-years and the clinical life table

The prospective study of prognosis in the last section was analysed in terms of a fixed follow-up for all patients. Each individual was known to be either alive or dead at 2 years from study commencement, and the 2 × 2 table (Alive/Dead by Continued/Stopped) formed the appropriate basis for analysis. Risks were calculated directly as the proportion who died over the period of follow-up. With many prospective studies however, a fixed period of follow-up is not available for each individual and special methods must be employed to estimate and compare risks. Use of the methods described in the last section are not valid. Two common situations where this arises are described below.

In a study of occupational mortality, for instance, employees of a particular firm may enter observation at the time of their first employment and be followed up until death or a particular point in calendar time. Of interest is mortality in relation to the type of work or exposure of the employees. Unfortunately, each individual will be followed up for different periods from the time of his/her first employment to the date the study has to be analysed. (Often the data for an occupational cohort study are collected retrospectively using employment records, though in essence the study design is prospective.) Thus, for an analysis undertaken now, an employee who started work 5 years ago would have only 5 years of follow-up, compared to a much longer period for an individual who commenced, say, 12 years ago.

The second common situation where variable follow-up arises is in the context of a clinical trial (see Chapter 11) or a prospective study of prognosis. Suppose a prognosis study of mortality commenced in 1980. (The end-point of interest can of course be an event other than death, but for simplicity mortality, or equivalently survival, will be discussed here.) Patients entered into the study at diagnosis, but, in calendar time, this occurred over a 10-year period. As in the occupational cohort study, however, the analysis must take place at a fixed point in calendar time. If analysis were being performed at the start of 1990, patients will have experienced various lengths of follow-up. The end-point for many patients will be known, because they have died, but an individual alive in January 1990 will die subsequently at an unknown date in the future. A follow-up terminated in this way due to the practical requirements of data analysis is referred to as a censored follow-up, and data from such a study are called *censored data*. Patients alive at the analysis stage of a study before experiencing the end-point of interest are called *withdrawals*. (Withdrawals should be distinguished from losses to follow-up — patients whose follow-up was terminated *before* the analysis date due to loss of contact, missed visit or whatever.)

Many erroneous approaches have been used to analyse prospective data arising from variable follow-up. The approach described in the last section of calculating mortality at a fixed time from study entry (e.g. 5 years) is only valid when each subject is known to be actually alive or dead at this time point. (This will be illustrated further in Section 10.12.) To use this fixed follow-up approach in a variable follow-up study requires that data collected on many patients be discarded. The calculation of a 'total study mortality', by dividing all the observed deaths by the total number studied, is not a mortality rate in any sense of the word since it takes no account of the time over which the events occurred. With a follow-up of everyone to death, this figure would eventually reach 100%! Sometimes, a mean 'length of survival' is calculated by averaging the time of death of the decedents and the time to last follow-up of withdrawals. The resulting figure, however, measures the average length of follow-up rather than anything else and is totally dependent on the study duration. It is not a suitable summary measure of survival either.

Apart from discarding much of the data and using the fixed follow-up approach, two techniques are available for the analysis of variable follow-up data. The first is used mainly for an occupational mortality study.

For such data a mortality rate per person-year of follow-up is calculated. (A person-year of follow-up, or a person-year at risk is one person followed for 1 year;

see Section 4.9.) For example, 20 deaths might be observed among 600 employees. The person-years of follow-up of these 600 is obtained by determining the length of follow-up of each employee and adding them up. If the total person-years of follow-up was calculated at 5400 years, the mortality rate would be expressed as 20/5400 or 3·7 deaths per thousand person-years, without explicit note of the number of individuals involved. A basic assumption of this method is that the mortality rate is not related to length of follow-up. Hypothesis tests and confidence intervals for such rates are described in Section 4.9. Risk comparisons between different groups can also be performed, and the methods for testing differences between groups are given in Section 7.14. Ratios of the mortality rates akin to a relative risk can also be analysed and this is covered below in Section 10.11.

For the analysis of variable follow-up data in a prognosis study or clinical trial the person-years of follow-up method can be employed, but in this situation what is called the *clinical life table method* is preferred. (See Chapter 13 for a discussion of the *population life table*.) Many variants of this are available and the *actuarial life table* is described below.

Essentially, the entire study period is subdivided into small intervals of time; usually years or months are employed, but some techniques require that the intervals be defined by the actual times of each event (death, loss or withdrawal). In each interval the number of patients alive at the start, the number of deaths and the number withdrawn alive or lost to follow-up are used to estimate a 'within-interval' mortality. These interval mortalities can then be combined to give a mortality risk (rate) for any time since study commencement. This method is described in detail in Section 10.12. The clinical life table approach gives an unbiased estimate of mortality at yearly intervals (or whatever size intervals are chosen) from study commencement, and thus gives a far more complete picture of what is happening than the usual 2×2 table which compares mortality at a single fixed time-point only. The clinical life table is either a table or graph showing the percentage mortality (or survival) at each time point from study commencement. These are sometimes called cumulative mortality or survival rates. Figure 10.1 shows the cumulative mortality over a 13-year follow-up of the continued and stopped smokers in the study of heart attack survivors discussed in the previous section. Although most of the patients were not followed for the full 13 years, the clinical life table method allowed calculation of the 13-year mortality, which was around 82% in the continued smokers and 37% in those who ceased. Mortality at all times from the start of the study can easily be read off the graph, and the visual presentation shows clearly how the two mortality curves diverge over time.

In addition to presenting a clear and unbiased picture of mortality over time, the clinical life table utilizes all the available data without discarding any of them. Losses to follow-up, as long as there are not too many, can also be accounted for by the method, given certain fairly reasonable assumptions. Statistical tests, the

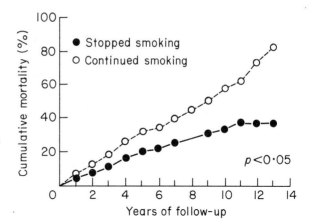

Fig. 10.1. Cumulative mortality in 157 continued smokers and 217 stopped smokers who survived a first heart attack by at least 2 years. Daly *et al.* (1983) with permission.

best-known of which is called the *logrank test*, are also available to compare the mortalities of two or more groups calculated by the life table method. Section 10.12 details the calculations for a life table analysis.

10.8 The case-control study

One of the purposes of the prospective study is to determine associations between risk factors measured at the start of the study and subsequent morbidity or mortality. In essence, a prospective study goes forward from a risk factor to the development of the end-point of interest. An alternative to the prospective study for the elucidation of associations between risk factors and disease is a case-control or retrospective study. As its name suggests, the retrospective study starts with the end-point and moves backwards in time to the identification of risk factors.

A group of persons with a particular disease (the cases) is studied as regards factors to which it was exposed in the past, and the results are compared with those obtained in a comparison group (the controls) without the disease. If the factor is associated with the disease, then it should appear more commonly in the cases than in the controls. The investigation of Herity *et al.* (1981) into the association between smoking and drinking and the development of cancer of the head and neck will be taken as an example of this type of study. A case-control study divides into four stages: the selection of cases, the selection of controls, the measurement of the risk factor, and the analysis of the association. To avoid bias, cases in a case-control study should be newly diagnosed. Although this will always reduce the numbers available for a study, a group containing a mixture of newly diagnosed cases and long-standing chronic cases can cause great difficulty in interpreting the results. The diagnostic criteria for defining a case must be explicit and clear. This will enable the study to be replicated elsewhere and avoid ambiguities of interpretation. Often persons with other concurrent disease will be excluded from the cases. Usually in a case-control study a presenting sample, to a particular hospital or unit, of newly diagnosed cases is taken. It must be remembered however that cases admitted to a hospital are not necessarily representative of all cases in the community at large. In the study of head and neck cancer, a presenting sample of 200 new patients attending a particular hospital over a two-year period for treatment of cancer of the head and neck formed the case group. The definition of head and neck cancer is given in the original report.

The selection of controls is, without any doubt, the most difficult part of a case-control study. Ideally, the controls should be representative of the general population without the disease, and thus be a random sample from the same population that gave rise to the cases. Practical considerations however usually dictate that controls are taken from a hospital population of patients who have neither the disease under investigation, nor a disease positively related to the risk factor being studied. One advantage of this approach is that the same factors that determined hospitalization of the cases in a particular hospital may also have been likely to determine the hospitalization of the controls. The problem is, of course, to what extent the controls may be judged representative of the general population.

Apart from the source of the controls, the next problem arises in their selection. A random sample from the hospital patients not affected by the disease in question could be taken, but it is then likely that cases and controls would differ as regards variables that might be related to exposure to the risk factors and development of the disease. Such variables, which would act as confounders of the association, could be controlled for in the analysis stage but are better adjusted for in the design of the study. Age and sex are two common confounders in case-control studies. To avoid the confounding effect of such variables, the controls are often chosen to have the same distribution as the cases in terms of characteristics such as age and sex. Two different methods are available to achieve this; the first has already been discussed and involves a paired sample (see Section 7.2). Typically, a control of the same sex and age (to within a specified number of years) is individually matched to each case, and the analysis proceeds as for paired comparisons, discussed in Chapter 7. Some studies however use *frequency matching* whereby the distribution of, say, age and sex in the controls is fixed to be identical to that in the cases, but not by individual matching. Usually this is achieved by determining the age/sex distribution of the cases in, say, 10-year age groups. If there are 15 males aged $45 - 54$ years in the cases, 15 males in the same age group would be chosen for the controls.* Although the overall

---

* Usually, in case-control studies, the numbers of cases and controls are taken to be equal.

distribution will be similar in the two groups, individual matching does not occur. What factors to match for in case-control studies often causes problems. Variables that are known to be associated with both the development of the disease and exposure to the risk factor are the prime candidates. As has been said, age and sex are two such factors. It should be noted, however, that to match for too many factors can, in practice, be a very tedious task and that any variables matched for cannot be analysed for a relationship with the disease. One can match on variables related to the disease but not to the risk factor of interest, if the influence of such variables is not to be analysed and a small effect of a different variable is being investigated. Matching must not take place on variables related to the risk factor only, since this will tend to ensure equal distribution of the risk factor in cases and controls, and hence no result.

Care must also be taken in the actual choosing of each individual control. Ideally, the person selecting the control should not know the nature of the risk factor being studied or subtle selection biases might occur. For instance, if cigarette smoking was one of the risk factors being studied, a potential control with a packet of cigarettes on his/her bedside locker might be deliberately avoided! In the study of head and neck cancer, the controls, frequency-matched to the cases for age (in 10-year age groups) and sex, were chosen from patients attending the same hospital 'for the treatment of non-smoking-related cancers and benign conditions' during the same period in which the cases were hospitalized.

Once cases and controls have been chosen, exposure to the risk factors must be determined. Unfortunately, this depends either on the patient's memory, or on available hospital records. It is important that cases and controls are interviewed in the same manner and by the same person. Ideally, that person should not know if the individual is a case or control in order to avoid a biased response as a result of leading questions or a more careful interviewing of cases. In practice, this is difficult to achieve. Also, if the case knows the purpose of the study, he or she might overemphasize or minimize exposure to the risk factors, thus biasing the results in this way. Some case-control studies are based on hospital charts and records only, and exposure information founded on these may be quite dubious. Often such records are incomplete, and no mention of a particular factor either means that the factor was not present, or that exposure was never ascertained or recorded. In the head and neck cancer study, a predesigned questionnaire was administered by one of the investigators, and details of sex, age, occupation, education, tobacco and alcohol consumption and dental care were noted.

After collection of the data, the association between the risk factor and the disease must be examined. From the significance-testing point of view, the methods outlined in Chapter 7 for the comparison of two groups will be adequate for examining the relationship of a single risk factor and a disease. It is important, however, to have a measure of the strength of the association between the risk factor and the disease. It has already been described how, in a prospective study, the absolute risks of disease in those exposed and not exposed to a risk factor can be calculated. Unfortunately, in a case-control study, no measure of absolute risk is available since there is no group that was followed forward in time. Table 10.4 shows a 2 × 2 table with the smoking results in the head and neck cancer study. The result is significant by the chi-square test,* showing a predominance of smokers among the cases. It cannot however be said that the absolute risk of a smoker getting head and neck cancer is 145/252, since 252 smokers were not followed forward over a period of time; in fact, if two controls per case had been chosen, a totally different answer would have been obtained. Absolute risks cannot be determined in a case-control study. It is possible, however, to calculate an approximate estimate of the relative risk if it can be assumed that the incidence of the disease in the population is small, that cases and controls are random samples from their corresponding populations, and that only new cases are included. This approximation to the relative risk is called the *odds ratio* (OR) and is calculated by dividing the 'odds' of a smoker getting head and neck cancer by the 'odds' of a non-smoker getting this cancer. The odds of an event are related to its probability; but the odds are defined as the number of persons who experience the event divided, not by the total number of persons, but by the number of persons not experiencing the event. Now, an individual odd cannot be calculated directly from a case-control study either. However, unlike the relative risk, the ratio of the two quantities ('odds') 145/107 and 55/93 = 2·29 estimates the true ratio of the odds and is not dependent on the number of controls taken per case, being the same for any sampling fraction of cases and controls. The 2·29 can then be interpreted as an estimate of the ratio of the odds, in the population, of a smoker developing

Table 10.4. Relationship between smoking and head and neck cancer in a case-control study. Abbreviated from Herity *et al.* (1981) with permission

	Cases	Controls	Total
Smokers	145 (72·5%)	107 (53·5%)	252 (63·0%)
Non- or ex-smokers	55 (27·5%)	93 (46·5%)	148 (37·0%)
	200 (100·0%)	200 (100·0%)	400 (100·0%)

$\chi^2 = 15\cdot487$; d.f. = 1; $p < 0\cdot01$

$$\text{Odds ratio (OR)} = \frac{145/107}{55/93} = \frac{145 \times 93}{55 \times 107} = 2\cdot29$$

* This illustrative analysis ignores the frequency matching, and treats cases and controls as independent samples.

head and neck cancer to the odds of a non-smoker developing this disease. Given the assumptions already mentioned, this odds ratio is a good approximation to the relative risk, and it can be said that a smoker has 2·29 times the risk of a non-smoker of developing head and neck cancer.

The above example dealt with (for illustrative purposes) two independent samples of cases and controls. If individually matched cases and controls were being analysed, the data in a 2 × 2 table would have to be laid out as described for the significance testing of paired proportions (Section 7.13). In this situation, the odds ratio is given by the ratio of untied pairs. The number of pairs in which the case and not the control is exposed to the risk factor is divided by the number of pairs in which the control is exposed and the case is not. These approximate relative risk calculations are summarized in Table 10.5 and confidence interval estimations are given in Section 10.10.

It was previously pointed out that the presence of a confounding variable such as age or sex, associated with both the disease and the risk factor, may distort an observed association between the risk factor itself and the disease. Such confounding can be controlled by study design through matching though the statistical analysis must take account of this. Other confounding variables may exist, however, and if

Table 10.5. Odds ratios in case-control studies

(a) Independent data

	Cases	Controls
Risk factor		
Present	a	b
Absent	c	d
	$a + c$	$b + d$

$$\text{Odds ratio (OR)} = \frac{ad}{bc}$$

(b) Paired data

	Case	
	Risk factor present	Risk factor absent
Control		
Risk factor present	a	b
Risk factor absent	c	d

$$\text{Odds ratio (OR)} \approx \frac{c}{b}$$

they have been measured, can be controlled in the analysis stage as indicated in Chapter 12. Essentially, the odds ratio is examined at each level of a qualitative confounder, and an average of these odds ratios is calculated. Methods for the analysis of frequency-matched data are also based on combining results obtained at each level of the matching variable(s). These methods are described in Chapter 12. It should be noted, of course, that matching is also possible in a prospective study and the above comments are relevant in that situation too. Sometimes one is also interested, not in controlling for a confounding variable, but in estimating the joint effect on disease occurrence of two variables acting together. The technique discussed in Section 10.6 for the measurement of synergistic effects can also be employed on relative risk measures obtained from a case-control study.

10.9 Comparison of prospective and case-control studies

Both prospective and case-control (retrospective) studies can be utilized to examine associations between risk factors and disease, and each approach has its advantages and disadvantages. The prospective study generally will require large sample sizes and extensive periods of follow-up. This is due to the fact that the incidence of many conditions is low, even in an exposed group, and many persons must be studied over a long-period to obtain even a few cases who develop the end-point of interest. The case-control study, on the other hand, utilizes existing cases with a large reduction in the required sample size. Case-control studies are thus cheaper to carry out and will provide results much faster. Such studies are especially useful in investigating the aetiology of rare conditions.

Unlike the case-control study however, the prospective study is not as open to bias in the measurement of the risk factors, and allows complete ascertainment and uniformity of measurement for the relevant data. The case-control study relies on memory or previously recorded data, and has many problems in this area. Proper choice of adequate controls in a case-control study is perhaps its greatest weakness, and it is probably true to say that very few case-control studies, in practice, have controls that satisfy the most stringent criteria for an unbiased comparison. The comparison groups in a prospective study, however, can usually be defined without bias, since they are formed without prior knowledge of which individuals will develop the disease being investigated. There is often no predefined separate control group in a prospective study; comparisons are just made between groups with and without the risk factor present as determined at the baseline examination. The prospective study also allows the calculation of absolute risks of disease, whereas only approximate relative risk measures are available with the case-control study. Further, the prospective study allows for the examination of the relationship of measured risk factors to many different end-points, whereas the case-control study is confined to one end-point and, usually, only a few risk factors.

Although the prospective study has many definite theoretical advantages over the case-control study in determining aetiology, the latter is more often encountered due to the sheer difficulty of setting up and following through the prospective study. Certainly, no prospective study should be started without a case-control study first, to check that a suspected association actually manifests itself. But, in many cases, the results of case-control studies only must be accepted as the method of determining disease aetiology.

The next sections in this chapter consider the formal statistical analysis of the study designs discussed so far.

10.10 Confidence intervals for relative risk type measures in 2 × 2 tables

When dealing with unmatched data in a 2 × 2 table, whether derived from a prospective, a cross-sectional or a case-control study, the appropriate significance test is the usual chi-square test of Section 7.10. The choice of a comparative measure for the table depends on the study design or the precise point one wishes to make. Comparative measures mentioned in this text include the excess (attributable) risk, the relative risk and the odds ratio, and confidence interval formulae are available for each of these measures.

The methods for calculating a confidence interval for a single absolute risk were discussed in Section 4.8 in the context of a single binomial proportion, and in Section 7.9 the confidence interval for the excess risk was given as that for the difference between two independent proportions. The confidence interval for the excess risk with paired data is given in Section 7.13. This could be an appropriate measure for a pair-matched prospective study (e.g. in a clinical trial; see Chapter 11).

This present section considers confidence intervals in the situation when relative risks or odds ratios are chosen as the comparative measure. Various approaches have been suggested for calculating confidence intervals for relative risk measures and only one will be described here. The method, first suggested by Miettinen (1976), has the advantage that it can be applied to relative risks and odds ratios derived from either pair-matched or independent data. The derivation is briefly described below but the next few paragraphs can be omitted if the reader does not wish to understand how the formulae arise and just wishes to be able to perform the calculations.

In general, for any statistic that has a normal sampling distribution (such as the difference between means or proportions for example) a 95% confidence interval is given by

$$\text{Statistic} \pm 1.96 \text{ SE (statistic)} \tag{10.1}$$

where SE (statistic) refers to the standard error of the statistic. Now the relative risk (RR) does not have a normal sampling distribution, but the natural logarithm of the relative risk — ln RR — does have.* Thus if the standard error of ln RR could be found it would be possible to obtain a 95% confidence interval for ln RR, and by taking the exponential of these limits the confidence limits for the relative risk itself would result. This is a good example of data transformation to achieve approximate normality (see Section 1.7).

Although an exact formula for the standard error of ln RR is not available an approximation can be obtained from the chi-square value on the 2×2 table on which the relative risk was calculated. Firstly one must note that for a statistic with a normal sampling distribution a significance test can be formulated as

$$z = \frac{\text{Statistic} - \text{null value}}{\text{SE (statistic)}} \tag{10.2}$$

where z has a standard normal distribution. For a two-sided 5% level of significance z must be greater than 1·96 or less than $-1·96$. As has been said above, the usual significance test for a 2×2 table is the chi-square test on 1 degree of freedom, and it so happens that the square root of a 1 d.f. χ^2 is in fact the corresponding z value from the normal distribution. For instance the 5% (2-sided) critical χ^2 value is 3·84 and its square root is 1·96 — the 5% critical value of the standard normal distribution. Similarly the χ^2 value of 6·635 corresponds to the z value of 2·576 (the 1% 2-sided critical value).

Now, in the context of a prospective mortality study in groups exposed and not exposed to a risk factor, a lack of association between mortality and the risk factor implies a relative risk (RR) of 1·0. Thus, for a significance test of a relative risk the null value would be 1·0, and for a test of ln RR the null value would be zero (the natural log of one is zero). Equation 10.2 could then be applied to the statistic ln RR giving

$$\chi = \ln RR / SE (\ln RR) \tag{10.3}$$

where χ is the square root of the chi-square for the particular table, which is equated with the z of a hypothetical significance test for ln RR. This gives an expression for SE (ln RR) based on the chi-square value

$$SE (\ln RR) = (\ln RR)/\chi. \tag{10.4}$$

---

* The 'ln' denotes the natural logarithm based on the constant $e = 2·71828 \ldots$ Usually logarithms are to the base 10, so that log 100 = 2 because $10^2 = 100$. Also since $10^{1·38} = 24$, log 24 = 1·38. Now for instance $e^2 = 7·39$ (referred to as the exponential of 2) so that the natural log of 7·39 (ln 7·39) = 2. Also $e^{3·18} = 24$, giving ln 24 = 3·18. Most good pocket calculators allow for easy calculation of e to any given power, or of the ln of any quantity.

Substituting this into Equation 10.1 gives the 95% confidence interval for $\ln RR$ as

$$\ln RR \pm 1\cdot96 \, (\ln RR)/\chi. \tag{10.5}$$

If the exponential of this is taken to transform the confidence limits for $\ln RR$ to limits for RR, the confidence interval for the relative risk becomes

$$e^{[\ln\ RR\ \pm\ 1\cdot96\ (\ln RR)/\chi]} \tag{10.6}$$

which simplifies to

$$RR^{(1\ \pm\ 1\cdot96/\chi)}. \tag{10.7}$$

The confidence limits derived in this way are called 'test-based limits' since they use the value of the χ^2 test statistic to derive the standard error. Limits obtained with this approach are reasonably good approximations to the exact limits, especially for relative risks not too far from unity.

An exactly similar argument applies for the odds ratio (OR), so that confidence intervals for the relative risk and odds ratio are given by

$$RR^{(1\ \pm\ z_c/\chi)} \tag{10.8}$$

$$OR^{(1\ \pm\ z_c/\chi)} \tag{10.9}$$

where χ is the square root of the appropriate chi-square for the 2×2 table from which the measures were calculated and z_c is the critical value from the normal distribution corresponding to the confidence level chosen. To find these limits it is necessary to have a calculator that calculates a number to a fractional power. Most scientific instruments now available can do this.

In the prospective study of smoking following a heart attack (Section 10.6) the relative risk of death for a continued versus stopped smoker was $RR = 1\cdot76$, and $\chi^2 = 3\cdot03$ on 1 degree of freedom. The 95% confidence interval for RR is then given by

$$1.76^{(1\ \pm\ 1\cdot96/1\cdot74)} = 1.76^{(1\ \pm\ 1\cdot13)}$$

or from $1\cdot76^{-0\cdot13}$ to $1\cdot76^{2\cdot13}$, which is from $0\cdot93$ to $3\cdot33$. Note that this interval overlaps the null value of $1\cdot0$, so that, on the basis of these data, at a 95% confidence level, there may not be a real mortality excess in continued smokers. (Remember, of course, that the chi-square for this table was non-significant leading to the same conclusion.)

Note that if the relative risk is greater than unity the plus sign in Eqns. 10.8 and 10.9 gives the upper limit of the confidence interval and the minus sign gives the lower limit. If the relative risk is less than unity the opposite holds. If the relative risk or odds ratio actually equal unity, the χ^2 value will be zero and the limits cannot be calculated using this method.

For the case-control study of head and neck cancer the odds ratio was OR =

2·29 with a χ^2 of 15·49 (Section 10.8; Table 10.4). The 95% confidence interval is given by

$$2\cdot29^{(1\pm1\cdot96/3\cdot94)} = 2\cdot29^{(1\pm0\cdot5)}$$

which is from 1·51 to 3·47.

For pair-matched data in a case-control study the odds ratio is estimated from

$$OR = c/b \qquad\qquad (10.10)$$

where c is the number of pairs with the case exposed to the risk factor but the control not exposed, and b is the number of pairs with the control exposed but the case not exposed (see Table 10.5 in Section 10.8). The appropriate chi-square for such a matched study is McNemar's chi-square (Section 7.13), and Eqn. 10.9 is applicable to calculate confidence limits for the paired odds ratio estimate if the square root of this chi-square is used in the formula. Sections C.12 and C.15 summarize confidence interval estimation for 2×2 table comparative measures.

10.11 Confidence intervals for the ratio of two rates based on person-years at risk

When rates are based on person-years of follow-up or person-years at risk (PYRS) in the denominator, statistical analysis relies on the Poisson distribution. Section 4.9 showed how to obtain a confidence interval for a single rate, and Section 7.14 described the confidence interval for the difference between two rates. This section describes a method for calculating confidence limits for the ratio of two rates.

The example of Section 7.14 will be used to illustrate the method. Table 10.6 repeats Table 7.13 which gives data relating to childhood deaths from cancer in two regions.

The ratio of these two death rates is $32\cdot10/22\cdot41 = 1\cdot43$, showing that the rate in Region 1 is nearly one-and-a-half times as high as that in Region 2. To calculate confidence limits for this, note that the rate ratio (which will be denoted RR)* can be expressed as

$$RR = (x_1/x_2)\,(PYRS_2/PYRS_1) \qquad\qquad (10.11)$$

where x_1/x_2 is the ratio of two Poisson variables — the numbers of deaths in Regions 1 and 2. The problem then reduces to determining a confidence interval for this ratio since the person-years can be considered fixed.

---

* RR was used previously to denote a relative risk as determined from a 2×2 table. The rate ratio is obviously a similar concept, though derived from a different data structure.

Table 10.6. Childhood deaths from acute lymphatic leukaemia in two regions

Group i	Region 1	Region 2
No. deaths (x_i)	11	17
Person-years at risk ($\times 10^6$) (PYRS$_i$)	0·3427	0·7586
Annual rate per 10^6 (r_i)	32·10	22·41

Unusually enough, use is made of the binomial distribution for this calculation. (Ederer and Mantel, 1974). The argument goes as follows. Out of a total of $x_1 + x_2$ events (deaths), x_1 were observed in Region 1. Thus,

$$p = \frac{x_1}{x_1 + x_2} \tag{10.12}$$

can be considered as a single (binomial) proportion calculated on a sample size of $x_1 + x_2$. With the methods of Section 4.8, using either the exact method (Table B.11) or the normal approximation (Eqn. 4.12), confidence limits for the population value of p can be calculated. Let p_l and p_u denote these lower and upper binomial limits. Noting that

$$\frac{x_1}{x_2} = \frac{p}{1 - p} \tag{10.13}$$

the binomial confidence limits can be substituted into this equation to give lower and upper confidence limits for the ratio of the Poisson events as respectively

$$\frac{p_l}{1 - p_l} \text{ and } \frac{p_u}{1 - p_u}. \tag{10.14}$$

Using Eqn. 10.11 the lower and upper confidence limits for the rate ratio (RR$_l$ and RR$_u$) are

$$RR_l = \frac{p_l}{1 - p_l} \frac{PYRS_2}{PYRS_1} \tag{10.15}$$

$$RR_u = \frac{p_u}{1 - p_u} \frac{PYRS_2}{PYRS_1} \tag{10.16}$$

where p_l and p_u are the lower and upper binomial confidence limits for the population value of $x_1/(x_1 + x_2)$.

In the example the relevant binomial proportion is 11/28 and from Table B.11 (see also Section 4.8) the lower and upper 95% confidence limits for this are 0·2150 and 0·5942. When these are substituted into Eqns. 10.15 and 10.16 the confidence limits for the rate ratio of 1·43 are

$$RR_l = \frac{(0 \cdot 2150)(0 \cdot 7586)}{(1 - 0 \cdot 2150)(0 \cdot 3427)} = 0.61$$

and

$$RR_u = \frac{(0 \cdot 5942)(0 \cdot 7586)}{(1 - 0 \cdot 5942)(0 \cdot 3427)} = 3 \cdot 24.$$

Thus, the 95% confidence interval for the ratio of death rates in Regions 1 and 2 is from 0·61 to 3·24. This procedure is summarized in Section C.16 of Appendix C.

10.12 The clinical life table: calculation and confidence intervals

This, and the following section, discuss the calculations required for the clinical life table using a simple example. Figure 10.2 shows, schematically, the follow-up of 14 male patients entered into a prospective study between 1980 and 1989. The left-hand side of the figure shows the 'lifespan' of each of the patients (labelled from A to N) in calendar time. Patient A, for instance, entered into the study in 1980 and died near the end of 1983 (between 3 and 4 years from study entry). Patient C was lost track of during 1985 but was known to be alive just over 4 years after study entry (a loss to follow-up). Patient E entered the study in mid-1983, and was alive at the start of 1990 (more than 6 years after entry into the study). Similarly, patients H, J, K, L and N were all alive at the time the study was being analysed, and are considered as withdrawals. The right-hand side of Fig. 10.2 shows the patient histories plotted from study entry, rather than in calendar time. The light lines refer to the potential periods of follow-up had the patients not died or been lost to follow-up. Suppose now that one wanted to calculate the 4-year mortality from time of entry into the study. Some of the incorrect methods already referred to in Section 10.7 will be illustrated first. Using the definition of number dead within 4 years divided by the total number of patients, the figure of 6 (patients A, D, F, G, I and M) divided by 14 = 42·9% would be obtained. This, however, is unduly optimistic, because it assumes that patients J, K, L and N, the withdrawals, who were not actually followed for as long as 4 years, would in fact have remained alive until the end of the 4 years. This is an untenable assumption. Alternatively a 4-year survival rate might have been defined, putting the number alive at 4 years over the total number in the study. This gives 4 (patients B, C, E and H) divided by 14, or 28·6%, which corresponds to a 4-year mortality of 71·4%. This is an unduly pessimistic figure, since its calculation assumes that the four withdrawals in the denominator would not have survived the full 4 years. In fact, the only unbiased estimator of a 4-year mortality rate is obtained by confining the analysis to only those patients actually followed for 4 years, or those who could have been followed if they had not died. This reduces the study cohort from

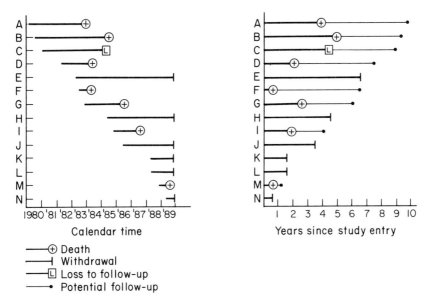

Fig. 10.2. Diagram showing follow-up of 14 male patients entered into a prospective study.

the original 14 to nine patients only (A to I) and gives a 4-year mortality of 5/9 = 55·5%. Because of the variable length of follow-up, the alternative to biased estimates of the mortality rate seem to require sacrificing much of the available information. It will now be seen how the clinical life table approach avoids this problem and provides an unbiased estimate of mortality.

As was said in Section 10.7, this approach requires a division of the total follow-up period into intervals. Supposing the 10 years of the study are now divided into 10 intervals of 1 year each; the data required for calculating a mortality rate using the clinical life table approach are then the total number alive at the start of the study and the numbers of deaths, withdrawals alive, and losses to follow-up observed in each interval.

The method is based on the law of combining conditional probabilities, discussed in Chapter 3 (Eqn. 3.3). To take a simple analogy, conditional probabilities combine like stages in a journey. To fly from Paris to New York via London, one must first get to London; when in London one has then to fly to New York. Take an example of this principle in terms of survival rates or probabilities. Table 10.7 displays a simple mortality study. One hundred persons enter the study at time zero. Fifty-five die in the first year (leaving 45 alive) and 15 persons die in the second year, leaving 30 survivors at the end of 2 years. The 2-year survival is then 30/100 = 0·3, expressed as the probability of surviving two years. Now the 1-year survival probability is, obviously, given by 45/100 = 0·45. Of these 45 persons who survived the first year, 15 die in the succeeding year, and 30 survive, so that

Table 10.7. Simple example of conditional probabilities. P (event) means the probability of the event

Time (years)	0		1		2
Interval no.		1		2	
No. alive	100		45		30
No. dying		55		15	

$P_1 = P$ (survival 0–1) = 45/100 = 0·45
$P_2 = P$ (survival 0–2) = 30/100 = 0·3
$p_2 = P$ (survival 1–2, given alive at 1) = 30/45
$\quad\ = 0·6667$
$P_2 = p_2 P_1$

the survival from the start of year 2 to the end of year 2, conditional on being alive at the start, is 30/45 = 0·6667. Note, however, that 0·45 × 0·6667 = 0·3. This is an example of the application of Eqn. 3.3. To survive two intervals of time it is necessary to survive the first interval, and given that, then to survive the second interval. If the probability of surviving from time 0 (study commencement) to time i (the end of the ith interval or year) is denoted by P_i, and the conditional probability of surviving the ith interval (from time $i - 1$ to i) by p_i, then the generalization of this is

$$P_i = p_i P_{i-1} \tag{10.17}$$

where P_0 is the probability of surviving to time 0 which must be 1. The P_i are called cumulative or unconditional survival probabilities.

The clinical life table utilizes this relationship by calculating the conditional probability of surviving each interval defined for the study, and then calculating the unconditional (cumulative) probabilities of survival from study commencement to the end of each interval. The cumulative mortality probabilities are obtained by subtracting the survival probabilities from 1, and can then be converted to percentages.

How then can the conditional probability of surviving each interval be calculated? First, some notation must be introduced. The intervals in the study are numbered from 1 to i, where 1 denotes the first interval, running from time 0 to time 1 (years or months). Table 10.8 displays the notation adopted. It has already been mentioned that the life table calculation requires that n_1, the number entering the study (and therefore the first interval), and the d_i and w_i, the deaths and withdrawals/losses in each defined interval, are known. No distinction is made between withdrawals due to study termination and losses to follow-up. It will now be shown how, starting with these data, an unbiased estimate of the 4-year mortality in the example discussed above can be calculated. Table 10.9 lays

Table 10.8. Clinical life table notation

Meaning	Symbol
Interval	i
End-points of interval i	$i-1$ i
Numbers entering interval i	n_i
Numbers dying in interval i	d_i
Numbers withdrawn or lost to follow-up in interval i	w_i
Adjusted number at risk at the start of interval i	n'_i
Conditional probability of death in interval i	q_i
Conditional probability of surviving interval i	p_i
Unconditional probability of surviving from time 0 to the end of interval i (i.e. to time i)	P_i
Unconditional probability of dying by the end of interval i (i.e. by time i)	Q_i

out the data. Fourteen persons entered the study, and in the first interval there were two deaths (patients F and M — see Fig. 10.2) and one withdrawal (patient N). If there were no withdrawals, the probability of dying in the first interval would be just 2/14, but the single withdrawal must somehow be taken into account. If it can be assumed that any withdrawals occurred on average halfway into the interval, it could be argued that each withdrawal only contributes a 'half person' to the number at risk, and that the denominator of the probability of death should be reduced accordingly. Instead of 14 persons being at risk of death in the interval, there would be only 13·5 persons, and the probability of death would be calculated as 2/13·5 = 0·1481. This is the total number of deaths in the interval, divided by what is called the adjusted number at risk. This is a central

Table 10.9. Clinical life table for data of Fig. 10.2 (males)

(1) Interval i $(i-1)-i$	(2) Numbers entering interval n_i	(3) Numbers withdrawn/ lost during interval w_i	(4) Adjusted number at risk n'_i	(5) Deaths during interval d_i	(6) Probability of death during interval q_i	(7) Probability of survival during interval p_i	(8) Cumulative probability of survival to end of interval P_i	(9) Cumulative probability of death by end of interval Q_i
1	14	1	13·5	2	0·1481	0·8519	0·8519	0·1481
2	11	2	10·0	2	0·2000	0·8000	0·6815	0·3185
3	7	0	7·0	1	0·1429	0·8571	0·5841	0·4159
4	6	1	5·5	1	0·1818	0·8182	0·4779	0·5221
5	4	2	3·0	1	0·3333	0·6667	0·3186	0·6814
6	1	1	—					

feature of the life table, that each withdrawal alive due to study termination or loss to follow-up only contributes one-half to the number at risk required to calculate a mortality probability in an interval. The adjusted number at risk is denoted n'_i (in the ith interval) and

$$n'_i = n_i - 0.5 \, w_i \qquad (10.15)$$

$$q_i = d_i/n'_i \qquad (10.19)$$

where q_i is the estimated probability of death in the interval. The (conditional) probability of surviving the interval is then

$$p_i = 1 - q_i \qquad (10.20)$$

which is given in column 7 of Table 10.9 as 0·8519 for the first interval. Equation 10.17 is now used to calculate the cumulative probability of survival from the start of the study (time 0) to the end of interval 1. This is, of course, the same as the conditional probability for the first interval, so $P_1 = p_1 = 0.8519$. The cumulative probability of death is then obtained by subtracting this from 1:

$$Q_i = 1 - P_i \qquad (10.21)$$

which is 0·1481 or 14·81%.

Now move to the second row of Table 10.9 to calculate the same quantities for the second interval. The number entering the interval is given by the number entering the previous interval less the withdrawals and deaths in that interval:

$$n_i = n_{i-1} - (w_{i-1} + d_{i-1}) \qquad (10.22)$$

which gives a total of 11. Check this with Fig. 10.2. The calculations proceed as before. Since there were two withdrawals in this interval, the adjusted number at risk is $11.0 - 1 = 10.0$, and the conditional probability of surviving the interval is 0·8000. The cumulative probability of surviving to the end of the interval is again obtained using Eqn. 10.17, multiplying this conditional probability of 0·8000 by the cumulative probability of surviving to the end of the previous interval (0·8519). This gives $P_2 = 0.6815$ and a cumulative probability of death by the end of the second interval at 2 years as $1 - 0.6815 = 0.3185$ or 31·9%. This process is continued for the next three intervals, as shown in the table. The 4-year mortality, calculated in this way, turns out to be 0·5221 or 52·21%. This is the best estimate of 4-year mortality available from the data. Usually, the cumulative probabilities of survival or death would be displayed graphically, as already illustrated in Fig. 10.1.

The main assumption underlying the clinical life table is that withdrawals due to study termination would have subsequently experienced a similar mortality rate to those actually followed for a longer period. Thus, the method does not allow for any secular changes in mortality and requires that all study participants, irrespective of when they entered the study in calendar time, are exposed to the same risks of death. It has been mentioned that losses to follow-up are treated in the same way as withdrawals, so it is also assumed that persons lost to follow-up are similar to persons with whom contact was maintained. This is unlikely to be so and the number of losses must be kept to a minimum.

A confidence interval for the cumulative proportion surviving to the end of interval i (P_i) is easily obtained. If there were no losses to follow-up or withdrawals, then the usual method using the normal approximation (Eqn. 4.12) could be applied giving for the 95% interval

$$P_i \pm 1.96 \; \text{SE} \; (P_i) \tag{10.23}$$

where

$$\text{SE}(P_i) = \sqrt{\frac{P_i \, (1 - P_i)}{n_1}} \quad \text{(no losses or withdrawals)} \tag{10.24}$$

with n_1 as the total number alive *at the start of the study*. (Note that the subscript i here refers to the time period in the life table and does not denote a particular group of patients.)

The problem is that n_1 is too large a figure for this standard error since the estimation of P_i is based on a smaller sample size due to withdrawals and losses to follow-up. To correct for this, n_1 is replaced by an 'effective sample size' (denoted $n_{(\text{eff})}$) for the entire study at the end of interval i. (This effective sample size should not be confused with the adjusted number at risk at the start of any particular interval; see Eqn. 10.18.)

Now, at the end of interval i, the actual number of persons alive is n_{i+1}, and in the absence of withdrawals or losses this, as a proportion of the total entering the study (n_1), would represent the cumulative survival proportion P_i of the entire study group. Thus

$$n_{i+1} = P_i \, n_1 \quad \text{(no losses or withdrawals)}. \tag{10.25}$$

With losses and withdrawals, however, an effective total study size which would have given rise to the same number alive at the end of the interval can be defined using Eqn. 10.25, giving

$$n_{(\text{eff})} = n_{i+1}/P_i. \tag{10.26}$$

Note that $n_{(\text{eff})}$ is dependent on the interval for which it is calculated but this is not explicit in the notation. This figure is then used in Eqn. 10.24 instead of n_1 to give a standard error for P_i which allows for losses and withdrawals:

$$\text{SE}(P_i) = \sqrt{\frac{P_i \, (1 - P_i)}{n_{(\text{eff})}}} \, . \tag{10.27}$$

When this is substituted in Eqn. 10.23, the 95% confidence interval formula for the cumulative proportion surviving to the end of interval i in the actuarial life table is

$$P_i \pm 1 \cdot 96 \sqrt{\frac{P_i\,(1 - P_i)}{n_{(\text{eff})}}} . \qquad (10.28)$$

The exact same formula can be used for confidence intervals for the cumulative proportion dead by the end of an interval (Q_i). Equation 10.28 is a fairly good approximation though it tends to give somewhat conservative values. It is possible too, with quite small numbers, that one of the confidence limits obtained may fall outside the range 0 to 1 and be essentially uninterpretable. In such an event the upper or lower limit, as the case may be, should be set at 1 or 0. It is important to note that, as for all calculations in this book, the proportions should be expressed in decimal rather than percentage form for correct use of the formulae.

Applying this method to the 4-year cumulative survival probability of 0·4779 (47·8%) obtained in Table 10.9, the effective sample size is, with $n_5 = 4$,

$$n_{(\text{eff})} = 4/0 \cdot 4779 = 8 \cdot 37$$

which is less than the actual sample size of 14. The 95% confidence interval is

$$0 \cdot 4779 \pm 1 \cdot 96 \sqrt{[(0 \cdot 4779)(0 \cdot 5221)/8 \cdot 37]}$$

which is 0·4779 ± 0·3384 or from 14·0% to 81·6%.

The method of calculating the life table described in this section is called the actuarial method and it is quite easy to do with the aid of a calculator. An alternative method, which would require a computer for large sample sizes, is called the *product-limit* or *Kaplan–Meier* life table. Essentially this approach does not predefine the interval in terms of months or years, but instead chooses the interval on the basis of the observed data. Interval end-points are chosen at the times of each death or withdrawal, so that the intervals are as narrow as possible given the data. The logic behind the method is similar to that described above but the somewhat arbitrary choice of interval widths is avoided. The actuarial life table, however, should prove adequate in most situations.

10.13 Comparison of two or more life tables: confidence intervals and the logrank test

When two life tables are being compared, the difference between the cumulative proportions surviving to the end of a particular interval (or equivalently dying before the interval end) can be calculated together with a confidence interval for the difference. Suppose that, in addition to the 14 male patients analysed in the last section, follow-up of 20 females was also undertaken. Table 10.10 gives the

Table 10.10. Clinical life table for 20 females

(1) Interval i $(i-1)-i$	(2) Numbers entering interval n_i	(3) Numbers withdrawn/ lost during interval w_i	(4) Adjusted number at risk n'_i	(5) Deaths during interval d_i	(6) Probability of death during interval q_i	(7) Probability of survival during interval p_i	(8) Cumulative probability of survival to end of interval P_i
1	20	2	19·0	4	0·2105	0·7895	0·7895
2	14	2	13·0	3	0·2308	0·7692	0·6073
3	9	1	8·5	3	0·3529	0·6471	0·3930
4	5	1	4·5	2	0·4444	0·5556	0·2183
5	2	0	2·0	1	0·5000	0·5000	0·1092
6	1	1	—				

life table for these patients. The 4-year survival in males is $P_4 = 0.4779$ (47·8%) and is 0·2183 (21·8%) in the females. To calculate a confidence interval for the 0·2596 (26·0%) survival advantage of males, the approach of Section 7.9 can be used, substituting the effective sample sizes in the appropriate formula. Using obvious notation (and dropping the subscript 4 denoting the end of the fourth interval) Eqn. 7.15 gives, for the 95% confidence interval,

$$(P_M - P_F) \pm 1.96 \text{ SE } (P_M - P_F) \tag{10.29}$$

where

$$\text{SE}(P_M - P_F) = \sqrt{\frac{P_M (1 - P_M)}{n_{M(\text{eff})}} + \frac{P_F (1 - P_F)}{n_{F(\text{eff})}}} \tag{10.30}$$

and $n_{M(\text{eff})}$ and $n_{F(\text{eff})}$ are the effective sample sizes in the males and females respectively at the end of year 4. Using Eqn. 10.26, these are 8·37 and 9.16 respectively. The confidence interval for the difference between male and female 4-year survival is thus

$$0.2596 \pm 1.96 \sqrt{\frac{(0.4779)\,(0.5221)}{8.37} + \frac{(0.2183)\,(0.7817)}{9.16}}$$

which is $0.2596 \pm 1.96\,(0.2201) = 0.2596 \pm 0.4314$. The 95% confidence interval for the survival advantage of males at 4 years is from -17.2% to 69·1%.

Obviously it is also possible to derive a significance test to compare the cumulative life table survivals (or equivalently mortalities) at a fixed point in time, but in general it is preferable to look at the life table curves in their entirety. Sometimes life table curves for two different groups may cross over each other, suggesting a survival advantage for one group at one point in time and a disadvantage at a second time point. In such a case also, it is useful to have an overall comparison which in some sense might compare the average experience over time.

The logrank test (also referred to as the Mantel−Haenzel test; see Section 12·5) and its related summary measure are the most commonly employed. Usually this method is applied to the Kaplan−Meier life table (mentioned above) but an adaptation of the technique suitable for the comparison of two actuarial life tables is described below. Essentially the logrank test involves the comparison of the observed number of deaths in each group with the number of deaths that would be expected if the groups had similar mortalities. These observed and expected deaths are calculated in each interval for each life table and summed over all the intervals. Table 10.11 details the necessary calculations for the comparison of the male and female life tables given in Tables 10.9 and 10.10.

Table 10.11. Layout for the logrank test comparing male and female life tables

Interval	Adjusted numbers at risk			Observed deaths (O)			Expected deaths (E)	
i	Male	Female	Total	Male	Female	Total	Male	Female
1	13·5	19·0	32·5	2	4	6	2·4923	3·5077
2	10·0	13·0	23·0	2	3	5	2·1739	2·8261
3	7·0	8·5	15·5	1	3	4	1·8065	2·1935
4	5·5	4·5	10·0	1	2	3	1·6500	1·3500
5	3·0	2·0	5·0	1	1	2	1·2000	0·8000
Totals				7	13	20	9·3227	10·6773

All calculations are based on the adjusted numbers at risk (see Eqn. 10.18) and the observed deaths for each interval. The expected number of deaths in each interval is obtained in the usual manner under the hypothesis that the mortalities in the groups being compared are the same. In the first interval, for instance, there was a total of six observed deaths in 32·5 persons at risk. Of these 32·5, 13·5 were male, so that one would expect

$$\frac{6}{32\cdot5} \times 13\cdot5 = 2\cdot4923$$

deaths among the males. Similarly, or by subtraction from the total of six deaths, one obtains 3·5077 expected deaths among the females in the first interval. Expected deaths in the remaining intervals are calculated in the same way and are summed to obtain the total expected deaths in males and females (E_M and E_F)*:

---

* Although the term 'expected deaths' is most often used, some statisticians prefer the term 'extent of exposure to risk of death' since in some situations these 'expected' numbers may actually exceed the total number of persons in the group.

$$E_M = 9\cdot3227; \quad E_F = 10\cdot6773.$$

Letting O_M and O_F represent the total observed deaths in the two groups,

$$O_M = 7; \quad O_F = 13.$$

The ratio of O/E in a particular group (called the relative death rate) represents the death rate, averaged over time, in that group relative to both groups combined. For the data above,

$$O_M/E_M = 7/9\cdot3227 = 0\cdot75$$
$$O_F/E_F = 13/10\cdot6773 = 1\cdot22.$$

Thus, males have a death rate 75% that of the entire group and females have a death rate 22% greater. The ratio of these two quantities estimates the death rate of one group relative to the other and thus is essentially a relative risk type measure. For this example,

$$RR = \frac{O_F/E_F}{O_M/E_M} = \frac{1\cdot22}{0\cdot75} = 1\cdot63 \tag{10.31}$$

showing that, averaging in some sense over the entire period of follow-up, the females have a $1\cdot63$ times higher mortality than males. The method used to calculate this gives a greater weight to mortality differences early in follow-up than differences towards the end of the life table.

The so called logrank test statistic which tests the null hypothesis of no group difference in mortality has a chi-square distribution with one degree of freedom (for a two-group comparison) and is given by

$$\chi^2 = \frac{(O_M - E_M)^2}{E_M} + \frac{(O_F - E_F)^2}{E_F}. \tag{10.32}$$

In this case

$$\chi^2 = \frac{(7 - 9\cdot3227)^2}{9\cdot3227} + \frac{(13 - 10\cdot6773)^2}{10\cdot6773} = 1\cdot084$$

which on 1 degree of freedom is non-significant.

Although other methods are available, a confidence interval for the ratio of the death rates in the two groups (the ratios of the two O/Es) is most easily obtained with test-based limits as described in Section 10.10 using the above chi-square value. Confidence limits of 95% for the RR of Eqn. 10.31 are then

$$RR^{(1\pm1\cdot96/\chi)} \tag{10.33}$$

where χ is the square root of the chi-square of Eqn. 10.32. In this case $\chi = 1\cdot04$ and the confidence limits are

$$1\cdot63^{(1\pm1\cdot88)}$$

Table 10.12. Confidence interval formulae for ratios of rates, odds and proportions (risks)

	Independent proportions		Paired proportions		Rates
	Disease		**Cases**		
Data layout	Exposure Yes No		Controls Exposed Not exposed		
	Yes $\quad a \quad b$		Exposed $\quad a \quad\quad b$		$r_1 = x_1/\mathrm{PYRS}_1$
	No $\quad c \quad d$		Not exposed $\quad c \quad\quad d$		$r_2 = x_2/\mathrm{PYRS}_2$
Hypothesis test	$\chi^2 = \sum \dfrac{(O - E)^2}{E}$ $\quad$ d.f. $= 1$		$\chi^2 = \dfrac{(c - b)^2}{c + b}$ $\quad$ d.f. $= 1$		(see Eqn. 7.28)
Ratio measures	$\mathrm{RR} = \dfrac{a/(a + b)}{c/(c + d)}$ $\mathrm{OR} = \dfrac{a/b}{c/d}$		$-$ $\mathrm{OR} = \dfrac{c}{b}$		$\mathrm{RR} = \dfrac{x_1/\mathrm{PYRS}_1}{x_2/\mathrm{PYRS}_2}$ $-$
Confidence interval	$\mathrm{RR}^{(1 \pm z_c/\chi)}$ $\mathrm{OR}^{(1 \pm z_c/\chi)}$		$-$ $\mathrm{OR}^{(1 \pm z_c/\chi)}$		$\mathrm{RR}_l = \dfrac{p_l}{1 - p_l} \dfrac{\mathrm{PYRS}_2}{\mathrm{PYRS}_1}$ $\mathrm{RR}_u = \dfrac{p_u}{1 - p_u} \dfrac{\mathrm{PYRS}_2}{\mathrm{PYRS}_1}$

p_l and p_u are binomial limits for $p = x_1/(x_1 + x_2)$

which is from 0·65 to 4·08.

Life table analysis is the most popular technique for mortality (or survival) comparisons in follow-up studies and is used extensively in the analysis of clinical trials (see Chapter 11). The methods described above can in fact be easily extended to the comparison of k groups. The calculation of the expected deaths is identical to that described, the logrank χ^2 has k terms, one for each group, of the form $(O - E)^2/E$, and the statistic has $k - 1$ degrees of freedom (see Eqn. 10.32). An excellent, readable and detailed discussion is to be found in Peto *et al.* (1976, 1977). A large advantage of the approach is that it makes no assumptions about the shapes of the mortality curves in the groups being compared. Mortality analysis can in fact also be performed by fitting the data to a parametric model in which a particular functional form is assumed to hold for the mortality curve. Estimated parameters of the model are then compared with one another.

10.14 Summary

In this chapter the scope and applications of the observational study in medical

Table 10.13. Hypothesis tests and confidence intervals for the clinical life table

Formulae	Eqn. nos.
Basic calculations	
$n_i = n_{i-1} - (w_{i-1} + d_{i-1})$	(10.22)
$n_i' = n_i - 0.5\, w_i$	(10.18)
$q_i = d_i/n_i'$	(10.19)
$p_i = 1 - q_i$	(10.20)
$P_i = p_i P_{i-1}$	(10.17)
$Q_i = 1 - P_i$	(10.21)

Confidence interval for cumulative survival

$$P_i \pm z_c \sqrt{\frac{P_i\,(1 - P_i)}{n_{(\text{eff})}}} \tag{10.28}$$

$$n_{(\text{eff})} = n_{i+1}/P_i \tag{10.26}$$

Confidence interval for difference between two cumulative survivals (at end interval i)

$$(P_\text{A} - P_\text{B}) \pm z_c \sqrt{\frac{P_\text{A}\,(1 - P_\text{A})}{n_{\text{A(eff)}}} + \frac{P_\text{B}\,(1 - P_\text{B})}{n_{\text{B(eff)}}}} \tag{10.29; 10.30}$$

Logrank test

$$\chi^2 = \frac{(O_\text{A} - E_\text{A})^2}{E_\text{A}} + \frac{(O_\text{B} - E_\text{B})^2}{E_\text{B}} \tag{10.32}$$

d.f. $= 1$

Overall relative risk and confidence interval

$$\text{RR} = \frac{O_\text{A}/E_\text{A}}{O_\text{B}/E_\text{B}} \tag{10.31} \qquad\qquad \text{RR}^{(1 \pm z_c/\chi)} \tag{10.33}$$

research have been outlined, and the basic elements of the design of cross-sectional, prospective and retrospective studies were considered. The important concepts of risk and comparative risk measures were introduced and the estimation of such measures, together with their statistical analysis, was described. Emphasis was placed on the estimation and significance testing of comparative risk measures in prospective studies, especially in the context of life table analysis. Tables 10.12 and 10.13 summarize the formulae used.

The next chapter considers studies of medical intervention or treatment, and is concerned not with the observational study but with experimental trials. The analytical techniques for prospective studies discussed above are, however, particularly useful in this situation also.

11

The Randomized Controlled Trial

11.1 Introduction

This chapter considers the design of the experimental trial in medical research. The purpose of the experimental trial is to evaluate the effectiveness of some intervention or therapy. What distinguishes the experimental trial from the observational study discussed in the last chapter is that the researcher has direct control over many aspects of the investigation, and in particular, over the allocation of individuals to different treatment groups. This chapter is not intended to be a handbook for the clinician wishing to undertake a trial, but merely a guideline to the principles and practices of such trials.

11.2 Treatment and control groups

One of the most important questions facing any practising physician or surgeon is 'What treatment shall I use?' It is vital that the doctor (and patient) knows the effectiveness of the different treatments available, and thus what may be best in a particular situation. Advances in medicine require a detailed knowledge of treatment efficacy, and the experimental trial provides the only valid procedure to achieve this. Many therapeutic regimes, commonly used in the past, were seen to be worthless or even dangerous when evaluated in such a proper and scientific manner. Any proposed new therapy, be it medical or surgical, should be tested by means of a trial, unless the results are so startlingly obvious that a formal evaluation is not necessary, as for example a successful treatment for a condition that was 100% fatal.

'I have a wonder cure for the common cold. If you take this preparation for one day only, your symptoms will be cleared within a week.' Faced with a claim such as this, the most important question is 'What would happen to my cold symptoms if I did not take this preparation?' The claim of effectiveness only stands up when a comparison can be made with the situation pertaining without the treatment. This is the foundation-stone for the evaluation of any therapy. Its effectiveness must be compared with the results of either no treatment or the best treatment available before its introduction.

To evaluate a new therapy, then, requires comparing results on a group of treated patients with the results on a group with the same disease not so treated. These two groups are usually called the treatment and control groups respectively. Many early evaluations of therapy used what are called *historical controls*. The results on a series of patients on the new treatment were compared with the results obtained on 'similar' patients in the past who did not have the 'benefits' of the newer approach. The word 'similar' is in quotations because the main problem with historical controls is that they are likely to be quite different from patients treated in the present. Historical controls may, in the first place, have had a better (or worse) outlook than the treatment group. Between the time when the historical controls were seen and treated and the present, there may have been changes in hospital admissions policy, general management may have improved, diagnostic criteria may have changed, and the historical controls may not have had as much attention and care as the treated group, who may be getting special attention because they are receiving the new therapy. For these and other reasons, a comparison between the results obtained on a treated group and a historical control group could be seriously biased, and any differences in outcome noted may not reflect a true treatment effect. A further problem with historical controls is that reliance is placed on past records to evaluate their prognosis, and missing or unrecorded information on some patients may further bias the results. In short, for a valid evaluation of therapy, a concurrent control group must be used. Note that, by its very nature an experimental trial is prospective, in that individuals must be followed forward in time to determine the effect of a therapy, and usually individuals are entered into a trial over what is sometimes an extended period of time.

11.3 Types of trials

The experimental trial in medicine may be employed in three main situations, distinguished by the type of individual studied and the effect of the treatment or intervention involved. In the *clinical* or *therapeutic* trial, the study groups consist of persons with a particular disease or condition, and the treatment is therapeutic. The purpose of such trials is to determine if treatment can effect a 'cure' or remove manifestations of a disease already present in the patients. The total sample size for such trials is often in the region of 20 to 100 patients if the treatment is even moderately effective. Examples of such trials abound in the medical literature. Trials, for instance, of antihypertensive agents to reduce blood pressure, and analgesics to alleviate pain, fit into this category.

In *secondary* and *primary prevention trials*, the treatment or intervention under investigation is prophylactic, in that its purpose is the prevention of a particular manifestation of disease which is not present at the start of the trial. In secondary prevention trials, the subjects already have the disease in question, or have suffered one event, and it is hoped to prevent or delay a further event. Examples are trials of chemotherapy regimes in patients with cancer, where the end-point is often cancer recurrence or death. Drug-treatment of patients who have had a heart attack, and coronary bypass surgery in patients with angina, can also fit into this category.

The primary prevention trial, on the other hand, is performed on subjects free of disease, with a view to preventing the first occurrence of an event. Cholesterol-reducing drugs have been tested in this manner to evaluate their effectiveness in preventing coronary heart attacks, and trials evaluating the usefulness of risk factor modifications, such as the cessation of cigarette smoking, have also been carried out in this area (see Section 11.7 which discusses community intervention trials).

Since both primary and secondary prevention trials are concerned with the prevention or delay of a particular event, rather than the elimination of a condition which is present, very large sample sizes and an extensive period of follow-up may often be required. This is because a reasonable number of events must occur in the study population before an evaluation of the intervention can be made, and often the rate of events that can be expected in the study group is so small that large numbers are needed for this. Secondary prevention trials can require up to and over 1000 subjects, while primary prevention trials (the few there have been) may require 10000 or more subjects in order to have any chance of detecting an important result. (Appendix D discusses the calculation of sample sizes in simple situations.)

Having examined the scope of the experimental trial, some of its salient features are now presented. Whether a clinical, a primary prevention or a secondary prevention trial is being conducted, the underlying requirements are the same, so that the discussion will, without loss of generality, be in the context of a secondary prevention trial evaluating a particular drug therapy (timolol — a beta blocker) in reducing mortality in patients who have had a heart attack (myocardial infarction). (The Norwegian Multicentre Study Group, 1981.)

Suppose now that a controlled trial has been performed with a treatment group and contemporaneous controls who did not receive the treatment, and suppose further that positive results (in terms of increased survival) in favour of the treatment are observed. What could explain these results? The first possible explanation is that there is really no difference between the two (population) groups* and that the observed difference is spurious, or due to chance (sampling variation). The whole purpose of statistical analysis is to answer this question at a

---

* See Section 11.4 for an alternative and more correct interpretation of statistical significance in a controlled trial.

specified probability level, so that either chance can be ruled out as the explanation (a significant result), or it can be accepted that it is a possible cause (a non-significant result).

If the observed difference between the treatment and control groups cannot reasonably be ascribed to chance, three further possibilities remain, either singly or in combination, which might explain the difference. The treatment and control groups may themselves differ appreciably in factors related to their prognosis, or the two groups may have been handled and looked after in different ways. In more statistical terms, these two possibilities relate to the existence of confounders of the treatment/outcome association (see Section 10.2). The third explanation, of course, is that the particular therapy being examined does indeed have a beneficial effect.

If chance is not the determining factor, the trial organizers will want to conclude that the effect of the intervention explains the observed results, and to do so they must be sure that the groups were in fact similar in all respects except for the intervention given, and were handled in the same fashion. A properly run clinical trial is designed in such a way that biases due to group differences of any sort (aside from the intervention) can be excluded as an explanation of any observed differences in outcome that might be found. Note that it is the design of the trial and the implementation of that design, not the statistical analysis, that ensure avoidance of these biases. The next few sections discuss procedures utilized in a controlled trial to achieve these ends.

11.4 Randomization

How then can it be ensured that the treatment and control groups are as similar as possible, regarding factors that may influence their eventual outcome? (Assume that only one treatment is being tested, although trials with more than two groups are possible.) The best method is by a process of *randomization (random allocation)*. After a patient is deemed to be eligible for entry into the trial (see below), a coin is tossed. If it lands heads, the patient is allocated to the treatment group; if it lands tails, to the control group. This process is the essence of randomization, although admittedly, if used in practice, it would probably irrevocably damage any confidence the patient may have had in his physician (but see the discussion of informed consent in Section 11.8).

Randomization by the tossing of a coin (or any equivalent method) ensures that the physician running the trial is not consciously or unconsciously allocating certain patients to a particular group. Thus, randomization can eliminate group differences due to selection bias. Without randomization for instance, trials of a surgical versus medical technique are wide open to this problem. Low-risk cases are much more likely to be assigned to the operative group, leaving high-risk patients to be managed by the physicians. Assigning volunteers to the treatment group, and those who do not volunteer to the control group, is also likely to result in a biased comparison — volunteers could be quite different in many respects from patients who do not volunteer.

Often it is suggested that patients be allocated to treatment or control groups alternately, or on alternate days. The problem with such methods is that referring doctors may know which day corresponds to which group allocation, and refer accordingly, or that the doctors running the trial may exclude certain patients if they know beforehand which group they are being assigned to. This latter problem can also arise if randomization according to birth date is employed (e.g. patients with an even birth year are assigned to one of the groups, and the remainder to the other). The process of randomization, embodied in the idea of tossing a coin (after patient eligibility has been determined), is the only way to ensure that there has been no bias in treatment allocation. Note that a bias may not necessarily be present with any of the other methods, but the problem is that it might be. The results of a controlled trial, based on a possibly biased method of group allocation, are always open to doubt.

It has been argued of course that the use of statistical methods to correct for group differences which could affect outcome (confounders) would obviate the necessity for randomization, and even allow for the use of historical controls. This is only true insofar as all the possible confounders are known and measured, and the statistical methodology is appropriate for the data being analysed. This leads to the second important reason for randomization: it ensures, in the long run, balance between the two groups as regards all factors, measured and unmeasured, that might confound the results.

Note it is not claimed that in practice balance will be actually achieved through randomization, but randomization does ensure that the two groups will differ only by chance. Significance testing, by its very nature, will allow for *chance* differences between the groups, and the *p* value allows for such differences when a significance level is assigned to a particular comparison. In a randomized controlled trial, it is wise however to check whether the measured confounders have similar distributions in the treatment and control groups, and a more powerful comparison (more likely to detect differences between the effects of treatments if they exist) is obtained if statistical adjustment is made for any observed differences. However, if a treatment effect is only apparent after such statistical adjustment, the results of the trial may not be widely accepted. As long as patients are randomly allocated to the two groups, possible differences in unmeasured confounders are still allowed for even without statistical adjustment.

In the trial of timolol which is being used as an example, randomization was employed to allocate the post-myocardial infarction patients to the timolol treatment or control group. Several hundred comparisons were made between the two groups, and the researchers concluded that the differences in these measured factors tended to be small. The final analysis did however include adjustments for the largest differences and other factors considered prognostically important, and it was noted that these adjustments did not materially affect the conclusions based on the unadjusted analysis. (See Chapter 12 for a discussion of statistical methods that can be used to adjust for confounders.)

The third and perhaps more subtle reason for requiring randomization in a controlled trial pertains to the assumptions underlying significance testing. Most trials are based on a presenting, non-random sample and the difficulties regarding the assumption that the treated and control groups are random samples from specified (hypothetical) populations have already been mentioned in Section 5.4. This assumption is no longer required if the groups were formed through random allocation. Suppose, for example, that a randomized controlled trial resulted in 12 persons being allocated into one group, and 13 into the other. These two particular groups can be viewed as being one of the many possible allocations resulting from the randomization of 25 individuals into two groups of 12 and 13 respectively. There is a total of 5 200 300 possible different outcomes from such a randomization, and for significance testing it is sufficient to determine, under a null hypothesis of no treatment effect, the chances of obtaining differences in measured outcome between the two randomized groups as large or larger than that actually observed. The 'population' is, then, the 5 200 300 possible allocations and the 'sample' is the specific allocation obtained in the actual study. If the difference observed is larger than that expected by chance alone, the effect of the treatment is implicated as causing the difference, assuming no other biasing factors were present. Thus, random allocation obviates the need for convoluted arguments concerning random sampling from larger populations. The statistical inference, however, relates only to the individuals entered into the study, and generalizing results to a larger population involves issues relating to the representativeness of the trial group to the general body of patients affected with the particular disease being studied. The generalizing of trial results is discussed in Section 11.6

Having cited the reasons for randomization — avoidance of bias in allocation, ensuring balance, in the long run, between the groups, and compliance with statistical assumptions — the practice of randomization must be examined. Obviously, randomization by means of a coin is impractical, and as any conjurer will know, bias is even possible here! What is done is to make use of a table of random numbers to simulate the tossing of a coin. The use of such tables to take a random sample from a defined population (Chapter 3) has already been discussed and the tables are used in a different context here. Usually the total sample size of a trial is fixed beforehand (see below) and a randomization schedule is made out before the trial commences. In practice a table of random numbers is entered at a random point. Start at the top of column 2 in Table B.1 for instance. Go down the column in order, assigning each consecutive patient to the treatment or control group according to whether the digit in the table is odd or even. Assigning even numbers to the treatment group, the first 10 patients would be assigned as follows (in order, where T = treatment, C = control): T, T, T, C, C, T, C, T, C, T, since the first 10 numbers in the column are 4, 4, 8, 3, 9, 6, 5, 4, 3, 6. Continue in this way until a schedule is made out for all the patients to be entered into the trial. Since even and odd numbers appear at random in the table, and since on average 50% of the digits are even, this satisfactorily simulates the tossing of a coin. (If there are more than two groups in the trial, or it is required, unusually, to allocate in a different ratio than 1 to 1, modifications of this procedure will have to be adopted.)

One problem immediately manifests itself: in randomizing the 10 patients, there are six in the treatment group and four in the control group. This type of result is to be expected with *unrestricted randomization* as described, and, using this method, it is not possible to ensure equal numbers in the two groups. This is not a major worry with large trials, but with a small total number of patients in a typical therapeutic trial such an imbalance of numbers is not desirable. A solution to this problem is to use a *restricted randomization* procedure. It is decided, beforehand, that of every *n* individuals randomized half will be in one group and half in the other. Suppose that of every 10 consecutive patients five are to be randomized to the treatment group and five to the control group. The tables of random numbers would be used as before, but after five persons are allocated to one group or the other the remaining patients in a block of 10 are assigned in such a way as to ensure that there are five in each group. Starting, for instance, at the top of column 5, the sequence C, T, T, C, C, C, C, is obtained from the numbers 7, 4, 8, 5, 9, 9, 3. Stop at this point, because five out of the seven patients have been allocated to the control group, and allocate the remaining three patients out of this block of 10 to the treatment group, obtaining finally C, T, T, C, C, C, C, T, T, T. This procedure, if continued, ensures balance of patients in multiples of 10 and is advisable even for large sample sizes. The timolol study used restricted randomization in blocks of 10. As well as ensuring balance of numbers in the trial as a whole, restricted randomization ensures, when interim analyses are being performed before the end of the trial proper, that if only a portion of patients has been entered, the balance is still achieved. Restricted randomization also guards against imbalances due to a time-trend in the type of cases admitted to a trial.

It has already been mentioned that randomization, in the long run, ensures valid comparability of groups and that any imbalance of confounding variables can be adjusted for at the end of the trial. However it is preferable to employ a design that aids comparability on known confounders than to adjust for these at the analysis stage. *Stratified randomization* achieves this purpose. If a few variables are known to be related to prognosis, then prior to randomization patients can be stratified into groups according to the values of these variables. Randomization then takes place separately within each group. This ensures balance with regard to these factors. In many trials too, the required sample size is so large that many different centres may have to participate. Such *multicentre trials* randomize separately within each centre to avoid imbalance of patients allocated from different centres who may differ in various respects. Too many strata should not be used in stratified randomization, however, because the trial may become administratively difficult to run and, paradoxically, with too many strata balance may be difficult to achieve. Restricted randomization should always be employed in each stratum to ensure that the numbers are balanced. In practice, stratified randomization is achieved by forming a separate randomization schedule for each stratum in the trial. If a stratified randomization has been used then the statistical methods employed in analysis should account for this (see Chapter 12).

In the timolol trial, eligible patients were first assigned to one of three risk groups, and randomized separately within each group. In risk group I, 178 patients were allocated to timolol and 174 to the controls. In risk groups II and III, the numbers in the treated and control groups were 547 and 543, and 220 and 222 respectively, giving 945 patients on timolol and 939 in the control group. Thus, the treatment and control groups were well balanced as regards numbers, and the distribution of the three risk groups. The timolol trial was also multicentre, with 20 centres participating, and the above procedure was carried out separately in each centre.

As has been stressed, the randomizing doctor must not know to which group the patient is to be allocated until after he/she has been judged eligible for entry into the trial. For this reason, the schedule of randomization should not be known beforehand. This is often achieved by a sealed envelope technique, where a separate pile of sealed opaque envelopes is prepared for each stratum within which randomization is to take place. The envelopes are marked consecutively, and inside each is a card, detailing the group to which each particular patient is to be allocated. Thus, in each centre of the timolol trial there were (presumably) three sets of envelopes for each of the three risk groups. If an eligible patient was in risk category I, the next envelope in the appropriate pile was opened and the patient's randomization group determined. As long as the size of the randomization block (for restricted randomization) is not known to the doctor, there is no way, without deliberate cheating, that the allocation group of a patient can be determined prior to the actual randomization. This implies, of course, that the randomization schedule is made out by an individual (usually the statistician or a member of the trial organizing committee) who is not directly involved in the actual process of the randomization. An alternative method of randomization, often employed in multicentre trials, is to telephone a central office once a patient is deemed eligible and to let them assign the patient from a prepared schedule. This has the advantage that at any time the actual number of patients entered into a trial is known by the central organizing committee.

The distinction between random sampling and randomization (random allocation) must be stressed. The purpose of the former is to choose a group which is representative of a larger population, and random sampling is not usually employed in controlled trials. The purpose of randomization, on the other hand, is to divide a single group into groups that differ only by chance. Randomization is the only way to ensure that individuals entered into a trial are not allocated to the treatment or control groups in a biased manner. (Although the above discussion has been in the context of randomizing individuals, it should be noted that some primary prevention trials have been based on the randomization of individual communities or factories into an intervention or control group. See Section 11.7.) The next section of this chapter discusses how to ensure that subsequent biases, arising from how the groups are cared for and evaluated, do not affect the validity of the final comparison.

11.5 Single and double blind trials

Once an individual has been entered into a trial, biases can still occur subsequent to randomization. If a patient knows to which of the two groups he/she has been assigned this, in itself, may introduce subtle biases in evaluating the eventual outcome. For instance, patients who know that they are on a 'new wonder drug' may for that reason alone, apart from any real effect of the treatment, experience a good prognosis. This is known as the *placebo effect* — in essence, this is the effect that an intervention may have on an individual, totally independently of the true pharmacological or surgical effect of the particular intervention. In the last world war, injured soldiers injected with saline only (because of lack of availability of morphine), who thought they were being given morphine, experienced considerable relief of pain. Also, if a patient knows which group he/she is in, the stated response to the treatment may be biased one way or the other, due perhaps to the desire to 'please the nice doctor'! A *single blind* trial is one in which the patient does not know to which of the two groups he/she has been allocated.

In a trial of a drug, for instance, single blindness can be achieved by giving persons in the control group tablets of a similar size, colour, taste and smell as the active treatment but which contain an innocuous or inactive substance, such as starch or flour. Such a preparation is called a *placebo*. It should have no pharmacologically active ingredient related to the drug being studied, and its only purpose is to 'blind' the patients as to their allocated group.* A placebo treatment is easiest in a trial comparing a new treatment with no treatment at all, and there have been trials carried out using placebo surgical procedures by making a small skin incision but not performing the operation. Needless to say, there would be many ethical problems using such an approach (see Section 11.8). If, as is often the case, a drug trial is designed to test a new treatment against the usual standard treatment, then if the trial is to be single blind, either the two drugs must be presented as similarly as possible, or a 'double placebo' procedure must be used, where each group receives one of the active drugs and a 'look-alike' placebo of the other. Single blindness, of course, should also mean that all the patients in a trial are managed similarly, with the same number of check-ups, out-patient visits and diagnostic procedures. In some situations, of course, a single blind trial is not possible, as for instance in comparing a surgical and medical intervention. If a trial is not single blind however, biases may result.

In addition to the patient being blinded as to treatment allocation, it is also desirable that the doctor be blinded. In a *double blind* trial, neither the patient nor the doctor managing the patient or evaluating any response to treatment is aware of which group the patient has been randomized into. The purpose of the double blind trial is to eliminate the possible biases caused by one group receiving better overall care (because they are known to be in the treatment group) or by the doctor unconsciously evaluating the patients in one group more stringently than in the other. In trying to be 'fair' for instance, a doctor may over-compensate, and thus judge individuals in the treatment group more harshly than if they were in the control group. For end-points that are subjective, in that they require a judgement in their interpretation, a double blind trial is definitely required. Thus, a trial of antidepressants, with an end-point evaluated by means of an interview concerning depressive symptoms, would need to be double blind to avoid possible biases in patient response, and doctors' evaluation of that response. It could be argued, if a trial had mortality as an end-point, that double blindness is not required. True, there is no room for bias in determining if an individual is dead or alive, but if a specific cause of death is the end-point there could be biases in assigning that cause to a decedent.

One obvious problem with a double blind trial arises if the doctor is worried about whether or not a particular symptom exhibited by the patient is a side-effect of the active treatment, and whether the treatment should be stopped and the

---

* In a placebo drug trial, randomization can be carried out, not through a sealed envelope method, but by preparing bottles of tablets to be given to consecutive patients. The bottles would contain either the placebo or the active treatment, as the randomization schedule required.

patient withdrawn from the trial. In such cases, the doctor may have to break the blindness of the study for the individual patient's welfare, and a record of the randomization schedule should be available. The term 'breaking the code' is sometimes used when a patient's group is determined in this manner, and should always be allowed for in the planning stages of the trial. In fact, a full list of the criteria for withdrawing a patient should be made out beforehand, and once a patient meets any of these criteria he/she should be withdrawn from the trial, even if it transpires that the patient was in the placebo group.

In the timolol trial, the controls received a placebo tablet similar in shape, size and colour to timolol, but differing slightly in taste. Although the end-point being evaluated was death, this trial was also double blind and the cause of death was classified by a steering committee who were unaware of the randomization group of any individual. Very definite criteria for withdrawing a patient from the trial were laid down beforehand, and the trial was analysed using life table methods (see Sections 10.7 and 10.13), counting trial withdrawals as losses to follow-up 28 days following their withdrawal.* Thus, events in withdrawals occurring a month later than the actual withdrawal were not included in the major analysis. A further analysis was performed, however, including all end-points observed in withdrawals, to check for biases due to different withdrawal rates in the two groups. Reasons for withdrawals, and the timing of these withdrawals were given in the trial report. This analysis did not materially affect the results.

The description of the design of the randomized double blind controlled trial in medicine is now completed and other aspects of experimental trials which deserve mention, particularly relating to patient selection and follow-up, are now discussed.

11.6 Applicability versus validity

The *validity* of trial results relates to whether or not the observed results of the trial are true, or whether bias of one form or another affected these results. Double blindness with stratified randomization is vital to achieving this end, but other factors are also relevant.

The sample size of the trial should be adequate to detect an important treatment effect at a given significance level. This question was discussed in Section 6.7 but its importance cannot be over-stressed. The sample size required for a trial must be estimated beforehand. Appendix D gives some sample-size formulae that will suffice in certain simple situations, but a statistician should be

---

* In this chapter the term withdrawal is used to indicate patient non-participation resulting from cessation of therapy, and not in the sense of Sections 10.7 and 10.13

consulted, concerning this and other aspects of a trial, at its planning stages. A note of warning to those planning a trial: the version of Murphy's law for the controlled trial states 'if bias can occur, it will', but another law also holds; 'if the annual supply of suitable patients when the trial is being designed is n, when the trial commences it will reduce to $n/10$' (Lasagna's law)! The trial organizers are invariably over-optimistic about how many patients will be available for a study.

Many trials are undertaken with sample sizes that are too small to detect even an enormous treatment effect, and such trials result in non-significant differences between the comparison groups. Again it must be stressed that statistical non-significance does not imply a lack of medical importance. If the confidence interval of the difference between the treatment and control groups is calculated in such trials, although overlapping the null value, it will often include at its extremes the possibility of large treatment effects. The treatment may have no effect, but it could have a large effect that has been missed, due to a small sample size. Often, sample sizes required for trials may seem excessive and in many cases will require many centres to enter patients. As already mentioned, the timolol trial entered a total of 1884 patients (945 on timolol and 939 on placebo) but the original report does not give details of how this figure was arrived at. The fact that the trial did however produce significant results suggests that care had gone into prior sample-size calculations.

In any trial, the end-points on which the effect of treatment is to be judged must be stated clearly, or the trial's validity may be suspect. These end-points, and there may be more than one, should be specified at the start of the trial; a particular end-point not considered at the start of the trial but which subsequently turns out to be greatly affected by treatment could relate to a chance occurrence, and positive results for such sought for end-points are always a little suspect. The more objective an end-point is, the better, but when necessary, subjective end-points have few disadvantages provided that the study is double blind. (See also discussion of measurement accuracy and validity in Chapter 15). As mentioned above, the major end-point for the timolol trial was mortality, both cause-specific and total, and non-fatal reinfarction. Events occurring when the patient was on therapy (active or placebo) or within 28 days of withdrawal from the study formed the basic end-points, although events in withdrawals were recorded up to the end of the study.

The validity of any trial is seriously compromised by inadequate follow-up of any of the patients entered. Many trials may run into years of patient entry and subsequent follow-up, and losses to follow-up can seriously bias the results. The follow-up of patients however is not an easy task, and its difficulty should not be underestimated. What happens to patients during follow-up is also very important. Withdrawals from the study due to adverse effects of treatment must be followed up as stringently as those who remain in the trial (see below). Treatments and interventions during follow-up, other than that being evaluated, should also be recorded. Some measure of patient compliance with the treatment (and placebo) regime is also required if treatment is long-term. Definite decisions as to what information is required at each follow-up must be made at the planning stage of the trial and, if a mortality end-point is included, cause and date of death must be ascertained from the appropriate sources. In the timolol trial, patients were seen at 1, 3 and 6 months following discharge from hospital, and thereafter every 6 months until the trial completion date. Patients were entered between January 1978 and October 1979, and analysis was based on a variable follow-up of all patients until October 1980. Thus, all participants had at least one year of follow-up with early entrants having just under 3 years. The withdrawal criteria were carefully determined beforehand and reasons for individual withdrawals completely documented. Compliance with the treatment regime was based on a count of remaining tablets in the supply given regularly to each patient.

Appropriate statistical analysis of trial data is a *sine qua non* for the validity of results. Many trials will necessarily involve a variable length of follow-up of trial participants, and thus life table methods will be appropriate for an end-point such as death, or other definite event (see Sections 10.7 and 10.13). In trials where the end-point may occur within a short period of time, each participant can be followed up for the same period, and more standard analytic techniques applied. Great care must however be taken in the analysis of data based on variable follow-up.

Even though the trial may have included stratified randomization, the two groups should be assessed in terms of comparability with regard to prognostic factors and, if necessary, statistical adjustment techniques used in the analysis (see Chapter 12). One must however be wary of over-analysing a clinical trial. By searching hard enough, subgroups of patients in whom the treatment appears to work well will always be found. Unless these subgroups are defined beforehand, and a stratified randomization is made within each subgroup, such treatment differences could easily be chance occurrences, or due to imbalances of other prognostic factors. Little credence can be placed on results in subsets of patients when the groups are retrospectively determined, even if such results are statistically significant. The timolol trial employed Cox's regression model (Section 12.9) to correct for possible confounding variables, but presented the final results in terms of unadjusted clinical life tables, since the adjustment did not materially affect the results.

In nearly all trials there will be individuals who, for one reason or another, did not receive any or all of the treatment required, in the group to which they were randomized. Patient withdrawals due to side-effects, poor compliance, and losses to follow-up all fit into this category. Should such persons, for analysis purposes, be included or excluded, or even changed from the treatment to the control group? The answer to this question depends on the purpose of the trial. If the purpose of the trial is to determine if the treatment can work or has an effect (an 'explanatory' trial), then non-compliers and withdrawals can be excluded from the analysis, and end-points counted only in the patients on active therapy or placebo. Although answering the specific question as to whether or not the treatment can work, the explanatory trial will not answer the perhaps more important question: 'Will this treatment work if employed in practice on a group of patients?' The analysis of such a 'management' trial requires that the groups be analysed as randomized (i.e. according to the intention to treat, rather than what actually happened) with all events in each group counted. This is the more true-to-life situation, where in any group of patients there will be drop-outs and withdrawals from treatment. The management trial is thus far more relevant to clinical practice. In the timolol trial, both methods of analysis were employed. The main analysis presented in the report only included end-points occurring when the patients were actually on treatment, or within 28 days of withdrawal from treatment; an analysis including all end-points, however, was also performed on the intention-to-treat basis, showing only a slightly smaller effect of timolol on survival. The results of the trial showed that timolol reduced total (cumulative life table) mortality at 33 months from 17·5% in the placebo to 10·6% in the timolol group — a reduction of 39·4% ($p < 0·001$). This effect of timolol was also significant in risk group II alone. When total deaths were analysed on an 'intention-to-treat basis', including all mortality end-points in those withdrawing from treatment, the mortality reduction was from 21·9 to 13·3% ($p < 0·001$) showing that there seemed to be no bias in the results due to selective withdrawals from treatment.

The most important of the factors that determine the validity of a controlled trial ('are the results true?') have now been covered. These factors include double blindness, stratified randomization, adequate sample size, and clearly defined end-points. Completeness of follow-up is essential in terms of the end-points being analysed and other factors which may relate to them. Finally, an appropriate statistical analysis must be performed. In all of this, only the suspicion of bias is enough to put a question mark on the results. The onus is on the investigator to show that bias was as far as possible avoided, not on the reader of the trial report to show that it actually existed.

The question now arises of the applicability of trial results, which relates to whether or not the results of the trial can be judged useful in clinical practice. This is determined almost totally by the type of patients selected for inclusion in the trial, and the type of treatment tested, although obviously it also relates to which end-points were studied. Many explanatory trials restrict patients studied to those at high risk of experiencing the end-points. This has obvious advantages in reducing the required sample size (end-points would be more numerous), but the generalization of results to subjects who are not high-risk is questionable.

Explanatory trials can show that the treatment works for some, but will not show that adopting this policy of treatment will have any real effect on the patient population at large. A management trial on the other hand is, as has been said, designed to see how the treatment works in practice, and thus low-risk cases should not generally be excluded.

In a trial, the patients entered are not a random sample of all patients. They are usually a presenting sample of such patients. The generalization of results to the patient population at large requires knowledge of how the patients were actually chosen for trial participation. Many trials will exclude patients with serious diseases other than that being studied, thus reducing the applicability of the end results, while ensuring on the other hand that imbalance of groups with 'awkward' cases is avoided. Diagnostic inclusion and exclusion criteria should however be clearly defined for any trial. The careful reading of a trial report may be a guide as to what kind of patient the trial may be generalized to. Trials based on volunteers are always suspect, because volunteers with a particular condition are likely to be quite unrepresentative of the full patient population.

Ideally a trial should carefully present the sources of the patients studied; if they are hospital cases or cases in a specialized centre, results may be hard to generalize. The presentation of the timolol trial is exemplary as regards this point. Male and female patients, aged between 20 and 75 years, who were admitted to one of the participating centres with a suspected myocardial infarct, were registered as potential trial entrants. Altogether, 11 125 patients were registered, of whom 4155 (37·3%) were diagnosed as having a definite myocardial infarction according to the defined criteria. Of these, 1884 (45·3% or 16·9% of the total registered) were eventually entered into the trial. Exclusions were due to early deaths, contra-indications to timolol treatment, requirements for concomitant treatment or other factors which could have caused problems in randomizing to a placebo group, together with likely difficulties with successful follow-up. It should be noted that the entry criteria should be satisfied prior to randomization, and exclusions made before this takes place. If this is not done, serious imbalance of the groups may result. In the timolol trial, even ignoring selection biases causing admission to the particular centres, only 17 patients out of every 100 with a suspected myocardial infarction could be judged suitable for timolol, and survive long enough to take it. The results must be interpreted in this light. Mitchell (1981) discusses this aspect of the timolol trial in great detail.

Another feature of trials relating to their applicability is the question of the actual treatment regime studied. Most trials use a fixed treatment dosage when drug therapy is in question, but to what extent this mirrors real clinical practice is a moot point. Often, in real life, the dose of a drug is adjusted to meet the individual patient's requirements or condition. Thus, a trial of a fixed dose of an antihypertensive drug may not prove instantly applicable to clinical practice. On the other hand, it must be said that trials allowing variable dosage are administratively difficult, and cause problems in determining the validity of the results. It is impossible for instance to adjust the dose of a placebo, so blindness is lost to a large extent. The timolol trial employed a fixed dosage of timolol and placebo, with treatment started immediately after randomization (5 mg, twice daily for 2 days, and then 10 mg twice daily until trial completion).

The timolol trial was, without any doubt, well designed, well executed, and well presented. Many trials do not fit into this category, or are so poorly presented when published that it is impossible to judge their validity or applicability. A clear and concise presentation of all the factors discussed so far in this chapter is required if the results of clinical trials are to be correctly interpreted, and needless to say, all the factors need to be considered when a trial is being designed in the first place.

11.7 Alternative trial designs

The secondary prevention trial of timolol described and discussed in the previous sections was based on a fixed sample-size design, to compare a single treatment and placebo in two separate groups of patients. Other designs for randomized controlled trials can be used, and three of the most common are described below. The non-randomized community intervention trial is also discussed.

The *sequential trial* design avoids the sample size being fixed beforehand in the comparison of two groups, and in general enables the trial to be completed with a minimum of patients consistent with a statistically significant result. The fixed sample-size trial, on the other hand, cannot be evaluated until all patients have been entered, unless allowances have been made in the sample-size calculation for interim analyses (see Section 15.7). Keeping the sample size in a medical trial at a minimum may be desirable on ethical grounds, but unfortunately a sequential trial can only be employed in certain situations. The more commonly used sequential trial design is described below. The basic idea behind the sequential trial is that patients enter in matched pairs, one member in each pair receiving (at random) the treatment to be tested and the other a placebo (or comparative treatment). Success or failure of the treatment is determined on each pair of patients sequentially as soon as the results become available and eventually, when a sufficient number of pairs have been entered into the study and evaluated, a statistically significant or non-significant result is obtained. At this stage, the patient entry is terminated with no greater number entering the trial than is required to achieve a definite result. Analysis of the data takes place continually throughout the period of the trial, instead of being contingent upon the entry of a fixed number of patients.

The usual sequential trial however can only be used to compare two groups, and one end-point only can be evaluated. This end-point is usually defined in terms of treatment success or failure, or in such a way that one of the treatments can be judged superior to the other in each patient pair. The sequential trial also will only achieve its aim of reducing the number of patients required if patient response to treatment can be determined fairly quickly after the commencement of therapy. If there is a long delay, many pairs of patients may already have been entered into the study unnecessarily when the trial is stopped. The statistical techniques involved in a sequential trial (sequential analysis) are somewhat complex and are not discussed here, but a brief outline of the method is given. Suppose it is wished to compare the effects of treatments A and B. As pairs of patients, suitably matched,* become available, one of the pair receives (at random) treatment A and the other treatment B. For each pair of patients, four outcomes are possible: both treatments a success; both treatments a failure; treatment A a success and treatment B a failure; treatment A a failure and treatment B a success. For the purpose of the sequential trial, the first two outcomes are described as 'tied pairs' and are discarded from analysis. Only the 'untied pairs' are used in the comparison of the two treatments.† Now, suppose a score of + 1 is given to an outcome in which treatment A is a success and treatment B a failure, and a score of − 1 to an outcome in which B is a success and A is a failure. As the trial proceeds, a cumulative score is kept. It is evident that if treatment A is markedly superior to treatment B, an increasing positive score will be cumulated, whilst an increasing negative score will cumulate in the reverse case. If there is no marked difference between A and B, then scores of + 1 and − 1 will occur in a random fashion, so that the total score will oscillate around zero. These three possible outcomes are then used to make a decision about the relative efficacy of the two treatments.

The application of sequential analysis makes use of a *sequential analysis chart*, and such a chart is shown in Fig. 11.1. This chart was used in the analysis of a clinical trial, set up to determine if the occurrence of a particular complication of a disease was increased when a particular therapy was employed. The end-point of the trial was, unusually enough, an unwanted treatment effect. The study was performed on premature infants with the respiratory distress syndrome. Diuretic treatment of such infants to reduce fluid retention and help alleviate their symptoms is often used. It had been suggested that a particular diuretic, furosemide — which shall be called treatment A — seemed to increase the incidence of a particular heart condition (patent ductus arteriosus), a complication in premature infants with the respiratory distress syndrome. It was decided to compare the

---

* On the basis of prognostic variables, or using each two consecutive eligible patients to form a pair.
† Note the similarity to McNemar's χ^2 test (Section 7.13).

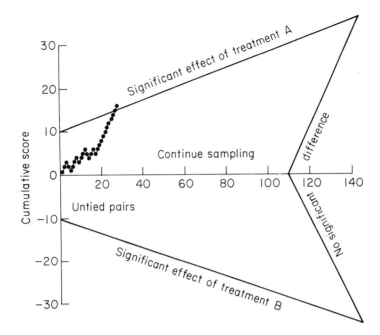

Fig. 11.1. Sequential analysis chart for comparing the effect of furosemide (A) and chlorothiazide (B) on a heart score in premature infants. Green *et al.* (1983) with permission.

heart functions of infants under treatment and infants on an alternative diuretic (chlorothiazide) which, for simplicity, shall be called treatment B. One of each member of consecutively admitted pairs of infants was assigned randomly to treatment A and the other to treatment B. After a specified period, a heart score, ranging from 0 to 6 (6 being a severe grading), was determined blindly on each infant and each pair was classified as 'favouring' treatment A or B (if not tied) according to which infant had the highest score. Whenever a pair of infants did not have an identical score (untied pairs), the results were entered into the chart in Fig. 11.1. The horizontal axis on the sequential analysis chart records the number of untied pairs included in the trial. The vertical axis records the cumulative score as the trial proceeds (a positive score indicating, in the example, that the treatment A infant had a higher heart score than the treatment B infant). In the figure, the cumulative score is shown by the zig-zag line. The meaning of the four 'boundary lines' marked on the chart can now be explained. A trial may be terminated as soon as the score line reaches one of the boundary lines. If the score line crosses the upper boundary line, this is interpreted to mean that treatment A resulted in a significantly higher heart score than treatment B. The opposite interpretation applies if the score line crosses the lower boundary line. Of course, the score line will not cross either boundary line unless a relatively high score has accumulated in favour of one or other of the treatments. If, on the other hand, the score line crosses either of the end boundary lines, this is interpreted to mean that there appears to be no difference between the two methods of treatment; the score is not high enough in relation to the number of untied pairs tested to indicate a statistically significant advantage of one treatment over the other.

The trial continues until the score line reaches one of the boundary lines, at which point a decision can be reached, at a predetermined level of significance and power, about the relative advantages of the two methods of treatment. In the example, the score line reached the upper boundary line after 28 untied pairs had been recorded. When the heart score was higher on an infant on treatment B, the score line would move downwards. When the score was higher in a treatment A infant, it moved upwards. Twenty-two of the untied pairs favoured treatment A, six favoured B, and, eventually, the cumulative score of 16 in favour of A was reached. This was sufficient to cause a rejection of the null hypothesis that there was no difference in treatment effects, and to declare that treatment A significantly increased the heart score in these infants. It can be seen that once the boundary lines have been fixed, plotting and analysing the results of the trial as they become available is quite simple. The complexity of the technique lies in fixing the boundary lines for the particular experiment being conducted, and details of this are not given here. The chart is set up, however, based on the same criteria for determining a fixed sample size in the more usual type of experiment. The chart in the trial discussed was based on a β error of 0·05 in detecting a twofold preference for one of the treatments at a two-sided significance level, α, of 0·05. If a fixed sample-size trial design had been used, the sign test for paired data (Section 7.7) or McNemar's test for paired proportions (Section 7.13) could have been employed.

A second alternative to the standard two-group randomized controlled trial is the *cross-over trial* which uses a matched design with each patient as his/her own control. Treatments are compared on the same patients in different time-periods. Self-paired experiments such as this ensure that the treatment or control groups are identical as regards patient characteristics, and thus require a smaller total sample size than an independent two-group comparison. In a comparison of two treatments (A and B again) the patient is first randomly assigned to, say, treatment A for a specified period. The effect of treatment is evaluated, and the patient is withdrawn from the treatment for a time until any residual effect disappears. After this washout period, the patient is 'crossed over' to receive treatment B, and again the treatment effect is evaluated after a second period. Patients entering the trial are thus randomized to A and B, or B and then A. The basic analysis is, of course, by means of a paired comparison of the two treatments.

Unfortunately, the cross-over trial can only be used in situations where the treatment effect is fairly immediate, and also disappears after the withdrawal of treatment. The cross-over trial can be used, for example, in testing antihypertensive therapy, or anti-inflammatory drugs for arthritis. In both these examples, the 'symptom' returns after treatment withdrawal, so that a second treatment can be applied after the first. It is sometimes difficult however, in the cross-over trial, to disentangle real treatment effects from a possible carry-over effect from the last treatment, even with a long washout period, or from changes in response with the passage of time.

The third randomized trial design which is considered in this section in a sense answers two questions for the price of one. If one wished to compare the separate effects of two different treatments (A and B) against a placebo, a *factorial design* should be considered. It might be tempting to design a three-group trial with, perhaps, randomization to A, B or the placebo, but it can be far more efficient to have four groups in such a comparison. Patients would first be randomized to receive either treatment A or the placebo. Within each of these groups, a second randomization would be made to either treatment B or placebo. Four groups would result: A and B; A only; B only, and neither A nor B. In the first International Urokinase/Warfarin Trial in Colorectal Cancer (Daly, 1991) patients with operable colorectal cancer were randomized into receiving post-operatively either an intravenous drip containing urokinase, or a saline drip (the placebo). Within each of these groups, patients were again randomized to receive either long-term warfarin therapy, or no such treatment. The trial design required 100 patients in each of the four groups, and the end-points were survival and recurrence-free survival. Table 11.1 shows the required number of patients in their randomized groups. A factorial design, such as this, is analysed for the effects of the two treatments separately. The effect of urokinase, for example, is determined by comparing the 200 persons on urokinase with the 200 persons not on this treatment, irrespective of their warfarin therapy. The comparison is not biased by the warfarin therapy, because half of each group is on this drug so that it cannot act as a confounder. Similarly, the effect of warfarin is analysed without reference to the allocation to urokinase. The sample-size requirements for a factorial design like this are the same as for a normal two-group comparison, so in

Table 11.1. A factorial design for evaluating the effects of urokinase and warfarin in colorectal cancer

	Urokinase	No urokinase	Total
Warfarin	100	100	200
No warfarin	100	100	200
Total	200	200	400

essence the extra result is free. The only problem arises if there is a synergistic effect (see Section 10.6) between the two treatments, and the group randomized to receive both has a better result than expected on the basis of either therapy in isolation. Apart from this, the factorial design provides a useful adjunct to the usual two-group trial.

It was mentioned in Section 11.3 that the randomized trial could be used for the evaluation of a primary prevention intervention such as the reduction of risk factors for coronary heart disease. An alternative to this approach is also used. The problem with primary prevention is that it generally requires individuals to change their behaviour or lifestyle. In practice, this can best be achieved by, in addition to individual counselling, a community approach through a process of health education and promotion, whereby the community adapts more healthy behaviour patterns. For example, cessation of smoking can be aided greatly by general publicity and the creation of 'smoke-free' zones. This type of intervention cannot be evaluated by the randomization of individuals because the intervention is in the population at large. Community intervention trials are an attempt to tackle this problem. Typically one community receives a health promotion pro- gramme supplemented by individual interventions. A control or comparison community does not receive such an intervention. The success of the intervention is judged by comparing random samples of each community to assess changes in risk factors and behaviour and by the careful monitoring of end-points (such as heart attacks) in the entire populations.

The difficulty with such evaluations is that there may be differences between the communities, other than the intervention, that give rise to variation in the end-points. The lack of randomization introduces the major problem of confounded effects. Some trials have randomized a number of communities to intervention and non-intervention groups but this does not overcome the difficulties. The community intervention trial, however, seems the only way to examine the effect of health promotion in primary prevention. The earliest community intervention trial in coronary heart disease was in North Karelia in Finland (Puska *et al.* 1981) and a current example is the Kilkenny Health Project in Ireland.

11.8 Ethical considerations

Many ethical problems are raised in the context of the randomized controlled trial in medicine, and in this section some of the issues involved are indicated. Such ethical issues are still hotly debated in the medical literature and there are no hard and fast answers to many of the problems raised. However, ethical questions are distinct from medico-legal ones, and no attempt to consider the latter is made. The Declaration of Helsinki, adopted by the World Medical Assembly in 1964 and revised in 1975, provides general guidelines on biomedical research involving human subjects, and is a cornerstone for the ethics of the randomized trial. The main points of this declaration are included in the discussion below.

To turn the basic question on its head, it might be asked whether it is ethical not to perform randomized controlled trials on proposed new therapies. In the history of medicine, many therapies commonly employed simply did not work or resulted in more harm than good. Most of these therapies could have been determined as useless far sooner if subjected to a formal trial and indeed many such therapies were abandoned as a result of their being tested scientifically. It is essential to know if a particular treatment is beneficial and the randomized controlled trial is, in essence, the only way by which this knowledge can be obtained. Clinical judgement on a haphazardly selected group with partial follow-up is not a firm basis for the evaluation of treatment. If the randomized controlled trial were to be considered unethical in all cases, then many patients would be condemned to unproven and worthless interventions and the advance of medical science would be halted almost completely.

Although one hopefully agrees with the above point, dilemmas still remain in accepting the existence of experimental trials in medicine. There are conflicts between an individual patient's welfare in the trial itself and the welfare of all patients with the particular condition in the future. There are conflicts between the doctor as healer and the doctor as investigator. In a trial patients are allocated into two groups, one of which will receive the new treatment under investigation, while the other will receive the best treatment available or, in certain instances, no treatment at all. The first question that is asked is whether it is ethical to withhold a potentially good treatment from some individual patients for the eventual good of a larger group. Herein lies the crux of the controlled trial; if the treatment is *known* to be good, a trial cannot ethically take place, but on the other hand, a trial cannot take place either without there being some suspicion that the treatment may be good. This leads to the conflict between knowledge and possibilities, and what may be firm 'knowledge' in one doctor's mind may be just a vague hope in another's. From the doctor's point of view, the individual patient's welfare must be of paramount importance, and if doctors have evidence that a new therapy is beneficial, they are not justified ethically in involving themselves in a trial of that treatment. Other doctors however may view the same evidence differently.

It would seem to be impossible to define universal criteria for what could be considered as evidence in favour of employing a particular therapy, apart from a well-designed and well-executed randomized controlled trial. On the other hand, there is no real argument against the doctor who says 'I tried it out on 10 of my patients, and it really worked. I won't allow any of my patients to be entered into a trial.' It is interesting, however, that some doctors may feel far less uneasy using a possibly inferior therapy through ignorance than they do in submitting a possibly beneficial treatment to the rigours of a controlled trial.

The subjective nature of what evidence is required to form knowledge is thus a major problem in determining whether or not a particular trial is ethical. As healers, doctors must do what they think best for the individual patient; as investigators, they also have a responsibility to that individual patient to determine what indeed is the best therapy. It would seem then that from the point of view of participating doctors a trial is only ethical insofar as those doctors accept that they do not know which of the two treatments is better, and have no preference for either.*

The question of exactly when a trial should be undertaken is relevant to this whole question. It is ethically easier to commence a trial at the introductory stages of a new therapy, since there would be little or no knowledge about its effects. However, a trial at the early stages of a new intervention is more likely to miss its full usefulness if it takes time (as with a new surgical procedure say) to get the treatment 'just right'. If on the other hand one waits too long, the procedure may become generally accepted as worthwhile (without formal evaluation), making a trial ethically difficult to perform.

A similar problem arises once a trial is underway. If particular doctors see the results as they accrue, and a trend in favour of one of the treatments becomes apparent, some may wish to change all their patients to that treatment because of their 'knowledge' of its better effect. Early trends in a trial, which will generally be statistically non-significant, may be very misleading; often an early trend will settle itself out after a time to give an entirely different result at the end of the trial when the validity and statistical significance of the results can be determined. It may in fact be unethical to stop a trial on the basis of early positive results which do not achieve significance, since the trial would not then have achieved its purpose. It must be stressed, however, that the patient's welfare comes first, and that if a doctor for any reason feels it better to withdraw a patient or change treatment, ethical considerations demand that this be done, irrespective of trial requirements.

In multicentre trials, this dilemma of early trends is often overcome by letting a steering committee, only, examine results as they come in. Trial participants will not be informed of results until the study has been completed, unless very definite trends are apparent. The ethical problem is thus switched from the participating doctors to a steering committee.

Patients have the right to expect individual and personal treatment from their

---

* One criterion for making this judgement has been suggested and that is the answer to the question 'Would I allow a member of my family to enter the trial and be randomized to one or other of the treatments?'

doctors and it must be asked if this individual right can be sacrificed for the benefit of humanity and the progress of knowledge. This right of the individual patient seems to be sacrificed if the doctor has no choice over which therapy is to be given, which, of course, would be determined by 'the toss of a coin'. However, when there is an honest lack of knowledge about which is the better treatment, the patients do not lose out. Outside of the trial, the chosen therapy would be, necessarily, at the whim of the doctor, and the fact that the treatment is chosen by the toss of a coin instead surely does not make a difference.

The question then of whether a randomized controlled trial is in itself ethical relates to the nature of evidence required to form knowledge. In most cases, a large body of doctors will agree on the necessity for a trial, although there will always be dissidents. As long as particular doctors are sure of their 'ignorance', the trial is, for them, ethically justified and patient's rights would not seem to be abrogated if they enter a trial. Indeed, rather than querying whether it is ethical to withhold a potentially good treatment from patients in the control group, it should perhaps be asked whether it is ethical to withhold the standard treatment from patients in the treatment group.

Once the hurdle of determining whether it is ethical to undertake a particular controlled trial in the first place is overcome, ethical problems still remain, relating to the design and conduct of the trial itself. Firstly, the treatment to be investigated must be safe. Safe, however, is a relative term, since no therapy is without risk. The right balance must be struck between potential benefit and possible harm. Nor can the design and analysis of the trial be divorced from ethical questions. It is not ethical to enter patients into a trial whose eventual results may never be accepted because of failure to avoid bias in the setting up and execution of the trial. Also, if the sample size of a trial is too small to detect important results, it should probably not have been started in the first place. Nor of course should more patients than necessary be entered into a trial. The sequential trial is designed to avoid some of these problems, but as already noted, its applicability is limited. Other little-used designs have also been proposed to reduce the number of patients on an inferior treatment. These *adaptive designs* require that a greater proportion of patients be randomized into the group showing the more favourable result at any time. Such trials, however, are limited in their scope and are in fact less appealing than they appear to be at first sight.

From the point of view of patient selection, ethical considerations will often demand certain exclusion criteria. The exclusion of pregnant women from most drug trials is universal, and ethical considerations must take precedence over the requirement of applicability of trial results.

The use of placebos and double blind procedures in a trial also raises ethical problems. Unless the condition being studied is fairly innocuous, like the common cold for instance, or no proven therapy is available, the control group should receive a standard therapy. Single blindness can still be achieved by using the double placebo procedure, and no control with a serious condition for which treatment is available should be given a placebo only. How far one should go with placebos is a moot question. There are some examples in the early literature of placebo surgery. Ligation of the internal mammary arteries, for instance, used to be a common procedure for the relief of angina, but a clinical trial showed this treatment to be useless. Those in the control group had a placebo surgical skin incision made, but without further operative intervention. Would the results of this trial have been accepted without the placebo procedure?

In general, blinding of patients to their particular treatment does not seem to raise serious ethical problems so long as informed consent has been obtained. As discussed previously, the double blind trial refers to the blindness of the patient and of the doctor managing the patient and evaluating any responses to treatment. There is no problem, however, in allowing the doctor who is managing the patients know to which treatment they have been allocated, so long as patients in the treatment and control groups are looked after similarly. In any case, if the patients' doctor is 'blind', the treatment code should always be easily available. The doctor evaluating the patients' response should, however, be 'blind'. Again it must be stressed that doctors have the right and duty to withdraw a patient from a trial if they see fit.

The largest ethical problem with the randomized controlled trial today is, however, that of informed consent. In most countries informed consent is a legal requirement of any trial in medicine. As with all ethical questions, that of informed consent does not have a simple 'yes' or 'no' answer. There is no doubt that patients have a right to know that they are participating in an experimental trial, and that the therapy being tested is unproven. The problem is, however, that many patients may not wish to exercise this right. Informed consent may demand that some patients know more about their illness and their prognosis than they wish to; many prefer to put trust in their doctor that the best possible care will be given them. Is it ethical to burden such patients with the knowledge that in fact it is not known what is the best treatment, and with all the ancillary information that would be required for them to give an informed consent? Seeking consent and the extent of it is a major question that must be decided by trial organizers in the context of the particular situation. The ever present possibility of legal action by a patient in a trial usually decides investigators in favour of seeking consent, but this is not why informed consent should be obtained. The patient's right to know what is happening is, surely, far more important than the doctor's legal protection.

If informed consent is to be obtained, what should it include?* This again is a

---

* It would seem that from the ethical point of view verbal informed consent is just as good as a written and signed statement. Written informed consent is often obtained for legal purposes only, though it does help to ensure that all points have been explained to the individual patient.

debatable issue. Patients cannot be expected to understand everything about their disease, and in fact one of the reasons for the trial in the first place is that doctors do not know the best therapy themselves. Informed consent however does demand that the relevant facts concerning the trial and its purpose be explained as fully and clearly as possible. The two treatments should be described, as should also their possible benefits and side-effects. If the study is blind, this should be explained also. Some doctors however balk at explaining that they will not be choosing the treatment, but that the patient will be randomized. This is of course central to the trial itself, but it may result in destroying the doctor−patient relationship. Whether randomization is to be included in the description of a trial, for the purposes of informed consent, must also be left to the individual trial organizers to decide.

An important element in the process of seeking informed consent is the pressure that the doctor may, unconsciously, place on the patient to participate. Patients must fully realize that they are under no obligation to do so, and that failure to become involved in the trial will not compromise their position with the doctor in any way whatsoever.

A trial design has been proposed by Zelen (1979) which neatly avoids the problem of obtaining informed consent to randomization and the consequent reduction of patient participation due to refusals. The resulting trial is controlled and (partially) randomized but its value is yet to be proven.

As has been seen, the randomized controlled trial poses many ethical questions, all of which are related to holding sacrosanct the welfare of individual patients and recognition of their rights. A very general principle could be proposed − that no patients in a trial be worse off than if they were not in the trial in the first place. The interesting fact is, however, that patients in a clinical trial often get better overall care and much more careful assessment and follow-up than the ordinary patient on standard therapy.

11.9 Summary

In this chapter the purpose, design, implementation and analysis of the randomized controlled trial in medicine have been discussed. The necessity of treatment evaluation with concurrent controls and the avoidance of bias with the randomization and blinding of trial patients and doctors were stressed; the distinction between therapeutic (clinical), primary prevention and secondary prevention trials was made, and designs other than the usual two-group comparative trials were discussed. Criteria were given for evaluating the validity (are the results true?) and applicability (are the results useful in clinical practice?) of trials, and the chapter concluded with a brief foray into the ethical problems raised by the randomized controlled trial.

12

Multivariate Analysis and the Control of Confounding

12.1 Introduction

So far in this book the statistical methods have concentrated on the analysis of the association between two variables only. For two quantitative variables the association is displayed by means of a scattergram with simple regression techniques to perform the statistical analysis (e.g. blood pressure and age). For a quantitative and a qualitative variable, the association can be examined by looking at the mean level of one variable in groups defined by categories of the other (e.g. mean blood pressure in males and females). The statistical techniques in this situation include t tests and analysis of variance. The final case of two qualitative variables is dealt with by contingency table analysis using one of the chi-square tests.

As has been pointed out, medical research is to a large extent aimed at determining associations between two variables, but in most cases account has to be taken of other variables which may act as confounders of an observed association. For instance, if one were to look at operative mortality from a particular procedure, one would find a very strong relationship between this and having grey hair. In such a situation it is obvious that the observed association would be due to a third variable — age. Older people usually have higher mortality, and there would be a larger proportion of grey-haired persons in this group. Thus, though grey hair has no causal association with mortality, a relationship is seen due to the confounding effect of age. In general, for a variable to act as a confounder of an association it must be related to both of the other variables. This chapter considers techniques that will correct for the existence of confounders and provide a valid statistical inference of confounded relationships.

Although control of confounders at the analysis stage of a study is important it must be remembered that confounding can also be controlled at the design stage. Thus, matching for potential confounders is used in case-control studies, and stratified randomization is employed in clinical trials. Control of confounding in study design is preferable to control with a statistical technique and should be done where feasible. However it is never possible to exclude all confounders at the design stage and the analysis of any data must include the search for and control of nuisance variables for which adjustment has not been made.

If some form of matching (frequency or paired) or stratification has been used in the study design to control for confounders, the statistical analysis should also take account of this. In Chapter 7 the analysis of paired data was discussed while the methods in this present chapter are suitable for the analysis of frequency matched or stratified data. Failure to take account of matching will result in a reduction of power, although the analysis will not be biased.

Some of the multivariate methods (particularly the multiple regression approaches) considered in this chapter are also used when one wishes to examine the relationship between one variable (the dependent variable) and a number of other explanatory variables considered simultaneously.

12.2 Multiple regression

In Chapter 9 simple regression and correlation were used in the examination of the association between two quantitative variables. Analysis which involves more than two quantitative variables can be approached in two ways. Using the first approach, the relationship between pairs of variables may be examined independently of the other variables. Thus, if there are three variables, say x_1, x_2 and x_3, the relationship between the pairs can be examined: x_1 and x_2, x_1 and x_3, and x_2 and x_3, in each case ignoring the third variable. An example of this kind of analysis is shown in Table 12.1. There are four variables in this example: cigarette and dairy product consumption in 1973, and male and female coronary heart disease mortality in 1974, determined in 14 countries. The figures in the table are the values of the correlation coefficient between any pair of variables. Thus, in the first line, the correlation between cigarette consumption in 1973 and dairy products consumption in 1973 is negative, with a value of $r = -0.36$. The correlation between cigarette consumption in 1973 and male coronary heart disease mortality in 1974 is 0.17 and so on. In the second line, the correlation between

Table 12.1. Zero-order correlation coefficients between cigarette consumption (1973), dairy product consumption (1973) and male and female coronary heart disease (CHD) mortality (1974) in 14 countries. Adapted and abbreviated from Salonen & Vohlonen (1982) with permission

	Cigarettes in 1973	Dairy products in 1973	Male CHD in 1974	Female CHD in 1974
Cigarettes in 1973	1·0	− 0·36	0·17	0·33
Dairy products in 1973		1·0	0·78*	0·70*
Male CHD in 1974			1·0	0·96*
Female CHD in 1974				1·0

* $p < 0.05$.

dairy products consumption and cigarette consumption in 1973 is omitted, since it already appears in the first line. The correlation between any variable and itself is necessarily unity, as shown in the diagonal of the table.

Each correlation coefficient is calculated between two variables quite independently of the other two variables. The table therefore consists of a number of separate bivariate correlation coefficients calculated by the method described in Section 9.3 and interpreted in the same way. Each correlation coefficient has been tested for significance, and those coefficients that are significantly different from zero at the 5% level are marked with an asterisk. A table of this kind, sometimes referred to as a matrix of bivariate correlation coefficients, is a useful method of summarizing the independent relationships between a number of variables, and of showing which relationships are significant. In Table 12.1 there are three significant relationships; the remaining correlations can be ignored. This example shows some of the problems in the interpretation of bivariate correlation coefficients. The relationships between dairy product consumption and male and female CHD deaths could possibly be attributed to a causal connection between the factors, while the association between male and female deaths is of little relevance in developing a causal hypothesis. This latter relationship is likely to be due, almost totally, to the influence of dairy consumption (and other factors) on the CHD deaths in both sexes.

The second approach to analysing relationships between more than two quantitative variables is quite different, involving the simultaneous analysis of the variables. This is called *multiple regression analysis*, as distinct from simple bivariate analysis, which deals with only two variables

In Chapter 9 the relationship of systolic blood pressure to weight in 10-year-old children was summarized by the simple linear regression equation

$$SBP = 79 \cdot 7 + 0 \cdot 8W$$

where SBP was the systolic blood pressure in mmHg and W was the weight in kilograms. In this study many other variables besides weight were examined for their influence on systolic blood pressure. The authors also presented a multiple regression equation with SBP again as the dependent variable, but with diastolic blood pressure and the time of day at which the measurement was taken as two extra variables in addition to weight. Such variables are often called independent variables to distinguish them from the dependent variable. Due to the fact, however, that some of these 'independent' variables may be highly correlated with each other, it is preferable to refer to them as explanatory or predictor variables.

Multiple regression is essentially a technique that examines the relationship between a single quantitative dependent variable and many quantitative explanatory variables. (The extension to qualitative explanatory variables is considered in the next section.) In the blood pressure study the authors presented the following multiple regression equation:

$$SBP = 39 \cdot 6 + 0 \cdot 45W + 0 \cdot 69 \; DBP + 0 \cdot 45T$$

where SBP and DBP are systolic and diastolic blood pressures in mmHg, W is weight in kilograms and T is the time of day measured in number of completed hours. In this multiple regression equation SBP is the dependent variable and DBP, W and T are the explanatory variables. The coefficients $0 \cdot 45$, $0 \cdot 69$ and $0 \cdot 45$ are called *partial regression coefficients*. For example, $0 \cdot 69$ is the average change in systolic blood pressure per 1 mmHg change in diastolic blood pressure when weight and the time of day are held constant. This shows how systolic blood pressure is related to diastolic blood pressure independently of the other two factors. The coefficient $0 \cdot 45$ is the partial regression coefficient for weight, which shows the relationship of systolic blood pressure and weight when diastolic blood pressure and time of day are held constant. The coefficient for T is also $0 \cdot 45$ and measures the relationship between systolic blood pressure and time of day when the other two factors are held constant. Note that the partial regression coefficient for weight ($0 \cdot 45$) is much less than the simple regression coefficient of $0 \cdot 8$ obtained when weight was the only explanatory variable included in the analysis. Thus, the relationship of systolic blood pressure with weight is not as marked when diastolic blood pressure and time of day are taken into account. For a fixed time of day and fixed diastolic blood pressure, systolic blood pressure will increase by $0 \cdot 45$ mmHg for every 1 kg increase of weight, compared to $0 \cdot 8$ mmHg when the other variables are not allowed for. Multiple regression can thus control for the confounding effects of other variables on any bivariate relationship.

The strength of the relationship between the dependent variable and the explanatory variables may also be estimated by calculating the *coefficient of multiple correlation (r)*. This is analogous to the simple correlation coefficient and, as before, its square measures the proportion of the total variation in the dependent variable which can be 'explained' by variations in the explanatory variables. The 'unexplained' variation may be due, of course, to other variables which have not been included in the regression equation. If these variables can be identified, then a new multiple regression equation can be calculated with these additional variables included. The value of r^2 will be increased, since the proportion of 'explained' variation in the dependent variable will be higher. The value of r^2 for the multiple regression equation above is $0 \cdot 53$ compared to the value of $0 \cdot 23$ in the simple regression equation with weight only included. More of the variation in systolic blood pressure is explained by inclusion of the extra variables. Moreover, by calculating what are called *partial correlation coefficients*, the strength of the relationship between the dependent variable and any *one* of the explanatory variables may be calculated, assuming the other explanatory variables are held constant. These partial correlation coefficients differ from the simple bivariate (or zero-order) correlation coefficients described earlier. In the former, the simultaneous influence of other variables is taken into account; in the latter, the correlation between two variables is calculated without any explicit attempt to remove the possible confounding effect of other factors.

Usually multiple regression analysis is performed on a computer as the calculations are, to say the least, fairly tedious. Computational details will not be given in this text. A multiple regression package will give as part of its output the constant term and the partial regression coefficients. As with simple regression, confidence intervals can be calculated for these coefficients (the coefficient $\pm 1 \cdot 96$ times its standard error for a 95% interval) and significance tests can be performed for the null hypothesis that the coefficient is zero (i.e. no association with the dependent variable).

When performing a multiple regression there is a limit to the number of explanatory variables that can be included and this limit is related to the sample size. From a practical point of view also, the number of variables should be kept to a manageable level. The choice of which variables to include is dictated by many factors. If one is controlling for confounders then variables should be retained in the equation if their inclusion materially alters the value of the partial regression coefficient of the principal variable of interest, even if they are not statistically significant. If one is looking for factors that best explain the variation in the dependent variable then there are a number of techniques available to choose the 'best' subset of the explanatory variables. *Forward (stepwise) inclusion* methods search through all the possible variables not already in the equation and add in, at each step, the variable that increases the coefficient of multiple correlation to the greatest extent. The process continues until either the increase in the coefficient is non-significant or a prespecified number of variables has been included. *Backward elimination* on the other hand starts with all possible variables in the regression equation and deletes them one by one to eventually obtain the 'best' set of explanatory variables. Variations on both these techniques are also available but most methods, depending on the criteria used for inclusion or exclusion, tend to give the same set of predictors.

When a number of explanatory variables are highly correlated, the effect of one of them on the dependent variable will often totally mask the effect of the others, resulting in some of these variables having small and non-significant partial regression coefficients. Usually, only one of a set of such variables will be included in the final equation because it will act as a proxy for the remainder. Variables excluded in this way may however be important predictors of the dependent variable and dealing with such *multicollinearity* can be a problem.

It must be stressed however that multiple regression techniques should not be used blindly to solve all problems with more than two quantitative variables. In essence a multiple regression analysis imposes a particular type of linear additive model on the interrelationships between the dependent and explanatory variables. The appropriateness of this model should be determined on theoretical grounds, if possible, and it should not glibly be assumed that nature obeys such constructs. (See Section 12.4 for methods that do not assume linear effects and Section 12.7 for methods to examine interaction.)

12.3 Analysis of variance

Chapter 8 explained how a one-way analysis of variance (ANOVA) could be used to compare the mean of one variable between more than two groups. The term 'one-way' was used because means were examined for their association with one qualitative variable only. ANOVA easily extends to the examination of the association of a quantitative variable with more than one qualitative variable.

Table 12.2 shows the results of a hypothetical study of serum cholesterol related to two qualitative variables — exercise (heavy or light) and sex. Note that in the total study group of 100 males and 100 females the mean cholesterols are the same in each sex. However, in both the heavy and light exercisers separately, cholesterol in males is 5 mg/100 ml greater than in females. The cholesterol relationship with sex is confounded by exercise. If exercise had not been examined in this situation one might conclude that cholesterols were identical in the two sexes — obviously a non-significant result! The further breakdown by exercise level shows that males really have higher levels of serum cholesterol than females, but because they exercise more (50% heavy exercisers compared to 25% in females) this association does not appear in the crude data. In this example the confounding effect of exercise masks the sex difference because exercise is related both to sex and to serum cholesterol. A confounding variable can either mask a real relationship (as in this example) or create an apparent association where none exists.

Note too that the exercise effect is only marginally confounded by sex — the difference between heavy and light exercisers in males and females combined is 18·67 mg/100 ml compared to 20 mg/100 ml in each sex group. Thus, when

Table 12.2. Mean serum cholesterol (mg/100 ml) by exercise level and sex (hypothetical data)

Exercise	Male (n)	Cholesterol	Female (n)	Cholesterol	Total (n)	Cholesterol
Heavy	(50)	220	(25)	215	(75)	218.3
Light	(50)	240	(75)	235	(125)	237.0
Total	(100)	230	(100)	230	(200)	230

associations are being examined, the degree of confounding is not a symmetrical property. The fact that the sex relationship with cholesterol is strongly confounded by exercise does not necessarily imply that the exercise relationship with cholesterol is strongly confounded by sex.

To test the sex/cholesterol association for statistical significance while allowing for the influence of exercise the usual technique would be a *two-way analysis of variance*, 'two-way' referring to the fact that cholesterol is classified by two qualitative variables — sex and exercise. The analysis is complicated by the fact that the data are what is referred to as 'unbalanced' — there are unequal numbers in each of the four sex/exercise categories. It was this, of course, that gave rise to the confounding in the first place. The computations for the analysis of variance in this case are quite complex and would usually be performed on a computer. The logic of the method involves comparisons of various estimates of variance as in the one-way case (see Chapter 8) but the output of any computer program requires careful interpretation and the advice of a statistician should be sought. (Note too that many computer programs cannot easily handle unbalanced data.)

In this example an analysis of variance would include significance tests comparing cholesterols between males and females, taking account of the differences within each category of the confounder (exercise), and would also allow the calculation of confidence intervals for the corrected or adjusted cholesterol differences. The estimate of the (corrected) mean cholesterol difference between males and females would be $5\,mg/100\,ml$ — the figure seen in each of the exercise groups. In general the corrected difference is some form of average of the differences in each category of the confounder. Analysis of variance should also be used when the data have been frequency-matched and is the usual approach for the analysis of a quantitative variable in such cases.

The analysis of variance can of course handle qualitative variables with more than two categories each and can be applied to quite complex data structures with more than two qualitative variables involved. The technique is much easier to apply when the data are balanced (usually meaning equal numbers in the various cells) and is a most powerful method for the analysis of experimental data, particularly in animal and laboratory experiments when balance can and should be achieved. The techniques are however too advanced for this text.

What happens when the effect of a quantitative variable is also to be allowed for — e.g. age in the above example? One possibility is to create age groups and treat age as a qualitative variable. The alternative is to use what is called an *analysis of covariance* which allows for the influence of both qualitative and quantitative variables. Thus, an analysis of covariance would handle the relationship between the dependent variable cholesterol and the explanatory variables age (quantitative), exercise and sex (both qualitative).

12.4 Analysis of variance, covariance and multiple regression

Analysis of covariance lies between multiple regression, where all the explanatory variables are quantitative, and analysis of variance, where they are all qualitative. In fact, although the approaches seem quite different, the three techniques are very closely allied and both the analysis of variance and the analysis of covariance can be formulated in a multiple regression framework with identical numerical results. The trick is to include qualitative variables in the multiple regression. This is done by means of 'dummy variables'. If the qualitative variable is binary (two categories only) then the use of this method is very straightforward. A binary variable is numerically coded for entry into a multiple regression using the value 1 for one category and 0 for the other. If the variable called MALE is coded 1 for a male and 0 for a female, and EXERCISE is coded 1 for heavy and 0 for light, the multiple regression equation formulation of the analysis of covariance discussed above would be

$$CHOL = a + b_1 \ AGE + b_2 \ MALE + b_3 \ EXERCISE.$$

Here b_1, b_2 and b_3 are the partial regression coefficients and a is the constant term. b_1 gives the change in cholesterol for a year's change in age, corrected for sex and exercise. b_2 can be interpreted as the difference in cholesterol between males and females corrected for the other factors. This is because the predicted cholesterol for a male (MALE = 1) is b_2 higher than the value for a female of similar age and exercise level. (With MALE equal to 0, the b_2 sex term disappears.) Similarly, the b_3 term is the corrected difference in cholesterol between heavy and light exercisers.

If the qualitative variable to be included has more than two categories the dummy coding scheme becomes more complicated. Suppose cigarette-smoking status with three categories of current, ex- and non-smokers were to be included in the above equation. Two dummy variables (CURR and EX) would be created as shown in Table 12.3 and both would be entered into the regression equation instead of the original three-category variable.

Table 12.3. Dummy coding

Smoking status	Dummy variable coding	
	CURR	EX
Current	1	0
Ex-smoker	0	1
Non-smoker	0	0

Arbitrarily, one of the categories of the original smoking status variable is considered as reference — in this case the non-smokers. The regression equation, including smoking status via the two dummy variables, would now read

$$CHOL = a + b_1 \text{ AGE} + b_2 \text{ MALE} + b_3 \text{ EXERCISE} + b_4 \text{ CURR} + b_5 \text{ EX.}$$

Note of course that the a, b_1, b_2 and b_3 coefficients would be unlikely to have the same values as in the previous equation because of the addition of the smoking variables. Using a similar argument as above in the case of binary variables, b_4 is the corrected difference in cholesterols between current smokers and non-smokers, while b_5 is the corrected difference between ex-smokers and non-smokers. Both coefficients measure the difference from the reference category. The difference between the cholesterols of current and ex-smokers would be given by $b_4 - b_5$. In general the number of dummy variables that have to be created to allow a qualitative variable to enter into a multiple regression is one less than the number of categories of the variable.

It was pointed out in Section 12.2 that a multiple regression approach to data analysis imposed a linear relationship between the dependent and explanatory variables. If the relationship is not linear the regression analysis may give misleading results. One way of examining if the dependent variable increases or decreases linearly with a particular quantitative explanatory variable is to categorize the latter (e.g. age into age groups) and enter it into the regression equation as a set of dummy variables. The partial regression coefficients for these dummy variables show immediately if a trend is present. If a linear trend is apparent it is quite legitimate to employ the original quantitative variable in the regression equation. If a non-linear trend is apparent, transformation of the original variable (see Section 9.6) may linearize it, and the transformed quantitative variable could be retained in the equation. Alternatively, the dummy variables could be used in the regression rather than the original quantitative one.

Although calculational details are not given here for either multiple regression or analysis of variance/covariance, it is hoped that the discussion above will guide the researcher as to what is possible with these techniques. The choice between a multiple regression or an analysis of variance in a particular situation often depends on the computer software available, but it can be argued strongly that the interpretation of the former is much more tractable, which is why it has been covered in more detail.

12.5 Contingency tables and stratified analyses: the Mantel—Haenzel χ^2

The previous three sections discussed the problem of confounding when the dependent variable was quantitative. When all the variables are qualitative the control of confounding can be achieved with contingency table analysis. Emphasis will be placed entirely, in what follows, on confounding in the analysis of two binary variables. As seen in the previous chapters on medical studies and the clinical trial, the 2×2 table with two binary variables is the starting point for many analyses, with the relative risk or the odds ratio as the usual measure of the association. The methods also have applications in vital statistics comparisons (see Chapter 13).

Computational details are included in this section because it is feasible to carry out the calculations without the use of a computer, and even if a computer package is used to generate the relevant tables, the output often does not include the statistics required and the actual statistical analysis may have to be performed by hand.

Table 12.4 shows the basic data from a prospective or follow-up study to examine reasons for females having a higher 24-hour mortality after coronary artery bypass surgery (CABS) than males. It is clear from this table that females have a significantly higher 24-hour mortality. The odds ratio (OR) is 1·96 and the relative risk (RR) is 1·93.* Using the usual chi-square test this result is statistically significant at the 5% level ($\chi^2 = 5\cdot24$; d.f. $= 1$). The confidence intervals (CI) are based on the methods of Section 10.10. This example is going to consider both the relative risk and the odds ratio as measures of the association between mortality and sex, though the former would be more likely to be used in practice since this is a prospective study. If the data had arisen from a retrospective (case-control) study then of course the odds ratio would be the measure of choice.

One possible confounder examined was body surface area (BSA). BSA can be taken as a proxy for body size and it has been suggested that bypass surgery may be more difficult in persons of small stature due to smaller coronary vessels. BSA was categorized into tertiles on the basis of the distribution in all 3910 persons;

Table 12.4. Twenty-four hour mortality after coronary artery bypass surgery, by sex. (Unpublished data from the Irish Cardiac Surgery Register, with permission)

Sex	Total	At 24 hours		OR (95% CI)	RR (95% CI)
		Dead	% Dead		
Female	544	15	2·8	1·96	1·93
Male	3366	48	1·4	(1·10 − 3·50)	(1·09 − 3·39)
Total	3910	63	1·6		

* The calculations in this section are based on the numbers in the tables and not the rounded percentages.

Table 12.5. Twenty-four hour mortality after coronary artery bypass surgery by body surface area (BSA). (Unpublished data from the Irish Cardiac Surgery Register, with permission)

		At 24 hours		OR	RR
	Total	Dead	% Dead	(95% CI)	(95% CI)
Low BSA	1250	35	2·8	2·71	2·66
High BSA	2660	28	1·1	(1·68 − 4·37)	(1·66 − 4·25)
Total	3910	63	1·6		

those in the lowest tertile were designated 'low BSA', and those in the top two tertiles were designated 'high BSA'. As might be expected, a much larger proportion of the females, 483/544 (88·8%), had a low BSA compared to 767/3366 (22·8%) of the males. Table 12.5 shows also that BSA (in both sexes combined) related very strongly to 24-hour mortality, those with low BSA faring much worse ($\chi^2 = 16\cdot38$; d.f. $= 1$; $p < 0\cdot01$). It would thus seem that the sex relationship with mortality might be confounded by BSA. The fact that low BSA is associated with a higher mortality, and that females tend to have a low BSA could explain the higher mortality in females. Table 12.6 shows that this is so.

In the low BSA group, males and females fared almost identically (OR: 1·06; RR: 1·06). In the high BSA group, though females did have a higher mortality than males (OR: 1·59; RR: 1·58), this was non-significant and a smaller difference than seen in the unadjusted analysis (OR: 1·96; RR: 1·93). Given this, it would seem legitimate to conclude that *within BSA categories* females do not fare worse than males, and that the lower BSA of females explains their observed higher mortality.

As was done in the last section for means, it would be useful to be able to

Table 12.6. Twenty-four hour mortality after coronary artery bypass surgery by sex within each BSA category. (Unpublished data from the Irish Cardiac Surgery Register, with permission)

		At 24 hours		OR	RR
Sex	Total	Dead	% Dead	(95% CI)	(95% CI)
Low BSA					
Female	483	14	2·9	1·06	1·06
Male	767	21	2·7	(0·54 − 2·10)	(0·54 − 2·10)
High BSA					
Female	61	1	1·6	1·59	1·58
Male	2599	27	1·0	(0·21 − 11·79)	(0·22 − 11·40)

adjust for BSA and to estimate an adjusted odds ratio or relative risk for females versus males, together with an appropriate significance test and confidence intervals. The first step is to perform a significance test, and the appropriate test is called the Mantel–Haenzel chi-square (Mantel & Haenzel, 1959). It is used to test the null hypothesis of no overall relationship in a series of 2 × 2 tables derived either from a cohort or case-control study. (In the CABS example there are only two tables in the series defined by the low and high BSA categories.) A series of tables could also be created for the categories of a factor employed in frequency matching — and this is the preferred method for the analysis of frequency matched data.

For a single table the usual chi-square would apply and the Mantel–Haenzel chi-square is a type of combination or average of the individual chi-squares for each table in the series. Suppose there are s 2 × 2 tables in the series and the ith table is laid out as Table 12.7 (note that the layout allows for either case-control or cohort data). The quantities required in each of these tables for the Mantel–Haenzel chi-square are the number with disease and exposed, a_i, the expected value of a_i, $E(a_i)$, and the variance (standard error squared) of a_i, $V(a_i)$. The expected value of a_i is obtained as for the usual chi-square by multiplying the totals in the appropriate margins and dividing by the total sample size for the table (n_i).

$$E(a_i) = \frac{(a_i + b_i)(a_i + c_i)}{n_i}.$$ (12.1)

The variance of a_i is given by the following formula

$$V(a_i) = \frac{(a_i + b_i)(c_i + d_i)(a_i + c_i)(b_i + d_i)}{n_i^2(n_i - 1)}.$$ (12.2)

It so happens that the quantity

$$\frac{[a_i - E(a_i)]^2}{V(a_i)} = \frac{(n_i - 1)}{n_i}\chi^2$$ (12.3)

Table 12.7. Layout of the ith 2 × 2 table in a series of 2 × 2 tables

Exposure	Disease	
	Yes	No
Yes	a_i	b_i
No	c_i	d_i

$n_i = a_i + b_i + c_i + d_i$ (total sample size for the table)

where χ^2 is the usual 2×2 table chi-square. For large enough n_i the difference between the two expressions is negligible. It may seem strange that the chi-square can be obtained by looking at the entry in one cell of the table only, but of course once the value in one cell of a 2×2 table is known the others are predetermined and can be obtained by subtraction.

Now, once the three quantities, a_i, $E(a_i)$ and $V(a_i)$ have been calculated from each of the 2×2 tables in the series, the Mantel–Haenzel chi-square (which has 1 degree of freedom no matter how many tables are in the series) is obtained by the following formula which sums up the individual components of the individual table chi-squares

$$\chi^2_{\text{MH}} = \frac{[\Sigma a_i - \Sigma E(a_i)]^2}{\Sigma V(a_i)}. \tag{12.4}$$

The calculation of this chi-square for the example is detailed in Table 12.8 below. In this case the a_i cell refers to female deaths, with disease corresponding to death and exposure corresponding to being a female. $\chi^2_{\text{MH}} = 0 \cdot 08$ on 1 degree of freedom and this non-significant result suggests that when allowance is made for BSA there is no real relationship of sex to 24-hour mortality in the post CABS patient.

As with the usual chi-square, however, there are some rules relating to when it is legitimate to apply the Mantel–Haenzel test. Essentially the criterion is that the sum over each table of the minimum and maximum possible values that the numbers in the a_i cell could take, assuming fixed margins, must be at least 5 away

Table 12.8. Calculation of Mantel–Haenzel chi-square

		Dead				
Sex	Yes	No	Total	a_i	$E(a_i)$	$V(a_i)$
Low BSA						
Female	14	469	483			
Male	21	746	767			
Total	35	1215	1250	14	13·524	8·072
High BSA						
Female	1	60	61			
Male	27	2572	2599			
Total	28	2632	2660	1	0·642	0·621
Summation:				15	14·166	8·693

$$\chi^2_{\text{MH}} = \frac{(15 - 14 \cdot 166)^2}{8 \cdot 693} = 0.0800$$

from the actual Σa_i. Taking the low BSA figures in Table 12.8, the minimum number that could have died among the females is zero (assigning all the 35 deaths to the males) and the maximum that could have died is 35 (assigning all deaths to females). In the high BSA table the corresponding minimum and maximum are 0 and 28. The two relevant sums are then 0 and 63, which are both more than 5 away from the observed sum of 15, showing the validity of the Mantel−Haenzel chi-square for this example. Usually the calculation of the maximum and minimum values are straightforward as in this example, but in some situations care must be taken when the minimum might not be zero. The maximum is always the smaller of the totals in the first row and first column.

The Mantel−Haenzel chi-square essentially tests for a consistent association in the series of 2 × 2 tables examined. A non-significant chi-square means that there is no overall association, or that there is no consistent association in the tables that predominates. Thus, if some of the tables suggest an association in one direction, and if others suggest the reverse of this association, the Mantel−Haenzel chi-square may end up non-significant. Such a case involves an interaction between the factors, and a summary analysis should probably not be attempted. This will be discussed further below.

The Mantel−Haenzel method can also be used with two or more qualitative confounders by forming a single composite variable and adjusting for that (e.g. age/sex groups from the single variables defined by age group and sex). It is interesting to note also that the logrank test for the comparison of two life tables (see Section 10.13) is in fact an adaptation of the Mantel−Haenzel chi-square.

12.6 The Mantel−Haenzel summary relative risk and odds ratio

Having described the significance test for overall association, an overall summary measure of association is now required. A summary measure of association must in some sense average the measure of association in each of the individual tables. In the CABS example the relative risks for female versus male mortality were 1·06 and 1·58 in the low and high BSA groups, and any summary measure of relative risk would be expected to lie somewhere between these two estimates. Remember, the crude relative risk was 1·93 and was excessively inflated due to the confounding effect of BSA. The summary or adjusted measure should correct for such confounding.

There are a number of different summary measures available for relative risks and odds ratios in a series of 2 × 2 tables but only one will be considered here. The measures to be discussed below are referred to as the Mantel−Haenzel estimates. Essentially they are a type of average of the component measures in each of the constituent 2 × 2 tables. Table 12.9 shows the layout of a series of 2 × 2 tables for which a summary measure is to be estimated.

Table 12.9. Definition of Mantel−Haenzel summary odds ratio and relative risk measures

SINGLE TABLE

	Disease		Odds ratio (OR)	Relative risk (RR)
Exposure	Yes	No		
Yes	a	b	ad/bc	$a(c+d)/c(a+b)$
No	c	d		

$n = a + b + c + d$

SERIES OF TABLES

	Disease		OR	RR
Exposure	Yes	No		
First table				
Yes	a_1	b_1	$\dfrac{a_1 d_1}{n_1} \Big/ \dfrac{b_1 c_1}{n_1}$	$\dfrac{a_1(c_1+d_1)}{n_1} \Big/ \dfrac{c_1(a_1+b_1)}{n_1}$
No	c_1	d_1		

$n_1 = a_1 + b_1 + c_1 + d_1$

ith table				
Yes	a_i	b_i	$\dfrac{a_i d_i}{n_i} \Big/ \dfrac{b_i c_i}{n_i}$	$\dfrac{a_i(c_i+d_i)}{n_i} \Big/ \dfrac{c_i(a_i+b_i)}{n_i}$
No	c_i	d_i		

$n_i = a_i + b_i + c_i + d_i$

MANTEL−HAENZEL SUMMARY MEASURES

OR_A	RR_A
$\displaystyle \sum \frac{a_i d_i}{n_i} \Big/ \sum \frac{b_i c_i}{n_i}$	$\displaystyle \sum \frac{a_i(c_i+d_i)}{n_i} \Big/ \sum \frac{c_i(a_i+b_i)}{n_i}$
(12.5)	(12.6)

The first part of the table shows the usual definitions of the odds ratio and relative risk for a single 2×2 table. The first and *i*th 2×2 tables in the series are then shown with the odds ratio and relative risks again given for each table. This time, however, the total sample size in the table is added in to both the denominator and numerator of the formula. (This does not affect the calculated value.) The last section shows how the Mantel–Haenzel summary measures are formed from the table components by summing the various quantities over all tables in the series. The calculations for the CABS study are shown in Table 12.10 where the data from the two tables in the example are summed.

Table 12.10. Calculation of Mantel–Haenzel adjusted measures

| Exposure | Disease | | | Odds ratio (OR) | Relative risk (RR) |
	Yes	No	Total		
Low BSA					
Yes	14	469	483	8·3552/7·8792 = 1·06	8·5904/8·1144 = 1·06
No	21	746	767		
Total	35	1215	1250		
High BSA					
Yes	1	60	61	0·9669/0·6090 = 1·59	0·9771/0·6192 = 1·58
No	27	2572	2599		
Total	28	2632	2660		
Summation = adjusted measure				9·3221/8·4882 = 1·1	9·5675/8·7336 = 1·1

Thus, we see that the Mantel–Haenzel adjusted odds ratio in this case is 1.1 as an average of the two component odds ratios of 1·06 and 1·59. Greater weight is given to the risk of 1·06 since it is based on much larger numbers of deaths. The conclusion of this analysis then is that 1·1 is the best summary estimate of the odds ratio between females and males within the low and high BSA categories. The crude odds ratio of 1·96 seen in the total group is due to the fact that females tend to have a much lower BSA. The relationship of sex and mortality was confounded by BSA. Males and females with similar BSA, in fact, have almost identical mortalities after CABS. Working with the relative risks instead of the odds ratios gives an identical conclusion.

It is also possible to put confidence limits on the Mantel–Haenzel adjusted odds ratios and relative risks. This is done with the 'test-based limit' method that was employed in Section 10.10 to obtain confidence intervals for the crude measures. The Mantel–Haenzel chi-square is used in the confidence interval formula for both the odds ratio and the relative risk. The 95% confidence limits are given by

$$OR_A^{[1 \pm (1.96/\chi)]} \tag{12.7}$$

$$RR_A^{[1 \pm (1.96/\chi)]} \tag{12.8}$$

where χ is the square root of the Mantel−Haenzel chi-square and RR_A and OR_A are the adjusted relative risks and odds ratios.

The Mantel−Haenzel chi-square was 0·08 so that $1 - (1.96/\chi)$ is -5.93 and $1 + (1.96/\chi)$ is 7·93. This gives the 95% confidence interval for the corrected odds ratio of 1·1 as 0·57 to 2·13. The confidence interval for the corrected relative risk of 1·1 is obviously the same.

12.7 Confounding versus effect modification

Note that, when performing an analysis to summarize a measure of association in any set of tables, the associations in the individual tables must be examined first. Otherwise, if the associations are in different directions, or are of very different magnitude, or no one pattern predominates, a summary significance test or a summary measure may not validly describe the situation.

In the CABS example, taking age as a potential confounder, suppose that in young patients females had a higher mortality than males, but that, in older patients, females had a lower mortality. A summary measure in this case might suggest that females had a similar mortality to that of males, obscuring totally the important fact that age modifies the sex relationship with mortality. In this case age would be referred to as an *effect modifier* of the relationship between sex and mortality. The concept of effect modification is the same as that of synergy or antagonism as described in Section 10.6. Effect modification is also referred to as *interaction*.

It is important to distinguish between an effect modifier and a confounder, though a variable may at the same time act as both. Effect modification relates essentially to differences between the measure of association at different levels of the effect modifier. The crude (unadjusted) measure of association obtained when the data are analysed ignoring the effect modifier is irrelevant to the concept of effect modification. Of course, the measure of association in practice is likely to vary between different tables in any breakdown and it is to some extent a matter of judgement whether there is effect modification or not. Statistical tests are available to determine whether the measure of association varies significantly between the tables, and these tests for homogeneity of the association can act as a guide to the presence of effect modification. When effect modification is present no summary or adjusted measure can adequately summarize the association found in categories of the effect modifier.

Confounding, on the other hand, essentially means that the crude or unadjusted measure of association does not reflect the measure in each of the component tables or does not average it in some reasonable way. When a variable acts as a confounder (and not as an effect modifier), the measure of association at each level of the confounder should be to a certain extent consistent and an adjusted measure is said to summarize the underlying association.

It is possible for a variable to act simultaneously as both a confounder and an effect modifier. Table 12.11 presents some hypothetical examples of different series of relative risks (the chosen measure of association) in three categories of a confounder/effect modifier (referred to as a control variable).

In Example A the crude relative risk of 2·5 does not reflect the underlying risks in the three categories of the control variable and is in fact larger than each of them. Thus confounding is present. The three risks are however not too dissimilar so that the control variable, though a confounder, is not an effect modifier. In Example B the control variable is still not an effect modifier but could not be considered a confounder either since the crude relative risk is in a broad sense representative of the three risks in the three categories. In Examples C and D the control variable would be considered an effect modifier since the relative risks are not consistent across the three categories. In fact, the heterogeneity is quite extreme in that the risk in the third category is in the opposite direction to that in the other two categories. When effect modification is present the question of confounding becomes somewhat academic since no single measure can *adequately* summarize the three component relative risks. However, in Example C, the crude risk of 1·5 might be said to be an average of the three risks and thus the result could be considered not to be confounded. In Example D the crude value cannot in any sense be considered representative of the three category values and thus confounding could be considered present in addition to effect modification.

Table 12.11. Examples (A–D) of confounding and effect modification

| Level of control variable | Relative risk at each level of control variable | | | |
	A	B	C	D
1	1·4	1·4	1·4	1·4
2	1·8	1·8	1·8	1·8
3	1·3	1·3	0·2	0·2
Crude relative risk	2·5	1·5	1·5	2·5
Confounder	Yes	No	(No)	(Yes)
Effect modifier	No	No	Yes	Yes

It must be pointed out, however, that the whole concept of confounding or effect modification of an association depends on the precise measure used to quantify the association. Concentration here has been on the relative risk-type measures, but of course in follow-up studies the attributable risk (risk difference or excess risk) might also be employed. A variable may be an effect modifier or confounder of the relative risk for example, but not of the excess risk (see also Section 10.6). Generally, in epidemiological analysis, concentration tends to be on relative risk-type rather than difference measures.

Effect modification can of course also be present when relationships between quantitative variables are in question, and one can determine the existence of effect modification with a regression approach also. This is done by introducing an *interaction term* into the regression equation. Suppose it was suspected that age was an effect modifier of the association of exercise with serum cholesterol in the example of Section 12.3. An interaction term for exercise and age would involve creating a new variable AGE × EXERCISE, which would have the value of the individual's age if they were heavy exercisers and zero otherwise. (Note that this is just the multiplication of the values of the component variables AGE and EXERCISE which is the general formulation of an interaction term.) The multiple regression equation might then be

$$\text{CHOL} = a + b_1 \text{ AGE} + b_2 \text{ MALE} + b_3 \text{ EXERCISE} + b_4 \text{ AGE} \times \text{EXERCISE}.$$

If the b_1 coefficient were significant or large enough it might be kept in the equation showing the effect-modifying action of age on the exercise/cholesterol relationship. A change in exercise level from low to high would result in a change in cholesterol of $b_3 + b_4$ AGE. The effect of a change in exercise depends on age, and if b_4 were positive in the example, the older the subject the greater the cholesterol change would be. If effect modification is suspected or to be looked for then it is necessary to include the relevant interaction terms in a multiple regression analysis. Three-way interaction terms are also possible though their interpretation becomes somewhat difficult. Again, either judgement or the results of significance tests will have to be employed to determine if such terms should be retained in the final model. It is worthwhile noting too that interaction or effect modification is symmetrical in that in the above example, for instance, one could talk about age modifying the effect of exercise on cholesterol or exercise modifying the effect of age. The degree of effect modification relative to the main effect will, of course, depend on the magnitude of the partial regression coefficients b_1 and b_3.

12.8 Multiple logistic regression

It was seen in Section 12.4 how multiple regression allowed for the analysis of the relationship between a quantitative dependent variable and both qualitative and quantitative explanatory variables. Multiple regression can be used both to determine the joint effect of the explanatory variables on the dependent variable, and to determine the association between the dependent variable and a single explanatory one corrected for the (confounding) effects of the remaining factors. Is there any way that multiple regression could be extended to cover the case of a qualitative dependent variable? Suppose for example that an analysis was to be performed relating the explanatory variables blood glucose level (G), age (A), systolic blood pressure (SBP), relative weight (W), cholesterol (C) and number of cigarettes per day (NC) to a qualitative dependent variable, measuring the presence or absence of major abnormalities on electrocardiographs. It is possible to imagine a multiple regression analysis with the presence or absence of an ECG abnormality as a dependent variable, obtaining an equation such as

$$P = a + b_1G + b_2A + b_3SBP + \ldots,$$

where b_1, b_2, etc. are the partial regression coefficients for the corresponding variables, and P has a value of 1 for the presence of the abnormality and 0 otherwise. The problem about this approach is that the predicted values for P from the equation, for given values of the explanatory variables, could quite easily be less than 0 or greater than 1 and would thus be totally uninterpretable. If P could be constrained to lie between 0 and 1, it could be interpreted as the probability of an ECG abnormality given the set of values for the explanatory variables. *Logistic regression* is a technique which achieves this. Basically, one works with a transformed dependent variable, running a multiple regression on the transformed variable

$$Y = \ln \frac{P}{1 - P} \tag{12.9}$$

obtaining a regression equation like

$$Y = \ln \frac{P}{1 - P} = a + b_1G + b_2A + b_3SBP \ldots, \tag{12.10}$$

where P is interpreted as the probability of an ECG abnormality. Given the form of this equation, P is constrained to lie between 0 and 1, and so has the required properties of a probability. If P is the probability of an event then $P/(1-P)$ is the odds of that event so that Eqn. 12.10 is a type of multiple regression equation with the dependent variable transformed to be the ln of the odds* (see Section 10.10 for a discussion of the natural log and exponential functions). Obviously,

$$P/(1 - P) = e^Y. \tag{12.11}$$

---

* It should be noted however that logistic regression cannot be performed using a standard least squares multiple regression package on a computer. A special program is needed.

The ln of the odds can be converted back to a probability giving a direct relationship between the probability of disease and the explanatory variables

$$P = \frac{e^{\hat{Y}}}{1 + e^{\hat{Y}}} \tag{12.12}$$

where

$$\hat{Y} = a + b_1 G + b_2 A + b_3 SBP \ldots \tag{12.13}$$

is the predicted value of Y for a given set of values for the explanatory variables. Table 12.12 shows the multiple logistic regression coefficients obtained for a study on ECG abnormalities using the variables already discussed. Coefficients significantly different from 0 are marked with an asterisk; relative weight was defined as the percentage of desirable weight based on standard weight tables. To show how the results of such an analysis might be employed, the equation will be used to predict the probability of an ECG abnormality for a male aged 50 years, with a blood glucose level of 98·2 mg/dl, a systolic blood pressure of 140 mmHg, a relative weight of 115%, a cholesterol level of 230 mg/dl and who smokes 25 cigarettes per day. The predicted $\hat{Y}$ value for this individual, using the values of the coefficients in Table 8.2, is

$$\hat{Y} = -12·1041 + 0·0009 \, (98·2) + 0·1339 \, (50) + 0·0178 \, (140)$$
$$-0·0079 \, (115) + 0·0034 \, (230) + 0·0075 \, (25)$$
$$= -2·768.$$

When this value is substituted into Eqn. 12.12, the value for P is found to be 0·059. (This P is not to be confused with p denoting significance level.) Thus, on the basis of this study, an individual with the listed characteristics would have a

Table 12.12. Multiple logistic regression coefficients for the relationship between six variables and ECG abnormalities in 3357 men aged 40–54. Abbreviated from Hickey *et al.* (1979) with permission

Variable	Logistic regression coefficients (b)
Glucose	0·0009
Age	0·1339*
SBP	0·0178*
Relative weight	−0·0079
Cholesterol	0·0034
No. of cigarettes	0·0075
Constant	−12·1041

* $p < 0·05$.

5·9% chance of having an ECG abnormality. The magnitude of the logistic regression coefficients gives some idea of the relative importance of various factors in producing the probability of an abnormality.

The coefficient for a particular factor can be interpreted as giving the amount of change in the ln(odds) for a unit change in that factor, holding all other explanatory variables constant. A partial multiple logistic regression coefficient for a variable expresses its relationship with the dependent variable corrected for the confounding effects of other explanatory variables.

When, however, there is a qualitative explanatory variable with 0/1 coding, the interpretation of the partial regression coefficient is particularly appealing. For instance, a logistic regression analysis on the CABS data of Section 12.6 gave the following equation for the odds of death:

$$\frac{P}{1-P} = e^{[-4.236 \; + \; 0.673 \; (\text{FEMALE})]}$$

where P was the probability of a 24-hour death and FEMALE was a binary variable coded 1 for a female and 0 for a male. From this the odds of death for a female are

$$e^{(-4.236 \; + \; 0.673)}$$

and that for a male are

$$e^{(-4.236)}.$$

The odds ratio for females compared to males is simply the first of these quantities divided by the second, which using the properties of exponents gives

$$\text{OR} = e^{(0.673)} = 1.96$$

where the constant term cancels out. Thus, the exponential of the logistic regression coefficient gives the odds ratio for that factor. The same value for the odds ratio was already calculated directly from the 2×2 table of sex by mortality in Table 12.4. This is a general result if there is only one explanatory variable. The logistic regression equation for the CABS example with two explanatory variables FEMALE and LOWBSA is

$$\frac{P}{1-P} = e^{[-4.546 \; + \; 0.095(\text{FEMALE}) \; + \; 0.961(\text{LOWBSA})]}$$

where LOWBSA is a variable taking on a value of 1 for those with low BSA, and 0 otherwise. Note first that the logistic regression coefficient for FEMALE is quite reduced compared to the situation when LOWBSA was not in the model − confirming the confounding effect of that variable. Using similar arguments to that above, the exponential of 0·095 can be interpreted as the odds ratio for females compared to males, corrected for LOWBSA:

$$OR_A = e^{(0.095)} = 1.1.$$

This is the same as the Mantel–Haenzel corrected estimate of Table 12.10. Logistic regression thus provides an alternative method for the control of confounding in 2 × 2 tables. With all binary variables in a logistic regression the numerical results for the adjusted odds ratios are usually quite close to the Mantel–Haenzel estimates. Ninety-five per cent confidence intervals for the odds ratio can be obtained by taking the regression coefficient plus or minus 1·96 times its standard error (given by most computer outputs) and taking the exponential of the result.

Logistic regression of course entails using the odds ratio as the measure of association and the method above can thus also be used for case-control data. Note, however, that the constant term in the regression has no interpretation in the case-control situation even though the computer package is likely to calculate it.

Logistic regression is a very powerful technique and, though not as easy to use as the Mantel–Haenzel approach, has a number of advantages in the analysis of a binary dependent variable. Firstly it can deal with a large number of variables when the Mantel–Haenzel adjustment may fail to work because of very small numbers in the component 2 × 2 tables. Logistic regression, too, can account for quantitative confounders without having to categorize them, and can examine effect modification (interaction) easily. Being a regression technique it examines many variables simultaneously, whereas the Mantel–Haenzel technique is specifically for the control of confounding on one particular association.

Logistic regression is often used for the analysis of mortality but it must be stressed that it can only analyse mortality determined at a fixed time point from study commencement. The dependent binary variable alive/dead must be defined for each subject at this specific time point and withdrawals or losses to follow-up cannot be accounted for.

12.9 Life table analysis and Cox regression

Confounding effects can of course also arise in the analysis of mortality in a variable follow-up situation. The logrank test of Section 10.13, however, can be extended to allow control of the confounding effect of other qualitative variables in life table comparisons. An alternative to this approach is to use *Cox's life table regression* model or, as it is sometimes called, the *proportional hazards* model (Cox, 1972). Essentially this is a multiple regression approach to the analysis of censored data. Remember that logistic regression discussed in the last section can only be used for the analysis of survival or mortality when the status of all subjects is known at a fixed time point and Cox's regression is to the life table what logistic regression is to the ordinary 2×2 table. An advanced text should be consulted for details of this regression method.

12.10 Multivariate analysis

The methods discussed so far in this chapter are often referred to as multivariate techniques since they are concerned with the variability of a dependent variable related to multiple explanatory variables. Technically , however, multivariate analysis is a body of methods designed to handle simultaneous variation in a number of dependent variables. Only a brief excursion through these techniques is attempted here, and the reader should be warned that the techniques are difficult to use and can easily be misapplied. An example of a multivariate technique is *discriminant analysis*. Suppose two populations are defined by a set of characteristics such as height, weight, serum cholesterol level, etc., and that for each characteristic the two distributions overlap so that, for example, the distribution of heights in population A overlaps with the distribution of heights in population B. Thus, although the mean height of individuals in population A may be less than the mean height of individuals in population B, one individual picked at random from population A may be taller than an individual picked at random from population B. Consequently, if an individual was encountered and it was not known which population that individual belonged to, he could not be definitely assigned to a particular population unless, for any one of the variables concerned, the distributions were known not to overlap.

The purpose of discriminant analysis is to enable individual units to be assigned to one or other of the populations with, in some defined sense, the greatest probability of being correct (or smallest risk of error). The techniques of analysis, which are not explained here, involve the specification of a discriminant function, in which the relevant variables are assigned a weight or coefficient. If the discriminant function is linear in form, it will 'look like' a multiple regression equation. For a particular individual or case, values of the variables (height, weight, etc.) are substituted in the discriminant equation and a value for the function calculated. On the basis of this value the individual is assigned to a particular population. As an indication of the possible application of discriminant analysis, suppose it is desired to allocate individuals to a 'high risk' or 'low risk' category for a particular disease, the allocation being made on the basis of certain diagnostic variables, e.g. blood pressure and age. Coefficients of the discriminant function are estimated using sample observations of those who have and have not contracted the disease in some past period. Individuals can then be assigned to one or other category using the discriminant function as the method of allocation. Discriminant analysis has very close theoretical connections with logistic regression, but can easily be extended to the case of more than two groups.

Other multivariate techniques do not require specification of group membership prior to analysis, and can classify individuals or allocate them to groups which are distinct in some sense. These groups are defined by the data structure, and may or may not be logical or natural in themselves. *Principal components analysis, factor analysis* and *cluster analysis* (numerical taxonomy) are different techniques used in this area. However, not many applications in the general medical literature are seen, although the techniques have, for example, been used to classify psychiatric diagnosis on the basis of patient symptoms.

12.11 Summary

In this section the analytic techniques for the control of confounding and examination of multiple explanatory factors for a variable have been considered. Many of these methods were also shown to be suitable for the comparison of frequency-matched groups as might be found in a case-control study or clinical trial. Table 12.13 summarizes the methods discussed and Table 12.14 repeats the formulae for the Mantel−Haenzel summary measures and chi-square.

Table 12.13. Summary of multivariate techniques for the control of confounding and for the examination of the effects of explanatory factors

Explanatory or confounding variable(s)	Dependent variable			
	Mean	Binary proportion (risk)	Rate	Life table Survival (mortality)
Qualitative only	ANOVA	Mantel−Haenzel techniques	Vital statistics methods (see Ch. 13)	Logrank methods
Quantitative and/or qualitative	Analysis of covariance Multiple regression	Logistic regression	−	Cox regression

Table 12.14. Summary of Mantel−Haenzel techniques for the control of confounding or the analysis of matched/stratified data

*i*th table in series of 2 × 2 tables			Formulae	Eqn. nos.
	Disease			
Exposure	Yes	No	$n_i = a_i + b_i + c_i + d_i$	
Yes	a_i	b_i	$E(a_i) = \dfrac{(a_i + b_i)(a_i + c_i)}{n_i}$	(12.1)
No	c_i	d_i	$V(a_i) = \dfrac{(a_i + b_i)(c_i + d_i)(a_i + c_i)(b_i + d_i)}{n^2{}_i(n_i - 1)}$	(12.2)

Mantel−Haenzel chi-square

$$\chi^2{}_{MH} = \frac{[\Sigma a_i - \Sigma E(a_i)]^2}{\Sigma V(a_i)} \tag{12.4}$$

$$\text{d.f.} = 1$$

Mantel−Haenzel summary measures

$$OR_A = \Sigma \frac{a_i d_i}{n_i} \bigg/ \Sigma \frac{b_i c_i}{n_i} \tag{12.5}$$

$$RR_A = \Sigma \frac{a_i(c_i + d_i)}{n_i} \bigg/ \Sigma \frac{c_i(a_i + b_i)}{n_i} \tag{12.6}$$

Confidence intervals

$$OR_A{}^{(1 \pm z_c/\chi)} \tag{12.7}$$
$$RR_A{}^{(1 \pm z_c/\chi)} \tag{12.8}$$

13

Vital Statistics

13.1 Introduction

A branch of statistics which is of particular interest to medical and social scientists is that concerned with the study of human populations, usually described as *demography*. Demographic studies involve *vital statistics* such as death rates and birth rates, the use and calculation of which are discussed in this chapter.

Vital statistics measures are commonly expressed in the form of *rates*; thus it is usual to speak of death rates, birth rates, bed-occupancy rates, and so on.* This is because absolute numbers are not very informative when, as is often the case, one wishes to compare, say, mortality conditions in two or more different countries or areas, or in the same area at different points in time. The larger the population of an area, the larger will be the expected number of deaths in any given interval of time. If, therefore, the mortality conditions of areas of different populations are to be compared it is necessary to use a measure such as the annual number of deaths per 1000 population, which is independent of the absolute size of the population.

13.2 Measures of mortality

The simplest measure of mortality is the crude death rate, defined as the number of deaths in a particular time period (usually a year) per thousand population. The annual crude death rate can be expressed as

$$\frac{\text{Annual number of deaths}}{\text{Mean population during the year}} \times 1000.$$

Note that since, typically, the population varies slightly during the year, the denominator is an estimate of the 'mid-year' population (often, however, this is difficult to estimate accurately unless there are regular and up-to-date population census data available).

---

* Although described as rates, some of the measures defined below are measures of risk rather than rates in the strict sense. However, this distinction is not pursued here.

Separate crude death rates can be calculated for males and females, for particular areas of a country, and for other subgroups in the total population, including particular age groups, to which reference is made below. The denominator would then refer to the mean population of the particular subgroup or area of interest.

For analytical purposes, crude death rates are of limited usefulness and may be misleading if used for comparisons. For example, country A may have a higher crude death rate than country B simply because, at the time of the comparison, the former had a higher proportion of elderly people. The death rate at every age may be lower and the expectation of life higher in A, and it would therefore be misleading to conclude, on the basis of a comparison of crude death rates, that country B's population is healthier or enjoys a higher level of medical care than that of country A. Comparisons must take into account the age distribution of the population. In addition, the overall crude death rate is also affected by the sex ratio in the population, since females generally have a longer expectation of life than males and, usually, separate death rates for females and males are calculated. Crude death rates for a number of countries are illustrated in Table 13.1, and a glance at the relative rates for different countries suggests the importance of age distribution as a determinant of the rate.

Table 13.1. Crude death rates (per 1000) for various countries (from *United Nations Demographic Yearbook (1987)*)

		Crude death rate	
Country	Year	Males	Females
Brazil	1984	7·4	5·1
Bulgaria	1984	12·6	10·0
Chile	1983	7·3	5·4
Denmark	1984	12·0	10·4
France	1983	10·8	9·8
Hong Kong	1984	5·2	4·3
Ireland*	1983	10·2	8·6
Israel	1984	7·2	6·2
Japan	1984	6·8	5·5
Mauritious	1984	7·6	5·5
New Zealand	1984	8·5	7·1
Thailand	1984	5·2	3·8
United Kingdom	1984	11·6	11·1
United States	1983	9·4	7·8
West Germany	1984	11·4	11·4

* In this and subsequent references, Ireland means the Republic of Ireland.

A way of neutralizing the effect of age distribution on the crude death rate is to calculate separate death rates for each age group in the population. These are called *age-specific death rates*, defined as

$$\frac{\text{Number of deaths in a specific age group}}{\text{Mean population of that age group}} \times 1000.$$

(Deaths and mean population relate to a specific calendar period, usually a year, although some rates are calculated at quarterly or even monthly intervals.)

Corresponding age-specific death rates for different populations can then be compared. An overall test for any significant difference in the mortality experience of two populations, allowing for differences in age structure, can be carried out using the Mantel–Haenzel χ^2 test (see Chapter 12). The comparability of these rates is also affected by the age distribution *within* each age group but, provided that the age group class intervals are fairly narrow, the influence of the within-group age distribution can be considered negligible. Five-year and 10-year age group intervals are commonly used. As an example, age-specific death rates for Scotland and for England and Wales are recorded in Table 13.2.

Table 13.2. Age-specific mortality rates (per 1000) in England and Wales, and Scotland in 1984 (from *United Nations Demographic Yearbook (1987)*)

Age group (years)	England & Wales		Scotland	
	Males	Females	Males	Females
All ages	11·6	11·1	12·4	11·9
0 − 1	10·8	8·5	11·9	9·1
1 − 4	0·5	0·4	0·6	0·5
5 − 9	0·2	0·2	0·3	0·2
10 − 14	0·3	0·2	0·3	0·2
15 − 19	0·7	0·3	0·8	0·3
20 − 24	0·8	0·3	0·9	0·4
25 − 29	0·8	0·4	1·0	0·5
30 − 34	0·9	0·6	1·3	0·6
35 − 39	1·3	0·9	1·6	1·1
40 − 44	2·1	1·4	2·8	1·8
45 − 49	4·0	2·5	5·4	3·3
50 − 54	7·0	4·3	9·1	5·6
55 − 59	12·7	7·3	16·1	9·6
60 − 64	21·6	11·5	25·2	14·8
65 − 69	35·0	18·4	41·4	22·4
70 − 74	54·5	29·1	63·5	34·2
75 − 79	84·6	48·3	96·5	59·9
80 − 84	129·9	82·1	140·0	89·2
85	211·3	169·0	221·5	177·8

Note that male mortality rates exceed female mortality rates in all (except one) age groups, a characteristic common to all developed and most developing countries. Note also, the relatively high mortality rates in the age group under 1 year (infant mortality) compared with subsequent age groups. This is further discussed below.

Although age-specific death rates provide an appropriate basis for comparing the mortality experience of different populations, it is useful to have a single overall measure of mortality which, unlike the crude death rate, allows for the effects of age distribution (assume throughout that males and females are considered separately). This is achieved by the calculation of one or more of a number of *standardized* mortality measures, the best-known of which will be described in the following section.

An age-specific death rate of particular interest is the *infant mortality rate*, which is often taken as an indicator of the level of medical and social standards in a community. It is defined as the number of deaths of infants under 1 year of age during a calendar period per 1000 live births during the same period:

$$\frac{\text{Number of deaths of infants under 1 year of age during a calendar period}}{\text{Live births during the same period}} \times 1000.$$

The infant mortality rate can be subdivided into two further rates, the *neonatal mortality rate* and the *post-neonatal mortality rate*. The neonatal mortality rate is defined as the number of deaths of infants under 28 days during a calendar period per 1000 live births during the same period:

$$\frac{\text{Number of deaths of infants under 28 days during a calendar period}}{\text{Live births during the same period}} \times 1000.$$

The post-neonatal mortality rate is defined as the number of deaths of infants 28 days and over and under 1 year during a calendar period per 1000 live births during the same period:

$$\frac{\text{Number of deaths of infants 28 days and over and under 1 year during a calendar period}}{\text{Live births during the same period}} \times 1000.$$

By definition, the sum of the neonatal and post-neonatal mortality rates provides the figure for the infant mortality rate. The reason for this subdivision of the infant mortality rate is that death in the early part of any infant's life is governed mainly by prenatal influences (e.g. congenital malformation, immaturity), while death in the later part of the first year is more generally environmental in origin (e.g. pneumonia, bronchitis). It is important then to calculate different rates for these periods of an infant's life.

A *stillbirth rate* may also be calculated. This is defined as the number of stillbirths during a calendar period per 1000 total (live and still) births during the same period:

$$\frac{\text{Number of stillbirths during a calendar period}}{\text{Total (live and still) births during the same period}} \times 1000.$$

The *perinatal mortality rate* has received increased attention in recent years. It is defined as the number of stillbirths, together with the number of deaths within the first 7 days of life, during a calendar period per 1000 total (live and still) births in the same period:

$$\frac{\text{Number of stillbirths} + \text{deaths within the first 7 days of life during a calendar period}}{\text{Total (live and still) births during the same period}} \times 1000.$$

There are several reasons for creating a perinatal mortality rate. Stillbirths and early neonatal deaths commonly have a similar aetiology, and the rate is regarded as an important index of the quality of obstetrical care. Further, since an infant who shows *any* sign of life is not regarded as being a stillbirth, the perinatal mortality rate overcomes the difficulty of deciding whether or not an infant is stillborn.

A *maternal mortality rate* is defined as the deaths ascribed to puerperal causes during a calendar period per 1000 total (live and still) births during the same period:

$$\frac{\text{Deaths ascribed to puerperal causes during the calendar period}}{\text{Total (live and still) births during the same period}} \times 1000.$$

The *case fatality (mortality) rate* is often of interest if one wishes to determine the proportion of patients with a particular disease or condition who die, e.g. in a pertussis outbreak. It is defined as the number of deaths from a particular disease or condition as a percentage of the total numbers suffering from the disease or condition:

$$\frac{\text{Number of deaths from a particular disease or condition}}{\text{Total numbers suffering from the disease or condition}} \times 100.$$

In concluding this section on the measurement of mortality it is pertinent to refer to the accuracy of death certification. A variety of studies on the accuracy of certified cause of death have been conducted. These include international comparisons of medical certificates of cause of death; comparisons of clinical findings with those found at autopsy; assessment, by means of a survey of certifiers, of the diagnostic evidence recorded on the certificate; comparison of the wording on the death certificate with the clinical diagnosis obtained from clinical case notes; and examination of the relation between certified cause of death and the age of the certifying doctor. All of these studies, using different approaches, have demonstrated considerable inaccuracies in certification and have shown it to be subject to various errors. There are three important reasons why accurate statistics of mortality are required: firstly, mortality data are frequently used to identify associated factors, e.g. occupation; secondly, mortality data are necessary to plan health services and later to evaluate these services, e.g. screening for cervical cancer; and finally, such data are of importance in research studies of an epidemiological type. For these reasons then, the medical profession must endeavour to determine accurately the condition from which a patient has died. It is not possible here to enter into a discussion of methods of improving accuracy of death certification but increasing autopsy rates would help considerably, although it should be emphasized that autopsies are not a complete answer. There is, among other things, a great need for education of medical graduates and undergraduates in the correct method of death certification and of the importance of determining the true cause of death.

13.3 Standardized mortality rates

As noted above, crude death rates for different populations cannot be properly compared because of the confounding effects of differing age distributions. Several methods are available for adjusting for age distribution in the calculation of mortality rates. As an example, suppose it is desired to compare the mortality experience of the populations of two different regions in a country. The *direct method* of standardization is as follows: the age-specific mortality rates of the first region, and then of the second region, are successively applied to the corresponding age groups of a *standard population*, yielding the number of deaths that would occur in that standard population if it were subject to the mortality rates prevailing in each region. The hypothetical numbers of deaths resulting from these calculations are denoted as D_1 and D_2 respectively. Any difference between these two figures can be attributed to differences in the mortality rates of the two regions, since the effect of age distribution has been eliminated by the use of a standard (common) population.

The hypothetical numbers of deaths, D_1 and D_2, can be expressed as a rate. If the size (number) of the standard population is denoted P, then the expression $(D_1 \times 1000)/P$ is called the *direct age-standardized death rate* for region 1, while $(D_2 \times 1000)/P$ is the direct age-standardized death rate for region 2. These statistics give the overall death rates that would occur in the standard population, if that population were subject to the age-specific mortality rates of regions 1 and 2 respectively.

As a slightly different example, Table 13.3 records mortality experience in 1986 for the population of Ireland, and for the population of travelling people, or

Table 13.3. Mortality experience of the Irish traveller (itinerant) population, 1986 (data aggregated and rounded; from Barry & Daly, 1988 and Barry *et al.*, 1989, with permission)

Age group	Population (000)	Deaths	Age-specific death rate (per 1000)
General Irish population			
0 − 24	1640	1200	0·7317
24 − 44	920	1300	1·4130
45 − 64	590	5500	9·3220
65 +	390	26000	66·6667
All ages	3540	34000	9·6045
Irish traveller population			
0 − 24	11·7	22	1·8803
25 − 44	2·8	10	3·5714
45 − 64	1·1	24	21·8182
65 +	0·3	28	93·3333
All ages	15·9	84	5·2830

itinerants, a small subgroup within the population. For simplicity of presentation (and also because of the small numbers of travelling people), wider than normal age groups are used for age-specific mortality rates, and the data refer to males and females taken together. From the aggregate data on population and deaths, the crude death rate for the population of Ireland is 9·60 per 1000, while that for travellers is 5·28 per 1000; age-specific death rates, however, are much higher for travellers in every age group. The crude death rate for travellers is lower because that population contains a much higher proportion of people in the youngest age group (in which age-specific mortality is lowest), and a lower proportion of people in the oldest age group (in which age-specific mortality is highest).

If the age-specific mortality rates for travellers are applied to the national (standard) population, the estimated number of deaths is 55 643, or an age-standardized death rate of 15·72 per 1000. This is much higher than the actual death rate of 9·60 in the standard population, and reflects the less favourable health status of travellers.

An alternative, though equivalent mortality measure is the *comparative mortality figure* (CMF). If the actual or observed deaths in the standard population is denoted as D, and the hypothetical or 'expected' number of deaths obtained by applying the age-specific death rates of the subgroup population to the standard population is denoted as D_E, then the CMF is calculated as $(D_E/D) \times 100$. The CMF is thus defined as the ratio of 'expected' deaths (i.e. the number that would occur if the standard population were subject to the mortality conditions of the subgroup population of interest) to observed deaths, multiplied by 100 to express it in percentage terms. A CMF less than 100 indicates that mortality conditions in a particular subgroup are 'better' than in the standard population, while a CMF greater than 100 indicates they are worse. Moreover, the CMFs for different subgroups can be compared.

From the travellers' example (Table 13.3), the actual number of deaths in the standard population is recorded as 34 000, while the 'expected' number of deaths, obtained by applying age-specific death rates for travellers to the standard population, was calculated to be 55 643. The CMF is therefore $(55\,643/34\,000) \times 100 = 163{\cdot}7$, confirming the much poorer mortality experience of travelling people.

The direct age-standardized death rate and the CMF are related. Defining the observed death rate for the standard population as $(D \times 1000)/P$, it is easily shown that

$$\text{CMF} = \frac{\text{Direct age-standardized death rate for the subgroup of interest}}{\text{Observed death rate for standard population}} \times 100.$$

The thoughtful reader may remark that, while the measures explained above have been standardized with respect to age, the numerical values of the measures will depend upon the standard population selected. In the example above, and in similar cases, the normal practice is to select as standard the national population, of which the populations of different regions, or occupations, or socio-economic groups form a part. For comparisons over time, however, there is a choice of standard populations, and the numerical values of the CMFs will vary, depending on which year is selected as the population standard. If the age structure of the standard population remains relatively stable over time, which year is chosen as standard will not make a great deal of difference, particularly since it is the relative rather than the absolute values of the CMF which are of interest. Nevertheless, this is a potential limitation of the CMF. Another feature of direct standardization which may cause problems is where the population of interest (of a region, or occupational group, or whatever) is small, or contains small numbers in particular age groups. In these circumstances, the chance occurrence of one or two individual deaths in a particular year may give rise to a much greater than normal age-specific mortality rate and hence distort the CMF. The converse (i.e. an atypically low mortality rate in a particular age group) may also occur.

In the *indirect method* of standardization, the age-specific mortality rates of a standard population are applied to the corresponding age groups of the subgroup population(s) of interest, to yield the number of deaths 'expected' if each subgroup experienced the mortality conditions of the standard population. Denoting the number of expected deaths in a particular subgroup as E, and the observed or actual number of deaths in that subgroup as O, the ratio of observed to expected deaths, usually multiplied by 100, is called the *standardized mortality ratio* (SMR). Thus,

$$\text{SMR} = \frac{O}{E} \times 100.$$

Referring again to the example in Table 13.3, application of age-specific death rates for the national population to the population of travellers yields 43 'expected' deaths (rounded to the nearest whole number). Actual deaths were 84. The SMR is therefore (84/43) × 100 = 195·4 and confirms again the much poorer mortality experience of travellers. An SMR less than 100, on the other hand, indicates a better mortality experience compared with the standard population.

Like the CMF, the SMR is based on a comparison of observed and expected deaths and is similarly interpreted. The former compares observed deaths in the standard population with the number that would have occurred if that population had been subject to the age-specific mortality rates of the subgroup of interest. The latter compares the observed deaths in a particular subgroup with the number that would have occurred if that subgroup had been subject to the age-specific mortality rates of the standard population. As with the method of direct standardization, the calculations involved in indirect standardization also permit the calculation of an overall age-standardized death rate; without further elaboration, this is obtained as the product of the SMR (defined here as a ratio rather than a percentage) and the crude death rate of the standard population. Thus, in the travellers' example the age-standardized death rate for travellers is 1·954 × 9·60 = 18·76 per 1000.

In many applications, the CMF and the SMR will be equal or very close in value, but this is by no means always the case. In the travellers' example, the CMF and the SMR are not very close in value because the age distributions of the two populations are significantly different, as already noted, but both measures point to the same conclusion. Like the CMF, the SMR has a number of limitations, but it requires less information to calculate. In particular, it is not necessary to know the age distribution of deaths in the subgroups of interest.

SMRs are commonly used in analysis of mortality in different socio-economic or occupational groups. As an example, Table 13.4 records a sample of standardized mortality ratios for males aged 20 − 64 in Great Britain, covering all causes of death.

The total population of men aged 20 − 64 is the standard population, and the (all causes) age-specific mortality rates of this population have been applied to each occupational population to estimate 'expected' deaths. The ratio of actual to expected deaths, multiplied by 100, gives the SMR. Figures over 100 imply a mortality experience worse than that of the standard population, while those less than 100 indicate a favourable mortality experience. Crude death rates are also recorded in the table. Although the pattern of crude death rates is rather similar

Table 13.4. Standardized mortality ratios (SMR) for selected occupations, men aged 20 − 64, Great Britain, 1979 − 80 and 1982 − 83, all causes of death (from Office of Population Census and Surveys, 1986)

Occupational group	SMR	Crude death rate (per 1000)
All persons	100	5·6
Economists, statisticians and actuaries	84	2·9
University academic staff	48	2·4
Medical and dental practitioners	65	3·5
Professional sportsmen	117	3·1
Publicans	152	9·9
Clerks	95	6·1
Police sergeants	159	5·1
Farm workers	112	6·0
Butchers	140	5·9
Bricklayers	106	5·8
Stevedores, dockers	168	11·1
Bus and coach drivers	119	5·9

to that of the SMR, the figure for 'professional sportsmen' is an illustration of how crude death rates can give a misleading impression of mortality experience. The crude death rate for this occupation is quite low, at 3·1 per 1000 (compared with 5·6 for all men aged 20−64), but the SMR is 117, indicating that when age distribution is taken into account, the mortality experience of professional sportsmen is worse than that of all males aged 20−64. The low crude death rate simply reflects the fact that the population of this occupation contains a large proportion of younger age groups, in which mortality rates are relatively lower.

Since SMRs are calculated by applying a standard set of specific mortality rates to each occupational population, SMRs for different occupations are not strictly comparable; the correct comparison is between the occupational SMR and the standard population. However, provided the age distributions of different occupations are similar, occupational SMRs can be compared.

Another application of SMRs is illustrated in Table 13.5. Here interest is in the mortality experience of different occupational groups with respect to a particular cause of death, in this case diseases of the respiratory system. Age-specific mortality rates for diseases of the respiratory system for all males aged 20 − 64 have been applied to different occupational groups, to determine the number of deaths expected if the mortality experience of the particular occupational group was identical to the standard (all males aged 20 − 64) population. The ratio of actual to expected deaths yields the SMR. The table shows, for

Table 13.5. SMR of men aged 20 − 64 from diseases of the respiratory system, by occupational order, Great Britain 1979 − 80 and 1982 − 83 (from Office of Population Census and Surveys, 1986)

Occupational order	SMR
Professional and related workers in education, welfare and health	40
Managerial	55
Clerical and related	85
Farming, fishing and related	114
Electrical and electronic workers	86
Transport and related workers	117
Materials storing and related	121

instance, that mortality from respiratory diseases is far lower amongst professional and managerial workers than in the total population, while workers in transport and materials handling, and farming and fishing, experience a worse than average mortality from these diseases.

Pursuing this a little further, Table 13.6 records SMRs for various causes of death for four of the occupational groups listed in Table 13.5. Management occupations display relatively low mortality in all five causes of death, and this is true also for other causes of death not listed here. Chemical workers experience relatively low mortality from mental disorders, but high mortality from congenital anomalies.

Table 13.6. SMR of men aged 20 − 64 by cause of death and occupational order, Great Britain, 1979 − 80 and 1982 − 83 (from Office of Population Census and Surveys, 1986)

	Infectious and parasitic diseases	Neoplasms	Mental disorders	Congenital anomalies	Diseases of the circulatory system
Managerial	66	83	50	65	86
Chemical and related	96	91	56	128	103
Farming, fishing and related	108	104	82	113	97
Transport and related	84	117	86	60	115

It is necessary to exercise caution in the interpretation of standardized mortality ratios for particular occupations or social groups. Firstly, in some cases quite small populations are being considered, and SMRs can change significantly from one period to the next, just through chance. Secondly, SMRs do not necessarily indicate the mortality risk of a particular occupation; in a pure experiment, individuals would be randomly allocated to particular occupations and their mortality experience then examined, but of course in reality the choice of occupation is not a random process. Professional athletes, for example, need talent and specific physical characteristics to make a success of such a career, while fishermen will usually be found amongst people who live on or near a sea coast with an established fishing industry. Occupational mortality may, therefore, be influenced not so much by the nature of the occupation as by other factors (education, area of work or residence, specific employment requirements and so on) which are associated with individuals who work in that occupation. In principle these factors, like age and sex, should also be standardized before valid comparisons of occupational mortality risk can be made, and more complex standardization techniques do take account of this.

The use of standardized mortality ratios is a well-established technique in analysis of mortality. Less well known, but attracting increasing attention, is the concept of *premature mortality*. Underlying this concept is the notion that death implies a loss of potential years of life, and that the younger the age at death, the greater the loss. For instance, suppose the average expectation of life in a particular population is 67 years. An individual who dies aged 40 can be said to 'lose' 27 years of potential life. If we know the age at death of every individual who dies in a particular calendar period, it is possible to calculate the total years of potential life lost (YPLL) for that population in the given calendar period. If we also know the cause of death, it is possible to calculate years of potential life lost for specific causes of death (in effect, to disaggregate by cause the overall YPLL). Alternatively, if we know the occupation or socio-economic status of each decedent, YPLLs for particular occupations or socio-economic groups can be calculated.

Before commenting further on the method of calculation, the distinctive feature of the premature mortality approach is the emphasis on mortality experience in younger age groups. The younger the age at death, the greater the years of potential life lost: hence, in the overall measure of YPLL, the mortality experience of the younger age groups is given greater weight. This contrasts with more conventional measures such as cause-specific mortality rates, which are dominated by the mortality experience of the elderly (since most deaths occur amongst the elderly). As a result, a ranking of causes of death by YPLL may be quite different from a ranking by cause-specific mortality, and this could have implications for health planning priorities. Moreover, comparisons of YPLL for different socio-economic groups may identify vulnerable or high-risk groups (e.g. ethnic minorities) to which additional health resources could be targeted.

Several different definitions and methods of calculation of premature mortality have been proposed. The most contentious issue concerns the selection of the upper end-point for the calculation of YPLL. As suggested above, one possibility is to take the average expectation of life at birth as the end-point (for further discussion of expectation of life, see Section 13.8). Thus, if the average expectation of life at birth is 67 years, the YPLL for any individual decedent is 67 minus age at death. For individuals who die at age 67 or above, the YPLL would be zero. An alternative method, which is less strongly biased towards younger age groups, is to take as the end-point the average expectation of life at age of death. For instance, supposing that the average expectation of life at age 40 is 30 years implies an end-point of 70 years; for an individual who dies at 40, the YPLL is therefore $70 - 40 = 30$ years. Since expectation of life varies at every age, this method involves the use of a range of end-points, and also ensures that every individual death, including the elderly, contributes to the calculation of the YPLL.

13.4 Statistical inference with vital statistics

Often, because vital statistics measures are based on very large numbers — thus reducing chance variation — statistical inference and significance testing tend not to be performed. However, when small groups are being analysed (as in the itinerants' example) or when there are only small differences, statistical analysis can be a useful adjunct. This section considers confidence interval estimation for some of the measures discussed.

Confidence intervals for age-specific rates and crude rates can be estimated using the methods of Section 4.9, assuming a Poisson distribution for the number of deaths. Now the directly standardized rate can be defined by

$$R_{(\text{adj})} = \frac{\Sigma N_i r_i}{\Sigma N_i}$$

where i represents the age group, N_i is the standard population in age group i and r_i is the age-specific rate in the study population. For example, in Table 13.3 for the first age group $0 - 24$, $N_i = 1\,640\,000$, and $r_i = 1\cdot8803$ (per 1000). The directly standardized rate was 15·72 per 1000. The standard error of a directly standardized rate is given by

$$\text{SE}\,(R_{(\text{adj})}) = \frac{\sqrt{\Sigma N_i^2\, r_i/n_i}}{\Sigma N_i}$$

where n_i is the number in the study population on which the age specific rate (r_i) is based. Note that n_i and r_i must both be expressed in the same form (e.g. in thousands and per 1000 respectively). The N_i may be expressed in any convenient unit and in this example is in thousands. Using the data on itinerants in Table 13.3

$$\text{SE } (R_{(\text{adj})}) = \frac{\sqrt{(1640)^2 \ 1 \cdot 8803/11 \cdot 7 + (920)^2 \ 3 \cdot 5714/2 \cdot 8 + \ldots}}{1640 + 920 + \ldots}$$

which turns out to be 2·11 (per 1000). A 95% confidence interval for the standardized rate is then

$$R_{(\text{adj})} \pm 1 \cdot 96 \text{ SE } (R_{(\text{adj})})$$

which is

$$15 \cdot 72 \pm 1 \cdot 96 \ (2 \cdot 11)$$

or from 11·58 to 19·86. Note that this interval does not include the death rate of 9.60 per 1000 for the (standard) population of Ireland, so that the itinerants can be said to have a significantly higher (age-adjusted) mortality.

Confidence intervals are available for the CMF which directly compares the itinerants to the Irish population, but are not considered. It is also possible, when there are two populations, to calculate a standardized rate for each and compare these rates. This can be done using a difference or ratio measure. The ratio measure is essentially the ratio of two CMFs. Confidence intervals (and significance tests) are available for such comparisons but confidence intervals for the SMR and ratios of SMRs will be given instead.

Because, for reasons which will not be gone into, the SMR has a lower standard error than the CMF, it is often preferable to work with indirect rather than direct standardization. The SMR is simply a ratio of observed to expected deaths (multiplied by 100), and the observed deaths can be considered to have a Poisson distribution. The methods of Section 4.9 can be used to obtain a confidence interval based on the observed deaths and if these limits are divided by the expected deaths and multiplied by 100 the confidence interval for the SMR results. The limits are

$$100 \ (x_l/E) \text{ and } 100 \ (x_u/E)$$

where x_l and x_u are the lower and upper limits for the observed number of deaths (O). In the example,

$$\text{SMR} = 100 \ (O/E) = 100 \ (84/43) = 196 \text{ (to the nearest whole number).}$$

From Table B.12 the 95% confidence interval based on a count of 84 is from 67·00 to 104·00, so that the 95% limits for the SMR are from 6700/43 to 10400/43 or from 156 to 242.

Although, as briefly mentioned in the previous section of this chapter, one must be careful in comparing SMRs for different groups, comparisons are frequently made and are acceptable provided that the groups being compared are broadly similar in age distribution. For instance, relative mortality in two groups A and B may be expressed as:

$$\text{SMR}_\text{A}/\text{SMR}_\text{B} = \left.\frac{O_\text{A}}{E_\text{A}}\right|\frac{O_\text{B}}{E_\text{B}} = \frac{O_\text{A}}{O_\text{B}}\left|\frac{E_\text{B}}{E_\text{A}}\right..$$

This is seen to be very similar to Eqn. 10.11 used to compare two (unadjusted) rates, and in fact the approach to the calculation of a confidence interval for the ratio of two rates can be used for the ratio of two SMRs. Section 10.11 explains the method which treats O_A as a binomial proportion on a sample size of $O_\text{A} + O_\text{B}$. Confidence limits for this proportion are obtained as p_l and p_u and the lower and upper limits for the ratio of the two SMRs are respectively

$$(\text{SMR}_\text{A}/\text{SMR}_\text{B})_l = \frac{p_l}{1 - p_l}\frac{E_\text{B}}{E_\text{A}}$$

$$(\text{SMR}_\text{A}/\text{SMR}_\text{B})_u = \frac{p_u}{1 - p_u}\frac{E_\text{B}}{E_\text{A}}.$$

13.5 Measures of fertility

The *birth rate*, or *crude birth rate*, is defined as the number of live births occurring during a calendar period per 1000 of the mean population during the same period:

$$\frac{\text{Number of live births occurring during a calendar period}}{\text{Mean population during the same period}} \times 1000.$$

The crude birth rate, like the crude death rate, is of limited value since it depends on the age and sex composition of the population. Specifically, the rate is influenced by the number of women of child-bearing age in that population, and because it relates to the total population it does not necessarily indicate the relative fertility of that population. For this reason, a *general fertility rate* is calculated. This is defined as the number of live births occurring during a calendar period per 1000 women of child-bearing age in the population during the same period of time.

Since the general fertility rate is based only upon the number of women of child-bearing age in the population (usually taken to be the age range $15 - 45$), it is clearly a better measure of fertility than the crude birth rate. However, the general fertility rate is also limited, because it does not take into account the age distribution of women of child-bearing age within the population of females $15 - 45$. For this reason *age-specific fertility rates* (similar to age-specific mortality rates) are calculated, from which a further measure called the *total fertility rate* is derived. The total fertility rate represents an estimate of the average number of children born to a woman throughout her child-bearing period, subject to prevailing age-specific fertility rates. Thus, a total fertility rate of 3700 per 1000 implies that, on average, 1000 women would be expected to bear a total of 3700 children throughout their child-bearing age span.

The concept of the total fertility rate is closely related to analysis of population trends. In analysis of population trends, the important factor to be determined is whether or not the female population is replacing itself from one generation to the next, for in the long run this determines the trend in total population. For this purpose, *gross and net reproduction rates* are calculated. The gross reproduction rate is similar to the total fertility rate except that it refers to *female* births only; thus, if it happened that male and females were born in equal numbers*, a total fertility rate of 3700 per 1000 would give rise to a gross reproduction rate of 1850 per 1000. The net reproduction rate is derived from, and is slightly less than, the gross rate — it takes account of mortality conditions as they affect women throughout the child-bearing span. In summary, the net rate measures the average number of female children born to a woman during her child-bearing life, subject to prevailing specific fertility and specific mortality rates.

13.6 Measures of morbidity

Morbidity, which is ill health or sickness, poses a variety of measurement difficulties. While death is an event that occurs at a point in time, sickness may last for a period of time, may recur within one period of time, and may be present with different degrees of severity. A person may have more than one illness; moreover, except for certain infectious diseases, most illnesses are not subject to notification, and sources of information on illness are necessarily partial and not recorded in such a way as to permit the derivation of measures of morbidity with the same degree of convenience and accuracy as mortality. Sources include hospital in-patient and out-patient records, general-practitioner records and, in many countries, information on illness or absence from work, collected as part of the administrative procedures of social security systems. The development of comprehensive systems of social security, the increased use of computers for processing and filing data, and the growing importance of preventive medicine are greatly improving the range of available data on morbidity, but much remains to be done.

It is not intended here to discuss morbidity statistics (which include virtually any information connected with health or ill-health) in any detail, but there are

---

* In fact, the ratio of female to total live births is slightly less than half.

two types of measure of morbidity which are in common use and will be explained. These are the *incidence rate* and the *prevalence rate* and they are often confused (see also Sections 10.4 and 10.6). An incidence rate is defined as the number of cases of a particular disease or condition *commencing* during a specified time per 100 of the average population at risk during the same period of time:

$$\frac{\text{Number of cases of a particular disease or condition } \textit{commencing}}{\text{during a specified time}} \times 100.$$

The prevalence rate that is commonly used is known as the *point prevalence rate*. The point prevalence rate is defined as the number of cases of a particular disease or condition *existing* in a population at a specified time per 100 of the population at risk at that time:

$$\frac{\text{Number of cases of a particular disease or condition existing in a population at a specified time}}{\text{Population at risk at that time}} \times 100.$$

Less commonly used is the *period* prevalence rate, which is the number of cases existing within a specified time period per 100 of the average population in that period. Incidence and prevalence rates are usually expressed as a percentage although other multiplying factors may be used. This of course presents no difficulty provided that it is stated clearly what the multiplying factor is. Incidence is concerned with the number of *new* cases of a disease or condition occurring, while prevalence is concerned with the total number of *existing* cases in a population.

Finally, reference may be made to *average duration of illness*, often in connection with the economic and social consequences of absence from work through illness. Average duration of illness (for specific, or for all illnesses) may be expressed in terms of the total population (at risk), or of persons who were actually ill during the period of time to which the measure refers. In the former case, the denominator of the measure is the total population at risk in a particular time period, while in the latter case the denominator is the number of persons who were ill during the particular time period. (If a particular individual was ill more than once during the period, he or she will be counted as a separate 'person' for each illness.) The numerator of the ratio in each case is the total number of days of recorded illness, which may be measured in calendar days, or in working days only. Data for these calculations derive mainly from Social Security statistics.

13.7 Hospital statistics

For legal, administrative and other purposes, hospitals maintain a considerable volume of statistical information relating to patients. In this section, a number of measures related to the utilization of hospital resources, which are commonly used for management and administrative purposes, are briefly discussed.

The *average length of stay* is designed to measure the average number of days spent (continuously) in hospital by a given group of patients. The arithmetic mean is typically used as the measure of the average. The simplest way of calculating the arithmetic mean length of stay is to record the length of stay of each patient registered in the hospital over a particular period of time, add these together and divide by the number of patients. An alternative, less direct measure is to calculate the total number of 'occupied bed-days' over a specific time period (say, a calendar month), and then to divide this total by the number of patients leaving hospital (by discharge, transfer or death) in the same period. This is not as precise a measure of the mean, since bed-days taken in earlier months by patients discharged in the current month will not be included in the numerator of the measure, and patients in hospital but not leaving during the current month will not be included in the denominator. The longer the period of time used for the calculation, the closer will this indirect measure be to the (true) average length of stay. The direct measure is to be preferred, since it is not only more accurate but also permits calculation of the standard deviation of the length of stay, which indicates the variability of length of stay around the mean; however, the form in which hospital records are maintained usually necessitates the use of the alternative, indirect method of calculation.

The *bed-occupancy rate* is a measure of the degree of utilization of available beds over an interval of time. This is often calculated as the ratio of the number of occupied bed-days in a particular period to the number of available bed-days over the same period, and multiplied by 100 to express it in percentage terms. Thus, if there are 100 beds, over a 30-day calendar period this gives 3000 available bed-days. If the number of occupied bed-days over that period is 2400, the bed-occupancy rate is $(2400/3000) \times 100 = 80\%$. Occupancy rates over 100% can occur if extra beds, over and above those usually available, have to be provided.

An alternative approach is to calculate the *daily* bed-occupancy rate, and then to calculate the average daily rate for the particular period. This will give the same average occupancy rate for a given period as the method described above (provided the number of available beds remains constant over the period), but has the added advantage that the standard deviation can also be calculated. The variability in the occupancy rate may be just as important as its mean.

The difference between the total available bed-days and the number of occupied bed-days in any period represents unoccupied bed-days and can be used to calculate what is called the *turnover interval*. This is defined as the number of unoccupied bed-days divided by the number of patients leaving hospital (by discharge, transfer or death) in a particular period. In the hypothetical example above, there were 3000 available bed-days in a 30-day period, and 2400 occupied bed-days. The number of unoccupied bed-days is, therefore, 600. If, during this period, there had been, say, 150 'bed departures' (discharges, transfers or deaths), the turnover interval can be calculated as 600/150 = 4 days. A truer measure of the turnover interval would be to calculate, for each of the 150 departures noted during the period, the actual time interval for which the bed is empty, and then to estimate the mean of these 150 time intervals. (This would also permit calculation of the standard deviation.) Usually, however, this method is not feasible, and the more indirect method is used. As with the measures of average length of stay, the longer the time period concerned, the closer will the indirect measure be to the true mean.

Another measure of resource utilization is the 'turnover' or *throughput* of patients per bed in any interval of time. Following the example quoted above, the average (daily) number of available beds in a 30-day period can be calculated as 3000/30 = 100. The number of patients departing during this period was 150, so that the average throughput of patients per available bed is calculated as 150/100 = 1·5.

13.8 Life tables

In an earlier section, a number of measures of mortality were described. One measure not covered in that section is the *mean expectation of life at birth*. The calculation of life expectancy involves what are called *life tables*, and is a special example of a form of statistical analysis termed *cohort analysis*. Other applications of cohort analysis involving so-called clinical life tables were discussed in Chapter 10 (Sections 10.7, 10.12 and 10.13). The life tables discussed in this section are often referred to as *population* life tables.

The disadvantages of the crude death rate as a measure of comparative mortality have already been pointed out. A comparison of crude death rates between countries A and B, or within the same country at different periods of time, may not be very meaningful because of differences in the age and sex compositions of the two populations. Ideally, it would be asked — 'What would the crude death rates be if the two countries had identical populations?' Another way of expressing this is to ask — 'What is the average expectation of life of an individual in each country?' It is to answer this question that life tables are constructed. To the extent that their purpose is to eliminate the effects of age distribution on measures of mortality, they have something in common with the standardized mortality measures described in Section 13.3.

The construction of life tables will now be explained with reference to Table 13.7. Suppose a *cohort* of 100 000 male births in a particular year is postulated. A number of the cohort will die during the first year of life (infant mortality). In Ireland, the number who die could be estimated by means of the current infant mortality rate. In the period 1980 − 82, the average male infant mortality rate for

Table 13.7. Irish life table no. 10, 1980 – 82, males (from Irish Statistical Bulletin, 1985, with permission)

Age x	l_x	d_x	L_x	T_x	e_x°	Age x
0	100000	1128	99029	7013928	70·14	0
1	98872	107	98818	6914899	69·94	1
2	98764	74	98718	6816081	69·01	2
3	98691	48	98667	6717353	68·06	3
4	98643	47	98620	6618686	67·10	4

Ireland was 11·28 per 1000, so that out of 100 000 male births the 'expected' number of deaths can be estimated as 1128. Thus, of the original cohort, 98 872 may be expected to survive to age 1. These figures are shown in the columns headed l_x and d_x in the table.

How many of the hypothetical cohort will survive to age 2? This can be estimated by using the actual $(1980 - 2)$ specific mortality rates for Ireland for the age group 1 and under 2 years of age. Thus, it is estimated that 107 of the cohort will die between the ages of 1 and 2, leaving 98764 to survive until age 2.

The general procedure will now be clear. At each age, the cohort is subjected to the specific mortality rates for that age group. Eventually, of course, the cohort will 'die off'. The number who die at each age is determined by the specific mortality rates, and these are usually based on the average mortality rates for the most recent period for which accurate statistics are available.

Consider now the column headed L_x. The figures in this column measure the estimated total number of years lived by the cohort at each age. To explain this, suppose the whole cohort had survived to age 1 (the infant mortality rate was zero). In this case, the total number of years lived by the cohort, between birth and age 1, would be 100 000 — each member of the cohort would have lived for 1 year.

However, it is estimated that only 98 872 of the cohort live for a year, while 1128 live for only part of a year. Thus, the total number of years lived by the cohort is 98 872 plus some fraction of 1128. The precise method of calculation will not be explained here.* In summary, it is estimated that the total number of years lived by the cohort, between the ages of 0 and 1, is 99 029.

Similarly, the total number of years lived by the cohort between the ages of 1 and 2 is 98 764 (the number of years lived by the survivors to age 2) plus a half of

---

* The simplest assumption would be that those who die live on average 6 months each, so that the 1128 of the cohort who die before reaching age 1 would live for a total of $1128/2 = 564$ years. This assumption is made for all age groups *except* the age group $0 - 1$, since most deaths in this group occur in the first month of life.

107 (those who die before reaching the age of 2). This is estimated to be 98 818. The interpretation of the L_x column should now be clear.

Turning now to the T_x column, the first figure in this column is the total number of years lived by the cohort at all ages — in fact, the sum of *all* the figures in the L_x column when the complete life table for all ages is constructed. Thus, the life span of all the members of the cohort is estimated to account for a total of 7 013 928 years. Since there were originally 100 000 persons in the cohort, the average number of years lived by the cohort is 7 013 928/100 000 = 70·14 years. This average, recorded in the last column of the table, is the mean expectation of life at birth of an Irish male. It indicates how many years an Irish male may be expected to live — or, alternatively, the average age of an Irish male at death — subject to certain specific mortality conditions.

The other entries in columns T_x and $e_x^{\,o}$ are also of interest. For example, the second figure in the T_x column measures the total number of years lived by the cohort from the age of 1 onwards; the second figure (69·94) in the $e_x^{\,o}$ column is derived from this, and measures the *mean expectation of life* at age 1. That is, a male who has survived to age 1 may expect, on average, to live a further 69·94 years. Thus, the figures in the $e_x^{\,o}$ column measure the average expectation of life at each age.

Incidentally, although not observed here, the mean expectation of life at 1 often exceeds the mean expectation of life at birth, though on *a priori* reasoning it would be expected that the mean expectation of life would fall with increasing age. This apparently perverse result is due to the effect of infant mortality on the life expectancy of the cohort at birth. From age 1, however, the expectation of life invariably declines with age, as expected.

There are many other features of life tables that could be discussed, but sufficient has been explained to demonstrate their relevance in analysis of mortality, despite their limitations.

Life tables can be constructed for different populations and comparisons made on the basis of life expectancy. Separate tables can be constructed for males and females, for different areas of the country (e.g. urban and rural) and for different occupations. Comparisons can be made that are independent of the effects of age and sex composition, and the mean expectation of life is a useful and simple concept to understand.

The most obvious limitation of life tables as described above is the use of *prevailing* age-specific mortality rates to calculate the *expected* mortality experience of the cohort. In the example above, age-specific mortality rates for 1980 – 82 were used. (There was a population census in 1981, so that the population of each age group could be ascertained with a high degree of accuracy, and this enabled firm estimates to be made of age-specific death rates.) If these are used to calculate the mortality experience of a cohort of 100 000 male births commencing, say, in 1981, then in the period 2010 − 15, the figures that will be applied to the survivors of the cohort are the age-specific death rates for males aged 30 − 34 that prevailed in 1980 − 82. As the cohort ages, the applicability of the 1980 − 82 age-specific death rates become increasingly open to question. In this respect, the concept of the mean expectation of life at birth (or indeed at any other age) must be heavily qualified, since the actual mortality experience of a cohort of male births in 1981 (and hence their life expectancy) is not known. Thus, the mean expectation of life and other measures* derived from a life table are purely hypothetical measures based upon prevailing (recent) age-specific mortality rates. It is, of course, possible to attempt to anticipate changes in mortality conditions by *predicting* changes in age-specific mortality rates, based perhaps on an extrapolation of past trends, but in certain respects this introduces a greater degree of ambiguity in the interpretation of the life table statistics.

13.9 Summary

This chapter has described a number of vital statistics which are particularly important in medicine. Different measures of mortality were defined, and it was explained how the mortality experience of different populations could be compared by means of so-called standardized mortality measures, which neutralize the influence of age distribution on mortality. In a later section of the chapter, the use of population life tables in analysis of mortality was also explained.

Other sections of the chapter covered measures of fertility (birth rates and reproduction rates), morbidity statistics and a variety of measures such as bed-occupancy rates which relate to the use of health care resources. Such measures can help in assessing the efficiency with which scarce health care resources are used, although they must be interpreted with care. With increased computerization, there is a growing availability of data on morbidity and on the utilization of health care resources, and the use of computers in medicine is the subject of the next chapter.

---

* It is possible to calculate, from the life table, a death rate called the *true death rate*, which is actually the reciprocal of the mean expectation of life at birth. In this example, the so-called true death rate is

$$1/70.13 \times 1000 = 14 \cdot 23.$$

14

Computers and Medical Research

14.1 Introduction

The development of microprocessors has been the most significant technological advance in this half of the 20th century and their application has profoundly affected — and will continue to affect — virtually every field of human activity, from grocery shops to space exploration. In recent years, computers have proved an invaluable aid to many aspects of medical research work (although in a very limited way in relation to their full potential), and are also extensively used for administrative purposes in hospitals. Although, in principle, the functions performed by a computer could be performed 'manually', in practice the immense amount of sorting and analysis that is involved in many applications would not be feasible without the aid of a computer. This is not simply because of the volume of manual labour required to replace the computer; in many applications no amount of manual labour could carry out the complex and interrelated calculations required in the time necessary. In speeding-up calculations by a factor of millions, microprocessors permit the introduction of more sophisticated process equipment.

In the past decade or so, the use of computers has been enormously enhanced by the development of microcomputers and, in parallel with this, the availability of 'user-friendly' computer software. A complete system can be purchased at relatively modest cost for personal use, and the necessary skills to operate the system can be acquired relatively painlessly. The following section describes, very briefly, the main components of a computer system (chiefly emphasizing micro-computers for personal use), while the following sections outline the principal types of application of computers in medical research.

14.2 Computer systems

Although a computer is capable of performing extremely complex operations, essentially it works by carrying out a sequence of simple arithmetic (add, subtract) and/or logical (if, then, or) steps, according to a sequence of instructions specified by the user. The series of related instructions required to deal with a particular problem or activity (like sorting data into tables, or calculating and comparing the means of two samples) form a *program*, which provides a step-by-step routine for the computer to follow. (Such programs are described as computer *software*; the pieces of physical equipment are the *hardware*.) Of course, if a problem cannot be defined and formulated in a detailed and logical way, then it is not possible to program it for solution by the computer. Quite often, it is the definition of the problem that creates the most difficulty. Special programs are required to control the activities of the computer system itself, and these are given the general name of 'system software'.

The set of hardware in a microcomputer system typically comprises a *processor*, which controls the system and provides the computer's 'memory'; a *keyboard*, which is the user's means of communication with the computer; and a *monitor* or visual display unit (VDU), which can display what is being entered and the results of applications. Since in many cases the user will want a 'hard copy' of data or results, the system will also commonly include a *printer*.

Attached to the processor will be one or more *disk drives*, by which instructions and data can be inputted to the system. With so-called 'floppy disk' drives, a disk is inserted into the machine for reading/writing, and is then removed; these disks are of varying capacity (in terms of the information or number of characters that can be stored) and size ($3\frac{1}{2}$ inches and $5\frac{1}{4}$ inches being the most common). Since disks can be damaged or lost, or can develop faults, it is important to make and maintain backup copies. A hard disk is a large-capacity storage disk which is usually fixed within the processor unit and has a much faster read/write capability than the floppy disk. It is used for storing data or programs which are frequently or commonly required by the user. Again, backup copies on floppy disks are recommended.

The list of instructions, or program, which tells the computer what to do, has to be written in a particular form or 'language'. The computer itself operates according to a so-called machine-code language, which is specified by the manufacturer (and which varies with each type of machine), but to make things easier for the user, programs are usually written in a so-called 'high-level' language which can then be 'translated' by the computer into its own machine code. Programming languages in common use include FORTRAN, C, and BASIC, all of which are written in a form designed for ease of use (and learning) by the user. (However, there is now available a wide range of user-friendly integrated software packages which require little or no programming knowledge on the part of the user.) The computer then translates the user-languages into machine code by means of a *compiler* (roughly analogous to a dictionary); a separate compiler is needed for each high-level language, and some machines will only operate on one user-language.

While similar in basic configuration, and performing similar types of work, mainframe computers differ from microcomputers in several important respects (including cost), although the distinction is less marked than it once was. Mainframes are larger and more efficient processors, have a greater memory base, and more sophisticated input−output devices and other peripherals. They can also cater for a large number of users simultaneously (strictly, in such a fast sequence that it appears simultaneous). Advances in technology are reducing these differences, but mainframes have obvious advantages (and may be essential) in handling large databases, such as census or large-scale survey data, complex scientific applications, and extensive but routine tasks such as payroll and administrative record-keeping, including the production of large volumes of hard copy.

14.3 Computer applications

There is an extensive and rapidly growing variety of applications of computers in medicine and health care, particularly related, but not confined, to the explosion in microcomputer technology. These include word processing (the fastest-growing segment of the market in recent years), fairly routine data-processing activities, such as invoicing and the preparation of payrolls, the organization of out-patient appointment systems, and so on, and quite complex mathematical models designed to 'simulate' particular physiological or environmental conditions. In this section some of the more important of these applications are briefly described.

In keeping with the subject matter of this book, an application of particular interest is the use of the computer for purposes of statistical analysis, including the recording and organization of data, the description of data, and their analysis using the techniques of statistical inference discussed in preceeding chapters.

As indicated in the previous section, the undertaking of a statistical analysis requires the user to supply the computer with the data and with the instructions (the program) necessary to analyse the data, which may include, for example, sorting them into frequency distributions, calculating the means and standard deviations for different groups within the sample data, and carrying out tests of significance on the sample statistics. Depending on the scale of the study, or its complexity, this may involve the assistance of a statistician/computer programmer However, for most computer systems there are now available a large range of prewritten statistical programs or 'packages' which can be used 'off the shelf' by the researcher, though statistical and/or programming advice may still be needed to determine the statistical techniques appropriate to the study, the capability of a particular computer system to handle the survey data, and so on. Nevertheless, the availability of such packages, along with the development of more user-friendly hardware and software have made it easier for researchers in all disciplines to undertake work on the computer using either a microcomputer or a remote-access terminal of a mainframe. Statistical packages, such as SPSS-X (Statistical Packages for the Social Sciences) or SAS, which are widely used in medical and social research, now contain a large array of subroutines for sorting, describing and analysing data (including means and standard deviations, regression, correlation, analysis of variance, z, t and χ^2 tests, discriminant analysis, etc.), any combination of which may be selected as appropriate for a particular study.

In many medical research studies the preparation and inputting of data is the most labour-intensive and time-consuming aspect of the work. Typically, the raw data will be recorded on a questionnaire or record form. Often it is possible to key in (assuming a microcomputer system with keyboard input) the data direct from the questionnaire/record form, but sometimes the data will be transcribed to a coding sheet, the layout of which will be designed to facilitate data entry and to conform with the characteristics of the software being used. For larger-scale studies and for other applications involving a large volume of data, a *database management package* can be used to organize, store and retrieve the information. A variety of database packages are available (and are constantly being improved) and selection of the most appropriate package depends on the user's requirements. Relevant considerations here include the use of variable or fixed-length records for data storage, the use of fixed or variable screen formatting for data entry and display, the compatibility of file structures with other programs, and the degree of flexibility in modifying the database. Moreover, database systems vary in the facility and flexibility with which data from different files or records may be combined, in data-entry procedures and branching facilities, and in data checks. This is a rapidly growing area of software development in which significant changes in technology can be anticipated.

Many database packages contain simple statistical programs. Whether or not a database package is being used, however, a specialized statistical package (as described above) is likely to be needed. Particularly for the non-specialist, it is worth purchasing a well established system; apart from other advantages that derive from an extensively used and tested package, user support, including regular updates, will be provided by the software manufacturer or their agents.

For the production of reports, including tables, results of statistical analyses, and text, a *word-processing package* is now a ubiquitous component of the microcomputer user's range of software. Word processing has been the fastest-growing microprocessor application in the past decade, and has revolutionized office technology. Standard or common features of word-processing packages include a wide range of editing functions (deletions, alterations, changes in layout), automatic pagination, alignment of margins (justification), standardized spelling, automatic indexing, and so on. Besides being able to produce reports and other substantive documents, a word-processing package is also useful in designing and producing questionnaires and record forms, regular standardized letters or memos, mailing lists, bibliographic references and so on.

Another useful software tool of growing popularity and with applications in medical research is the *spreadsheet program*. Essentially, a spreadsheet comprises a tabular array, or matrix, each cell of which contains an item of data; this is the basic 'worksheet' which is displayed on the screen and is then subject to manipulation by the user. A key feature of spreadsheet programs is their ability to assess the effect of changes in one or more cells on all the other cells of the matrix, in the manner of a forecasting or simulation model. Results of particular model runs can be printed out or stored for later reference. In addition, a spreadsheet package will typically contain a range of simple arithmetic and statistical functions (means, standard deviations, etc.) and, increasingly, graphics software for the display and printing of charts and graphs.

Use of a spreadsheet program is one example of the application of computers to *modelling and simulation*, a science whose scope has been greatly enhanced by the microprocessor. Briefly, this involves the formulation of a mathematical model of a system (which may be based on actual or hypothetical data) and the use of the model to 'simulate' the consequences of particular events or decisions which are specified by the user. These are designed to reflect 'real-life' possibilities and to indicate, with varying degrees of probability, what might happen in particular situations. Some of the best-known examples of simulation models occur in the social sciences; economists, for example, construct computer-based models of the economy and use them to predict what might happen to output, employment and so on if, say, the government were to reduce taxes. As another example, flight-simulation models are used to train airline pilots, including the simulation of emergencies (such as engine failure) which would be risky (and possibly disastrous) to replicate in actual flight training.

The use of simulation models in medicine and health care includes analysis of the effects of epidemics under varying assumptions about population movement and rates of infection; determination of 'queuing' or waiting times at clinics, under varying assumptions about rates of referral, treatment times and patient throughput; training of health care administrators or managers in resource-allocation decisions through simulation of the operation of health care systems (e.g. hospitals). Simulation techniques are also being developed for training in diagnosis. A hypothetical patient with specific diagnostic characteristics is simulated on the computer, and the student asked to diagnose and prescribe treatment; it is possible to some extent to simulate response to treatment. Clearly this development offers considerable possibilities, although as a complement to, rather than a substitute for, traditional clinical training methods.

The diagnostic checks and procedures used in simulation may also be used with real patients, the computer in this case undertaking the evaluation on the basis of the patient information with which it is supplied and printing out its diagnosis or, more likely, a list of possible diagnoses. For the general physician, automated diagnoses of this kind may be a particularly useful form of assistance in cases of unusual or uncommon diseases and/or symptoms since, in effect, he or she is calling upon the diagnostic skills of specialists involved in the diagnostic programming of the computer facility.

In a more comprehensive way, medical record linkage provides a continuous record of individual patients from birth to death, including illnesses, hospitalization, operations, allergies and so on. Prior to the use of computers, the linking together of different events in an individual's medical case history was extremely difficult, since individual events (treatment by family doctor, stay in hospital, etc.) were, and indeed usually still are, recorded separately at different locations with no systematic procedures for bringing together these elements of case history into a single record. With computer-based recording systems such linking becomes more feasible. Medical records can be put to better use and information stored efficiently. Moreover, this information can be retrieved more rapidly than before; cumulative files for individuals can be compiled and assembled into family groups, socio-economic categories, and so on, for purposes of analysis. Longitudinal studies, which involve following up a given group or cohort over a period of time, are a well-established application of the concept of medical record linkage, and the large and comprehensive computerized databases built up through record linkage offer a wide range of potential research studies. It must be noted here, however, that the development and use of such data raise issues of confidentiality in patient records, and touch upon the much broader question of the protection of individual privacy in conditions in which many details of personal circumstances (financial status, social security history, and so on) are on computer files and may be vulnerable to unauthorized access.

A somewhat related but more specific use of computerized records and data processing arises in screening the results of routine examination of large numbers of individuals, often at regular intervals (e.g. airline pilots, military personnel, schoolchildren, or simply groups drawn from the general population). Test results can be examined and collated, results for individuals compared with standard or average results or with those of earlier tests for the same individual, and summaries printed out, including reference to potentially significant, unusual or unfavourable test results that call for priority attention. This may be seen as a special but particularly useful application of the computer for diagnostic purposes.

Substantial use of computers is now being made in clinical laboratories, in the control and monitoring of equipment and in the evaluation of results, and this has been one of the most successful and intensive areas of computer applications related to health care. Clinical data (blood pressure, temperature, respiration, etc.) can be evaluated, warning signals indicated, and printed and/or graphical output produced. For continuous monitoring of patients in intensive care, the patient may be directly linked to computer-controlled equipment which will alert staff to any significant change in conditions.

Finally, computers are extensively used on the administrative and planning side of health care, and applications here are many and varied. They range from maintaining computerized-payroll, staff-scheduling and stock-control systems, similar to those used in industry and commerce, to more specialized applications including the monitoring of hospital waiting lists, recording and analysing bed occupancy and average length of stay in hospital, and comparing bed-utilization rates between different units and over time. Cost data may be used to estimate the true resource cost of various forms of health care delivery, and to identify critical areas where more efficient resource allocation would improve health care productivity. On a larger scale, within national health care systems such as the British National Health Service, computer-based models of the system can be used to estimate, for example, the optimal location pattern for specific health care facilities, the areas to be served by each hospital within an administrative region, and the probable demand, and hence recommended capacity, for specific facilities (surgical, obstetrical, etc.) within a newly planned hospital.

As is clear from the foregoing, the scope for the application of computers in medicine and health care is enormous. Realization of this potential is at an early stage, although progress has been rapid. Earlier experience of computer applications has been mixed, with some projects abandoned and others not obviously more efficient than the 'manual' systems that they replaced. As is invariably the case with new technologies, there is a learning-by-doing process, which requires adaptation and the acquisition of new skills and practices, and — most of all — an understanding on the part of the user of what a computer can and cannot do, and how best it can fulfil its task in the particular application for which it is installed. Too often, purchasers have ambitious but vaguely articulated expectations of a computer's possibilities and are subsequently disappointed; perhaps the computer cannot perform the tasks expected of it because it is not powerful enough or because the wrong system has been purchased.

14.4 Summary

This chapter has provided a simple introduction to computers, including a description of the basic configuration of a typical computer system. In medicine, as in other fields, the development of microprocessors is revolutionizing traditional practices, and Section 14.3 contains a brief review of the application of computers in medicine. Developments in hardware and software technology continue apace, however, and the frontiers of what is possible today will surely expand in the future.

15

Bias and Measurement Error in Medical Research

15.1 Introduction

Bias may be defined as any factor or process which tends to produce results or conclusions that differ systematically from the truth.* Any research study in a medical field is open to bias from many sources, and it is important that the researcher be aware of these biases, and in designing, executing and analysing a study avoid them where possible. Many of the biases that can arise in the planning and execution of the study are avoidable, but a badly run study cannot be rescued by clever statistical manipulation of figures. For this reason, study design is a far more important aspect of research than pure statistical analysis.

In the body of this book, it has been indicated at various stages how bias may interfere with the eventual outcome of a study, and this chapter brings together some of these ideas and introduces some new ones. Particular forms of bias are more likely with some study designs than others, and the discussion below indicates which pitfalls are more likely in which studies.

Sackett (1979) has identified 56 sources of bias in medical research, and although all these biases are not considered individually here, the article makes for fascinating reading. This chapter considers the different biases that can arise in the context of the different stages of a study execution — the design stage, patient selection, data collection, data analysis and interpretation of results. Many of the biases, of course, fit into more than one of these categories.

15.2 Study design

The previous chapters outlined the four main study designs often used in medical research — the cross-sectional, the prospective (cohort) and retrospective (case-control) observational studies and the experimental trial. Chapter 11 considered, in some detail, the avoidance of bias in the experimental trial by the use of randomization and double blind procedures. These arguments are not repeated

---

* This broad definition of bias thus includes errors in analytical methodology and errors of interpretation.

here, but, instead, points relating to the design of studies in general are considered.

Perhaps the first question to ask about any study is whether a comparison or control group is required. In most cases, the answer will be yes, and indeed many research studies are uninterpretable without a comparison group. The fact that, for example, 80% of a group of lung cancer patients smoke does not in itself suggest a relationship between smoking and lung cancer. It is necessary to know what the percentage of smokers is in the general population (the comparison group). This fact is often overlooked. Similarly, in evaluating a preventive or therapeutic measure, there must be a comparison group against which to evaluate the results. Some studies, of course, will not require a specific comparison group. In a prospective study, for example, the comparison groups are usually defined by the variables measured at the start of the study, and an explicit comparison group need not always be built into the study design. A sample survey to estimate some parameters may also fit into this category. For instance, a study to determine the factors relating to birth weight would not require a control group.

Given, however, that many studies will require an explicit control group, it is necessary to ask if, at the end of the day, like is being compared with like. If this can be achieved by designing a study in a particular way, it is far better than adjusting for extraneous differences between groups at the analysis stage. Thus, in a case-control study, some form of matching may be employed or, in an experimental trial, randomization (stratified or simple) may be used.

An important source of bias in many situations relates to the number of individuals studied. This is discussed in the context of interpreting the results in Section 15.7, but in general, professional advice should be sought in determining the appropriate sample size for any investigation (see also Appendix D). Obviously, the design of a given investigation depends critically on the question to be answered and it must be ascertained whether the study as designed will answer that question.

15.3 Selecting the sample

The selection of individuals or items to be included in a study is the area with the greatest potential for bias and relates to a large extent, but not exclusively, to whether the results of a study are generalizable. As already mentioned, for example, studies based on volunteers can cause great difficulties in this area. If, however, those studied form a random sample (in the strict sense of that term) from the population of interest, then selection bias should not be a problem, as long as results are generalized only to the actual population from which the sample was taken. Studies based on hospital admissions are not generalizable to all patients with a particular condition. Comparisons between admissions to different hospitals are also often biased for the same reason. The type of patient admitted to a particular hospital will depend on, among other things, the catchment population for the hospital, admission criteria, the fame of the doctors and surgeons, the facilities and diagnostic procedures available, and the intensity of the diagnostic process. These, and other factors which determine admission to a particular institution or hospital, are even more important when it is remembered that many studies are based on a presenting sample of patients. Admissions to a hospital will of necessity exclude, for example, patients managed in the community and patients who do not survive long enough to be admitted to hospital in the first place. A further bias (Berkson's bias) can result in spurious associations between an exposure and disease in a case-control study if the admission rates to hospital differ in different disease/exposure categories. The mechanism of this bias, which is complex, is explained by Sackett (1979).

A general rule relating to studies of any particular disease is to commence the study in all patients at some fixed point in the natural history of the disease. Failure to do this properly can be a further source of bias. This is why it is suggested in a case-control study, for instance, to include newly diagnosed (incident) cases only — diagnosis being usually a fixed point in a disease's history. Evidence of exposure to a particular factor may be masked if the disease is present for some time. A problem does arise however if some patients are diagnosed earlier than others, and the bias is often called *lead time bias*. Suppose a group of breast cancer patients, diagnosed when they presented with a definite lump in the breast, had been studied and that it is wished to compare their subsequent survival with a group of cases diagnosed by mammography (X-ray) at a screening clinic. This latter group would enter the study at an earlier stage in the natural history of the disease (before an actual lump was detectable) than the former group and thus would be likely to have a longer survival anyway, due to this earlier diagnosis. Some correction for this lead time bias would have to be made when analysing or interpreting the results.

Selecting patients at a fixed point in the natural history of a disease in a survival study is not achieved, however, by retrospectively determining the date of disease onset. Apart from problems in patient recall and adequacy of available records, such a process would result in a biased group with a spuriously long survival. A researcher who determined the survival of a group of cancer cases attending a clinic by measuring the time from their diagnosis (in the past) to the present would necessarily exclude patients who had died earlier, and would thus load the group with those who survived the longest. Such an investigation can only be performed if the survival of *all* patients is determined from diagnosis, and is best done by means of a prospective study.

For any study of disease, the diagnostic criteria must be clear and explicit. Different centres may label different conditions with the same name, and it is important (as discussed in Chapter 11) to know precisely what patients were studied, and thus to which population results can be applied. The exclusion of cases because of concomitant disease or other factors may affect the general applicability of findings, although it is usually necessary to avoid contamination of the study groups. In addition to these selection biases, the problems raised by a large number of patients refusing to participate in a study must not be forgotten. This question of non-response bias has been discussed before, and it is best reduced by making the study as simple as possible, and not in any way daunting to potential participants.

15.4 Data collection — accuracy (bias and precision)

Every study in medicine must involve some data collection or measurement, and an interaction between the observer and the patient or object being observed. Measurement bias, or measurement error as it can be called, is a factor that every researcher must be wary of. All studies should employ a predesigned data collection form with the information required, whether it be based on interview, case records, or direct measurement, laid out neatly and comprehensively. If data are to be processed by computer, the form should be laid out in a manner suitable for easy transferral of the data to machine-readable form, and a computer programmer should be consulted (see Chapter 14). The specific problems of questionnaire design are not considered here, except to note that it is much more that just writing down a list of questions which require an answer. Bennett and Richie (1975) give a detailed account of the use of questionnaires in medical research.

Some of the biases of data collection, in the context of the case-control study and the experimental trial, have been discussed, emphasizing the necessity, where possible, of blinding the observer to the particular group (case/control, treatment/control) from which information is being collected. This is to avoid biases in the observer's elicitation and interpretation of a response. Measurement bias can also, of course, be due to non-response and lack of complete follow-up, when missing items of information can cause very definite problems.

The problems of measurement go deeper than this, however, but unfortunately there is no standardized terminology in this area. The definitions given are widely, but not universally, accepted and represent an attempt to put the subject into a realistic framework. In this chapter an *accurate* measurement will be defined as one which is *precise* and *unbiased*. Perhaps the best way to illustrate these two terms is by reference to Fig. 15.1. This shows the hits obtained on four targets by four individuals using different air guns. Mr A's shots are closely grouped around the centre of the target. From this, it might be assumed that the sight of the gun was properly aligned, so that the shots went where they were aimed, and also that he was a 'good shot', and had a steady hand, because of the close grouping around the bull's eye. Ms B did not however achieve a close bunching of her shots,

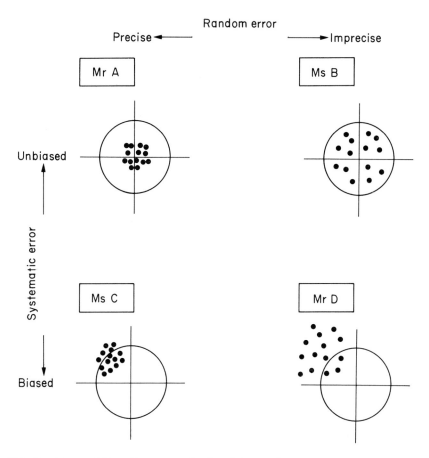

Fig. 15.1. Precision and bias. Target practice in a fairground.

although obviously, 'on average', she was hitting where she was aiming for. It might be assumed that the sight of her rifle was well-adjusted, but that her hand was not too steady, resulting in a wide spread of shots. Ms C, on the other hand, obviously had a steady hand, since her shots were grouped closely together, but she was consistently off target; either the sight of her gun was badly adjusted or there was, perhaps, a strong wind. Mr D is most unfortunate; not only is his hand a bit shaky, but by looking at where his shots are grouped, it would appear also that his sight was out of alignment.

Precision relates to the scatter of shots caused by, for instance, the random shake in an individual's hand, while bias refers to whether or not the shots are hitting the target on average. A faulty sight, or cross wind, causes a *systematic error* in one particular direction away from the bull's eye. In terms of a measurement, bias is a result of a systematic error which tends to make the actual recording of a measurement consistently above (or below) the true value. The term error in this context should only be used if the true value of the measurement is known and, in general, the term variation will be used instead. The precision of a measurement relates to the amount of *random variation* about a fixed point (be it the true value or not). An imprecise measurement will sometimes be above this fixed point, sometimes below it, and will vary randomly about it.* If the error is defined as the observed reading minus the true value, then random errors have a zero mean but any standard deviation and can be assumed to have a normal distribution. Random errors can also be considered independent of each other.

An accurate measurement, then, is one which can vary very little (precise) around the true value (unbiased) of what is being measured. For the correct classification of an individual into one group or another, on the basis of a single measurement, it is necessary that it be accurate. If a measurement is biased, the only way to solve the problem is to correct for this bias by adjusting the observed value. Thus, if an investigator were to classify individuals on the basis of a random blood glucose level, and used a small finger-prick drop of capillary blood for assay purposes, the measured values would have to be adjusted upwards by about 10% to enable estimation of the level of glucose in the venous blood.

If a measurement lacks precision, repeated measurements of the same characteristic, finally using an average of all these readings, will reduce the problem. Repeated measurements will not of course correct for bias.

What then can affect the accuracy of a given measurement? Different factors affect both precision and bias, and Fig. 15.2 displays some of these. Remember, to define bias it is necessary to know the true value of the measurement, and for the moment it will be assumed that the factor being measured is actually the factor about which information is required. (See discussion of validity below.) Thus, in evaluating measurements of blood pressure, what is being evaluated is the measurement's capability of determining the pressure exerted by the artery on the cuff of the measuring device.

Observer variation has a major impact on measurement accuracy, and can be split into two components — *within- (intra-) observer variation* and *between- (inter-) observer variation*. Within-observer variation refers to the variation between different recorded measurements by one observer, when the observations are made on different occasions. In theory, this assumes that the true value is constant, and that the differences in the measurements are due only to the observer. In practice, it is impossible to distinguish such observer variation from that of subject variation (if it exists; see below) when the same individual is tested

---

* Sometimes, the term precision is used in the sense of 'a height of 2·544 m is a more precise measurement than that of 2·5 m'. The two usages are similar, however, in that a measurement with a large amount of random variation cannot be expressed with the same degree of exactness as one with little such variation.

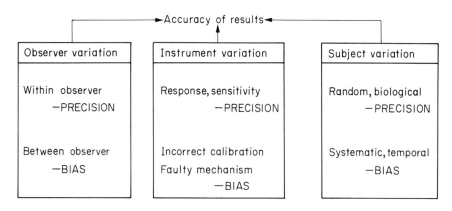

Fig. 15.2. Sources of variation in measurement results.

more than once. However, if an observer is interpreting, for example, an ECG tracing or an X-ray, 'pure' within-observer variation can be detected. Within-observer variation may be caused by factors such as reading a dial, or the height of mercury in a sphygmomanometer at slightly different angles each time, or just failing to judge exactly the reading required. Slight errors in diluting a sample for assay, slightly different inflections in the voice in administering a questionnaire, or just misinterpreting a result, all contribute to within-observer variation. The important point is that within-observer variation in itself does not cause bias, but does affect precision. The variation within-observer is assumed to be random.

Between-observer variation, on the other hand, can bias results and can cause great difficulty in combining measurements recorded by different individuals. Between-observer variation is the variation in a recorded measurement performed by two or more different observers. The results of between-observer variation can be severe ('doctors differ and patients die'), and in any study should be allowed for. Between-observer variation can be caused by different criteria for making a measurement (phase 4 or phase 5 in measuring diastolic blood pressure, for instance), by different techniques (blood pressure taken supine or standing), and by differing observational methods (the angle from which the level of mercury is read in a sphygmomanometer affects the observed height).

Different methods of actually recording a measurement can also lead to between-observer variation. In blood pressure again, *digit preference* is a large problem. A blood pressure of 117/89 is rarely recorded; observers tend to have a preference for certain values, or end digits, especially 5 and 0. Thus, readings of 120/85 mmHg and similar are far more common in recorded blood pressures than would be expected on any reasonable distribution of the variable. Again, whether measurements are rounded up or down to the nearest even value or to values ending in 5 or 0, for instance, affects between-observer variation. In administering questionnaires, between-observer variability can be due to different ways of asking questions, and even the general demeanour of the interviewer. Between-observer variation due to such factors can be reduced substantially by very careful standardization of methods, and training of observers. In any study where observations are to be made by different individuals, this must be done to avoid spurious differences between groups. This is particularly so in multicentre trials for instance. Observer variation too is always a problem when clinical records or charts are being employed to gather data. Between-observer variation can also be due to unconscious bias on the part of the observer who knows the group in which the individual has been classified. This can be avoided, as has been discussed, by blinding the observer. Between-observer variation, in essence, biases results insofar as two different observers cannot both be right. This bias is avoided, as has been said, by standardizing the methods of measurement.

A second major influence on the accuracy of observed measurements is *instrument variation*. The precision of an instrument may be low insofar as an actual reading is difficult to determine. The term instrument is used in the widest possible sense and includes physical measuring devices (weighing scales, sphygmomanometers, thermometers), questionnaires and interview schedules, and even biological assays. The precision of an instrument depends on its 'sensitivity' or response to the quantity being measured. An instrument from which a measurement is recorded by reading a pointer on a dial would be considered imprecise if the pointer hovered around but never actually stopped at a particular reading. The response or sensitivity of an instrument, however, can often not be distinguished from the effects of observer variation, or indeed (as with questionnaires for instance) from the effect of subject variation also.

Instrument variation resulting in bias is usually a result of a faulty machine or incorrect calibration. If the scale of a mercury sphygmomanometer slips down, a blood pressure reading will be higher than its true value. Careful maintenance of equipment, and testing in a situation where the true value of a measurement is known, will reduce this bias enormously.

Subject variation also affects the accuracy of test results but, of course, in one sense, it is often subject variation which is being measured — for example, a drop in blood pressure due to treatment. Random or biological subject variation relates to the fact that an individual's blood pressure, say, may vary in a random way around some fixed value. This of course affects the precision of a blood pressure's determination, and such subject variation is the main cause of the phenomenon known as regression to the mean (see Section 9.8). Random subject variation is best controlled for, of course, by repeat measurements. Systematic subject variation will cause a measurement bias. Many parameters can be affected by the subjects' mood, the conditions under which the measurements are taken, the time of day, the season and even the very fact that the subjects know that they are being observed. Such bias is of course intrinsically linked to observer variation, in that standardization of measurement technique can reduce some of the systematic variation in this area. Bias can also be due to the subjects' awareness of why they are being studied. *Recall bias*, for instance, can occur if subjects in a case-control study ruminate overmuch concerning exposure to possible causal factors, and thus remember more than if they were, in fact, controls without the disease. In a clinical trial an individual's response may be affected by his knowledge that he is in a group on a 'new wonder drug' which he knows should work (the placebo effect).

An interesting bias that can affect study results in different ways is *compliance bias*. For convenience, it is mentioned under the general heading of subject variation. If, in a controlled trial, participants in a treatment group fail to comply fully with their therapy, the apparent effect of that therapy in the full group is diluted. Also, it has been noted in some clinical trials that compliers with the placebo therapy can fare better than non-compliers with this therapy − even though there is no direct effect of the placebo. This is an interesting variation of the placebo effect. If the proportion of the compliers in the treatment and control groups differs, a biased comparison may result.

In the final analysis, however, whether variation in a measurement is random or systematic is far more important than its source. Systematic variation in any measurement is a problem; individuals will be wrongly classified on the basis of such measurements, which is serious in screening programmes or actual clinical practice. Sometimes, however, a measurement which is systematically biased (in the same direction and by the same magnitude) in each of two groups can be useful for comparative purposes. However, the size and direction of a bias is not often known, and between-group comparisons can be highly distorted if the biases occurring in each group are different.

Random variation, on the other hand, causes less of a problem. For the individual, of course, random variation can cause misclassification, but it can be controlled by taking repeat measurements on the same individual. In statistical-type investigations, analysis is performed on groups, and random variation will tend to cancel out. Thus, the mean blood pressure of a group of 100 individuals may represent the true situation of the group very well, while lacking precision for any one individual. Random variation in a measurement increases its standard error, but increase of sample size can allow for this, once the amount of random variation is known. Random variation, in general, will tend to obscure group differences and reduce the magnitude of correlations between groups.

The *repeatability (reliability, reproducibility*, or *consistency*) of a measurement can be specifically determined by making replicate observations. A measure is repeatable if the same (or very nearly the same) result is obtained each time. If the same observer makes all the measurements, the repeatability of a test is directly related to its precision (amount of random variation involved) and the standard deviation of all the readings about their mean is a good measure of this random variation. Quantification and identification of the source of random variation (within-observer, instrument, or subject) is sometimes possible, depending on whether the measurements are repeated on the same individual (e.g. blood pressure) or repeated on the same test material (e.g. an ECG tracing or blood sample). When repeatability is being determined by repeated tests on the same individual or test material, by different observers, it is essentially a measure of between-observer variation. As has been said, it is important to identify, quantify and rectify this, if biased comparisons are not to result.

15.5 Data collection — validity

The last section discussed, in terms of precision and bias, problems with measurement relating to the question, 'Is the observed result the same as the true result of the measurement?' This section considers the other important question, 'Are we actually measuring what we are trying to measure?', which relates to the *validity* of a procedure. For instance, what is really required to be measured in using a sphygmomanometer is the intra-arterial pressure exerted by the blood. This can be measured directly, and the question is whether or not the indirect measurement obtained by deflating a cuff placed on the right arm, and noting the height of a column of mercury at the appearance and disappearance of sounds is a valid method of doing this. The validity of any procedure is, thus, only determinable if some 'gold standard' of absolute truth exists, and the results of the measurement are gauged against this. Sometimes, such a gold standard may not exist and the operational definitions of the variable being measured themselves become a standard. If intelligence is defined as what is measured by an IQ test, then an IQ test is a valid measure of intelligence. The validity of a test or measurement can only, in a sense, be considered in the context of an accurate test because, obviously, problems with bias and precision will reduce a test's validity. An accurate test, however, is not necessarily a valid one. An especially important area in which validity merits attention is in the process of making a diagnosis. The 'true' diagnosis is usually made on the basis of a history, clinical examination, signs, symptoms and the results of one or more biochemical, electrical, radiological or other measurement processes. Although it may be difficult to lay down exactly what the criteria are for the diagnosis of a given condition unless autopsy reports are available and relevant, a clinical diagnosis based on all available information is, perhaps, the best available 'gold standard' for diagnosis.

Obviously, validity has important consequences in categorizing individuals. A single diagnostic test will misclassify some individuals, and this is extremely important in screening studies and in clinical practice. A *false-positive* result is a result which suggests an individual has a disease, whereas, in terms of some 'gold standard', he/she does not. A *false-negative* result categorizes an individual as disease-free, whereas, in reality, he/she has the disease. Table 15.1 shows the classification of 1000 individuals by whether or not a particular diagnostic test gave a positive result, and by their actual disease status. In general, the entries in the cells of the table are labelled *a*, *b*, *c* and *d* as noted. In the example, there are 180 false-positives and 10 false-negatives.

The *sensitivity* of a test measures its ability to detect true cases, and is defined by the number of true-positives as a percentage of the total with the disease, or in this case, 90/100 = 90%. The *specificity* of a test, on the other hand, measures its ability to detect disease-free individuals, and is defined as the number of true-negatives divided by the total without the disease, or 720/900 = 80%. Ideally, a test should have high sensitivity and high specificity. One without the other is useless. For example, a test which defines bowel cancer to be present in all persons with a height above 0·25 m is 100% sensitive, in that, certainly, all cases of bowel cancer will be detected. The test which diagnosed bowel cancer as present in all persons over 2·5 m high would be 100% specific. Unfortunately, however, sensitivity and specificity are not usually independent, and in any particular test, as one increases the other is likely to decrease. Fig. 15.3 shows the hypothetical distribution of a symptom score obtained by questionnaire in a group of psychiatric cases with a diagnosis of neurosis, compared to a normal control population. The normals have a mean score of 4 and the neurotics a mean score of 10. If a cut-off point of 6 in the symptom score was used to determine a diagnosis of neurosis, the sensitivity of the test would be fairly high, only missing neurotics with a symptom score of less than 6, as shown by the dark shaded area.

Table 15.1. Measures relating to the validity of test results

	Disease		
Test result	Present	Absent	Total
Positive	90 (*a*)	180 (*b*)	270 (*a* + *b*)
Negative	10 (*c*)	720 (*d*)	730 (*c* + *d*)
	100 (*a* + *c*)	900 (*b* + *d*)	1000 (*n*)

Sensitivity: $a/(a + c) = 90/100 = 90\%$
Specificity: $d/(b + d) = 720/900 = 80\%$
Predictive value: $a/(a + b) = 90/270 = 33\cdot3\%$
(False-positive rate: $b/(a + b) = 180/270 = 66\cdot7\%$)
False-negative rate: $c/(c + d) = 10/730 = 1\cdot4\%$

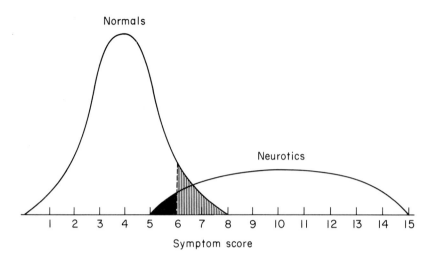

Fig. 15.3. Distribution of a symptom score in neurotic patients and normal controls.

The specificity of the test would not be so great, however, since it would misclassify any persons in the normal population with a score of 6 or over as denoted by the lightly shaded area in Fig. 15.3. Moving the cut-off point down to a score of 5 would give a test with a 100% sensitivity, while a test based on a score of 8 would achieve 100% specificity. Any intermediate point would result in the sensitivity and specificity indices increasing and decreasing in tandem. In a situation such as this, the best cut-off point to use can be determined only by the relative costs (to the investigator and to the patient) of the two types of misclassification. This is, obviously, a subjective judgement.

Reality is never as clear-cut as this example however. Diseased persons may just have higher values of a particular quantitative variable in a unimodal distribution and it could be questioned whether the presence of some diseases can ever be determined as definite. The grey area of uncertain diagnoses should always be allowed for. The sensitivity and specificity of a diagnostic procedure can be altered by the inclusion of more than one test to determine disease status. A diagnosis may be made only if the results of two different tests are both positive. This is called *testing in series*, and tends to increase specificity at the expense of sensitivity. Alternatively, a diagnosis might be made if either of two tests showed a positive result. Such testing *in parallel* would increase the sensitivity of the diagnostic procedure.

A word of caution should be inserted here on the question of *normal ranges*, particularly for biochemical tests. It is usually not very clear what these normal ranges represent. The first and common definition of a normal range (and for simplicity a test will be discussed in terms of abnormal values being above a specific cut-off point) is that in a general population only a certain proportion (usually 5%) of persons will have higher values than this upper limit of normal. This is a statistical definition of normality and has no relationship whatsoever to disease status. Conclusions based on such a definition will give a disease prevalence of 5% for any condition. An upper limit of a normal range could also be defined as that level above which some pathology may be present in an individual. Normal ranges based on this approach, which might be described as clinical, can be difficult to determine. A prognostic normal range, on the other hand, might define a test level above which an individual's prognosis is poor and an operational or therapeutic normal range might define that point above which medical intervention is likely to be of benefit. Prognostic or therapeutic normal ranges can only be determined on the basis of prospective studies. These four possible definitions of normal are however totally distinct and may bear no relationship to each other.

In general, individual tests not having 100% specificity and sensitivity will distort any estimates of disease prevalence. For example, in Table 15.1 the true prevalence of the disease is 10% (100 per 1000) while, on the basis of the test results, the prevalence is 27% (270 per 1000). If the validity of a test is different in two population groups being compared, spurious differences between the groups may occur. A real difference may be magnified, or it may be masked. If the validity of a test is consistent across comparison groups, the effect is always to dilute or weaken any association which may be observed between the disease and a factor.

A common error, which can lead to serious bias, arises in studies where the validity of a test is incorrectly adjusted for. In many studies, the often small number of individuals with a positive test result are examined further to try to reduce the number of false-positives. Unfortunately, no corresponding effort is made in those with a negative test result to reduce the number of false-negatives; this will tend to result in a spuriously low prevalence estimate.

Although sensitivity and specificity may seem adequate in determining the validity of a diagnostic test, there are two further measures which are perhaps even more important in describing the effect of misclassification errors. Sensitivity and specificity can be determined independently by studying separate groups of diseased and non-diseased individuals. However, the usefulness of a diagnostic test also depends on the true prevalence of the condition in the population being studied. For the practising clinician or organizer of a screening programme, the *predictive value (diagnostic value)* of a test is a most important parameter. The predictive value of a test is the proportion of true cases among all those with a positive test result; in other words, it relates to what a clinician sees − those individuals with positive tests. In Table 15.1, the predictive value of the test is 90/270 or only 33·3%. Thus, although the sensitivity and specificity of the test are 90% and 80% respectively, only one-third of the persons for whom the test results were positive actually had the disease. The usefulness of the test would be quite questionable.

The predictive value of the test can be calculated if, in addition to the test's sensitivity and specificity, the true prevalence of the disease is known, or if, as in the example, the test is performed on a sample from the population in which it is to be applied. The predictive value of a test of given sensitivity and specificity increases (decreases) as the true prevalence of the condition increases (decreases). Thus, a test with a high predictive value developed in a hospital setting (where a high prevalence of any condition is to be expected) may be quite inapplicable when applied to a general population.

The *false-positive rate* for a test is calculated as the number of false-positives as a percentage of all positive test results, and is 66·7% in the example. It is, of course, 100% minus the predictive value, and is another way of looking at that parameter. The *false-negative rate* for a test is the false-negatives as a percentage of the total negative test results, and has, in the example, the low value of 1·4%. Note that the false-positive and false-negative rates are calculated with, respectively, the number of positive and negative test results as denominator, *not* the total number with or without the disease.*

Although the sensitivity and specificity of a test are measures of its validity, high values for these parameters do not in themselves make for a usable test in clinical practice. The usefulness of a test depends also on the prevalence of the condition being studied and in any evaluation of a diagnostic test predictive values and false-negative rates should be calculated if it is to be judged adequately. If the true prevalence of the condition is unknown, these calculations could be done for a series of prevalences that might be observed in practice.

15.6 Statistical analysis and interpretation

If a study has been well designed and well executed, the main hurdles have been overcome. Errors in the statistical analysis and interpretation of results can of course still occur, but can be corrected. That such errors do occur is highlighted by, among others, Gore *et al.* (1977) who, in reviewing 62 reports in the *British Medical Journal* which included statistical analysis, showed that over half had statistical errors of one kind or another, that just under 30% had serious errors, and that five articles (8·1%) made claims that were not supportable when the data were examined carefully. Errors of interpretation can of course be on the part of the investigator, or the reader of a published paper. Errors related to the statistical

---

* Some sources define the false-positive and false-negative rates with denominators of all diseased and non-diseased persons respectively. The definition given here is more generally used.

analysis can arise in various ways, and most relate to failure to use appropriate statistical techniques. Errors of omission mean that a technique that should have been used on the data was not; errors of commission mean that a technique was applied incorrectly. Some of the more common errors are detailed below.

Failure to distinguish between independent and dependent observations causes many problems. If measurements are repeated on the same individual, they are not independent, and it is totally invalid to analyse them as if they were. For instance, if 20 diabetic patients were studied to determine pancreatic activity, and five observations were made on each patient, the data cannot be analysed for a sample size of $20 \times 5 = 100$ observations. The most important factor is the number of different individuals, and in such a case, the analysis could be performed on the 20 mean levels calculated on each individual. Analysis of variance also provides a very useful technique that can handle replicate observations in comparative studies. Failure to distinguish between independent and dependent data often arises also in clinical trials or case-control studies, where the two groups are paired or matched. The use of the independent t test or χ^2 test, instead of the paired t test or McNemar's χ^2 test, is a common error in paired comparisons.

Many errors relate to ignoring the assumptions underlying the parametric significance tests. The assumptions of approximate normality and equality of variances in group comparisons (homoscedasticity) are important in many cases, and although some tests are fairly robust (departures from some of the assumptions do not seem to matter a great deal), biased analyses can result from misapplication of tests to highly skewed data for instance. Transformation of the data may iron out such problems. With small sample sizes in particular however, assumptions can often not be checked and the non-parametric tests should perhaps be used more frequently.

Problems also arise with repeated use of significance tests. If a set of data is dredged for any significant relationships without reference to the purpose for which the study was set up, some relationships will appear statistically significant purely due to chance. A similar problem arises in a fixed sample size experimental trial, where interim analysis of results takes place before the requisite number of patients have entered. In such situations, spurious differences may appear by chance, and the p value required to declare a significant result should be decreased to allow for multiple testing. This of course will usually require an increase of sample size if the conventional levels of statistical significance are to be claimed.

Lack of understanding of the significance tests available and the type of data they can be applied to can result in biased analysis. This is particularly true in prospective studies of survival, where the problems of variable follow-up and losses to follow-up cause much difficulty. Clinical life table methods or, less preferably, the person-years at risk concept can be used to great advantage in such situations.

In many studies, failure to adjust for confounding variables can result in a totally biased analysis. As has been said, however, controlling for the confounders at the design stage through randomization or matching is preferable to statistical adjustment, although the latter is often necessary.

Over-interpretation of the data is a problem that can also arise. The erroneous assumption that sensitivity and specificity, on their own, are good indicators of the usefulness of a particular diagnostic test has already been discussed. The problem also occurs when appropriate denominators are not available for the calculation of rates. For example, it is not possible to estimate absolute risk in a case-control study. Also, if a study of causes of death is being performed, only proportional mortality analyses can be carried out, unless the population from which the deaths arose is known. Thus, it might be determined that 2% of all deaths under the age of 1 year were due to infectious diseases, while the proportion among deaths in those aged 1 − 2 years was 8%. This would not mean that the death rate (per 1000 of the population in these age groups) from infectious diseases was greater in the older age group. In fact, the death rate would be much higher in those under 1 year. When the number of deaths, only, is available for analysis the large number of deaths from all causes under the age of 1 year results in the proportional mortality for any single cause being considerably reduced.

Misinterpretations of the meaning of statistical significance abound. The confusion of statistical association with causation must be avoided and the results should not be generalized to inappropriate populations. Also, a non-significant result does not mean a negative result; it means only that chance is a possible explanation of an observed association. Important results may be non-significant, due mainly to small sample sizes. On the other hand, a statistically significant result does not necessarily mean a medically important result. A trivial difference between two groups can always be made statistically significant with a large enough sample size.

15.7 Critical reading of the literature

One of the purposes of this book is to enable doctors to approach the medical literature with a critical mind. Many published studies are not all they seem to be at first reading, and it is up to the reader to judge a study's conclusions in the light of its design and analysis. Many biases can be detected if a report is approached with a logical mind, and if the important question 'What else could have produced the results obtained?' is asked. Errors in statistical analysis are often difficult to spot, but flaws in design and execution are more easily detectable. It goes without saying, of course, that a report must describe the study adequately in order for a judgement to be made, and many published reports fail to give sufficient information in this respect.

A report in the medical literature is usually given the following headings: 'Introduction'; 'Materials and Methods'; 'Statistical Techniques'; 'Results'; 'Discussion' or 'Conclusions'. In the introduction, there should be a clear statement of the objectives of the study, and the population to which the findings are to be related. Without this, it is difficult to see if the study design and analysis are appropriate to the question being asked. The materials and methods section, usually in small print, should give in some detail the design of the study, whether a cross-sectional retrospective or prospective observational study, or an experimental trial. Precise definitions of inclusion and exclusion criteria should be given, together with the description of the population from which the study group was formed. If random sampling was employed, this should be stated, as should also the procedure used for randomization. If matched groups are involved it should be clear whether frequency or paired matching was employed. From these descriptions it should be possible to detect any sources of selection or other biases, and to see if the researchers have made any attempt to allow for them.

There should be clear definitions of all the variables studied; this is particularly important for the major end-points of the study, and details of how the measurements were made, whether from case records, interview, direct measurement or official sources, should be indicated. If necessary, comments on the accuracy and validity of the data should be included. If patient follow-up is involved, the methods of tracing patients should be stated and an indication as to whether complete follow-up was achieved should be given.

The statistical techniques section of a paper, which is often included in 'Materials and Methods', should state, at least, which tests were performed, the significance level adopted, and whether one- or two-sided tests were used. If less common techniques were used, references, or a full description, should be given. It should be asked if appropriate techniques were actually employed, and if in fact the data were worthy of statistical analysis. This book has attempted to cover a fair proportion of the statistical techniques employed in medical research, but techniques will be encountered that have not been detailed. In such cases, the adequateness or appropriateness of an analysis may be difficult for the general reader to judge. This section of a published paper should also, ideally, give an indication as to how the study sample size was arrived at — was any attempt made to use statistical methods, or was the size of the study group decided totally on the basis of convenience?

The results section of a paper is, without any doubt, the most important. Are the results presented clearly and in a comprehensible manner? A problem with many reports is that the results section is incomprehensible, with too much detail, too many large and complex tables, and a totally inadequate explanation as to how the results were actually arrived at. If a study is to be widely read and understood, simplicity of presentation is vital. This must be balanced, however, by the necessity to present sufficient detail for judging the adequacy and applicability of the results to the problem under investigation. The results of a study may have arisen from an extremely complex and comprehensive analysis; all aspects of this cannot be presented, and extensive summarizing may be necessary to present the kernel of what was found. There is a danger of swamping the reader with too much detail. The procedure adopted in some reports relegates such detailed results to an appendix, or to 'mini-print' tables. The results section should at least include a simple description of the distribution of the important variables studied in the different comparison groups, so that the reader may make a judgement about any confounding effects. Any statements made in a results section, such as 'males did better than females', should be backed up by summary statistics of the comparison. If confounders have to be adjusted for statistically, it is advisable that both adjusted and unadjusted results are given, to enable the actual effect of the confounding to be seen.

Significance test results, or preferably confidence intervals, should be presented for comparative measures. If a study is reporting statistically non-significant results, then calculations should be presented as to whether or not the study was powerful enough (in terms of sample size) to detect medically important findings.

It is surprising sometimes how often numerical inconsistencies appear in published reports. Often there are discrepancies between figures given in tables and figures given in the text, or numbers in tables or percentages do not add up to the required totals. These should be checked by the reader, because although such errors are easy to make (with retyping of drafts, bad proof-reading, etc.) they may indicate more serious deficiencies in the study.* Do the numbers in the tables and text differ because some patients with missing observations were omitted from the final report but were included originally? Inconsistency may often be due to missing data (refusals, lost records, losses to follow-up), and the paper should state clearly how these problems were dealt with.

The discussion section of a paper should highlight the main results, show how they throw light on the research question being studied, and put the results in context by referring to the relevant literature.

In any study, bias may not be actually present, but the possibility of bias may put a question mark on the acceptance of final conclusions. No study can be perfect however. The important factor is whether the results do give new information which, of course, may be examined in a different way in a further investigation. If the authors of a paper identify possible sources of bias and discuss their potential influence on the results, any conclusions are all the more worthwhile. Finally, if you do discover inadequacies in a published study, ask yourself 'Could I have

---

* The astute reader may discover some inconsistencies in this text!

done it better?' In many situations it will be found that there is no feasible alternative to that of the approach adopted, and it will be concluded that an excellent piece of research has indeed been performed.

15.8 A note on research procedures

For those who may become involved in setting up a research project, or for those who are involved in analysing or writing up a study, a few simple words of advice are offered below. Firstly, do not rush into any project. A good research project may take months, or even years, of planning before any individual is actually studied. Some statistical advice should be sought at a very early stage, especially as regards an appropriate sample size and the design of data collection forms if a computer analysis is even a possibility. A good literature survey is essential, to give an idea of what has already been done in the area of interest and to provide insights into the particular problems the study might face. It must then be decided whether the study is to be observational or experimental and what design features can reasonably be included.

The sections in this book on study design and bias in research provide an overview of the areas which must be considered, but further reading will most probably be necessary. A preliminary *pilot study* on a smaller number of individuals is often very helpful, to test data collection procedures and to provide preliminary estimates on the distribution of some variables as an aid to sample size calculations.

It is often difficult in a study to decide what variables should be measured. Do not be tempted to measure everything. The literature review and knowledge of what is being studied should be a guide to the relevant variables. A good procedure to judge what variables are really needed is to plan out in a rough way what tables would, ideally, be presented in a final report, and thus to determine the variables which are most likely to be related to the study outcome; use only these. Avoid, too, taking measurements which will have missing information in a large number of subjects.

It is worthwhile, in the planning stages of a project, considering the type of statistical analysis that might be undertaken. This also may be a guide as to which variables to include in the data collection. It is advisable in any project to describe the complete study design, and all ancillary information in a written *protocol*. This will greatly aid in the final write-up of a study, and help ensure that the original design is strictly adhered to. Where many persons are involved in a project, and for multicentre trials, this is particularly important. This protocol can then be consulted by anyone involved in the project if there are any doubts about exactly what should be done in a particular situation. A written protocol is also necessary for submission to funding agencies (if funds are required!) and most hospitals require that research proposals be submitted to an ethics committee for approval before study commencement. A good research protocol should include a precise statement concerning the objectives of the study and its importance in the light of current medical knowledge. The actual design of the study should be given in great detail with careful attention paid to the selection of study participants (including the sample size) and potential sources of bias arising therefrom. Ethical problems must also be considered. Clear and concise definitions of the variables to be measured and the measurement techniques to be employed are essential, as are considerations of the relevance, accuracy and validity of these measurements. Data collection forms and questionnaires should be included, as should an indication of the type of statistical analysis that will be performed.

The protocol must be a practical document and should include far more than will ever appear in a published report. It should detail the manpower required for successful implementation of the study and estimate costings in terms of diagnostic tests and other procedures, stationery, printing, etc., travel, computer costs and all the administrative overheads that will accrue. The likely duration of the study must be indicated and a timetable for completion of the various stages (e.g. study group selection, data collection and follow-up, analysis) should be given. How the study is to be implemented in practice, together with an outline of the responsibilities of those involved, should also be presented. Much thought should go into this area.

The execution of a study design demands careful adherence to the written protocol. All individuals involved with any of the subjects being studied should know that a special investigation is being carried out and should have read the protocol. Often, departures from the protocol may be necessary for ethical or other reasons, and careful note should be taken of such departures. Often, as a study progresses certain decisions, especially as regards exclusion or admission criteria, may have to be made in situations not considered in the original design. These too should be noted.

Once the study data have been gathered, a statistical analysis will have to be undertaken. For a large study, this may require the use of a computer and professional advice may be required. Many analyses can be undertaken by computer that would be impractical by hand, but pencil and paper methods are no more outmoded than the wheel. The statistical methods detailed in this book should be sufficient to enable a fair proportion of the data in any reasonably sized study to be analysed with the use of nothing more than a pocket calculator. This book, also details some of the methods used for the control of confounding which are not implemented on many computer systems, and the description of multiple regression techniques may help in the interpretation of such analyses.

At the end of the study, the results must be written up for publication. Choose a journal appropriate to the subject matter of the study, and read a good few articles in that journal to gauge the requirements in presentation. Also, pay careful attention to the 'instructions for authors' which are usually published in each journal on a regular basis. It is not easy to write up a research report, and a fair amount of time and effort is required. The previous section in this chapter, on the critical reading of the literature, should provide some guidelines as to what should be included in an article. Apart from that, it is all up to you.

15.9 Summary

The purpose of this chapter has been to bring together and expand on the subject of bias in medical research. Bias can arise in every stage of a research project, from design, subject selection and data collection to statistical analysis and interpretation. The chapter highlighted some, but not all, of the problems which can arise and it is hoped that it may prove useful to the reader of the medical literature and to the individual involved, for the first time, in the setting up, execution or analysis of a project.

Appendices

A

Computational Methods

A.1 Introduction

Unless you have a computer, you will need a calculator to perform statistical computations. Your calculator should have a square root function at least, and functions for the natural logarithm, exponentiation and the raising of a number to a decimal power are needed for some of the confidence interval calculations. Some models automatically calculate means and standard deviations,* but these are not essential.

This appendix outlines some short-cut computational formulae that will simplify some of the calculations discussed in the text. In particular, simple formulae for the standard deviation, for the χ^2 test for 2×2 tables, for regression and correlation coefficients and for analysis of variance are presented.

A.2 The standard deviation

The calculation of the standard deviation using Eqn. 2.3

$$S = \sqrt{\frac{\Sigma (x - \bar{x})^2}{n - 1}}$$

is fairly cumbersome and an easier computational formula can be derived, which gives the same numerical answer. The sum of squared deviations in the numerator can be expressed

$$\Sigma (x - \bar{x})^2 = \Sigma x^2 - \frac{(\Sigma x)^2}{n} \tag{A.1}$$

so that

$$S = \sqrt{\frac{\Sigma x^2 - (\Sigma x)^2/n}{n - 1}}. \tag{A.2}$$

---

* Usually two different standard deviation functions are provided, one dividing the sum of the squared deviations by $n - 1$ and the other by n. The former should always be employed.

This involves squaring each observation, taking their sum (Σx^2), and subtracting from this the square of the sum of all the observations $(\Sigma x)^2$ divided by the total sample size (n). This is then divided by $n - 1$ and the square root taken.

Table A.1 illustrates the layout for this calculation. Column 1 gives six observations (x) for which the standard deviation is to be calculated. The sum of the observations (Σx) is given at the foot of the column. Column 2 is the square of each value (x^2) with the sum of these squares (Σx^2) at the foot of the column. These values are then substituted into Eqn. A.1 to give the standard deviation.

It is advisable to keep as many digits in the intermediate steps as are displayed on the calculator. The final computed standard deviation need however only be expressed to two decimal places more than the original observations, unless it is to be used in further calculations. Most calculators display only eight digits and sometimes an intermediate computed quantity may exceed the display capacity. In such cases, the original observations can be rescaled to a size more manageable on the calculator. If the original units are too large, either a constant should be subtracted from each observation, or each observation should be divided by some constant. If the units are too small then each observation should be multiplied by a constant. The calculations as described are carried out on the rescaled observations. If subtraction of a constant was employed in the rescaling then the computed standard deviation needs no adjustment and is the same as would have

Table A.1. Calculation of the standard deviation

1 x	2 x^2
530	280900
518	268324
572	327184
595	354025
527	277729
548	300304
3290	1808466

$$n = 6$$
$$\Sigma x = 3290$$
$$(\Sigma x)^2 = 10824100$$
$$(\Sigma x)^2/n = 1804016 \cdot 7$$
$$\Sigma x^2 = 1808466$$
$$\Sigma x^2 - (\Sigma x)^2/n = 4449 \cdot 334$$
$$\frac{\Sigma x^2 - (\Sigma x)^2/n}{n - 1} = 889 \cdot 8668$$
$$S = \sqrt{889 \cdot 8668} = 29 \cdot 83$$

been obtained on the original data. If multiplication (or division) was employed, the computed standard deviation must be divided by (multiplied by) the chosen constant to obtain the correct result. The example in Table A.1 is recomputed in Table A.2 using rescaled values obtained by subtracting 500 from each observation and then in a separate calculation by dividing each observation by 100. The same final standard deviations are obtained. Although rescaling was not necessary in this example, the advantages of the smaller numerical quantities at each step are clear.

If a series of observations has many repeat values, or if the standard deviation of grouped data is being calculated, again there are some short-cut computational methods. In grouped data, remember that all the observations in an interval are assumed to have a value equal to the midpoint of the interval. If there are f occurrences of the value x then the standard deviation is defined

$$S = \sqrt{\frac{\Sigma f (x - \bar{x})^2}{\Sigma f - 1}} \qquad \text{(A.3)}$$

where the sample size is given by the sum of the frequencies in each class (Σf). A computationally easier formula is given by

$$S = \sqrt{\frac{\Sigma f x^2 - (\Sigma f x)^2 / \Sigma f}{\Sigma f - 1}}. \qquad \text{(A.4)}$$

The application of this to calculate the standard deviation of the birth weight data discussed in Chapter 2 is illustrated in Table A.3. Column 1 gives the midpoints of each class interval which correspond to the observations x. Column 2 gives the

Table A.2. Example of rescaling in calculating standard deviations

	Original units	− 500	÷ 100
	530	30	5·3
	518	18	5·18
	572	72	5·72
	595	95	5·95
	527	27	5·27
	548	48	5·48
Σx	3290	290	32·90
$(\Sigma x)^2$	10824100	84100	1082·41
Σx^2	1808466	18466	180·8466
$\Sigma x^2 - (\Sigma x)^2 / n$	4449·334	4449·334	0·4449334
$\sqrt{\dfrac{\Sigma x^2 - (\Sigma x)^2 / n}{n-1}}$	29·8306	29·8306	0·298306
S	29·83	29·83	29·83

Table A.3. Standard deviation for grouped data (birth weight data of Table 1.3)

1 Class midpoints x	2 No. of observations f	3 x^2	4 fx^2	5 fx
1·88	4	3·5344	14·1376	7·52
2·13	3	4·5369	13·6107	6·39
2·38	12	5·6644	67·9728	28·56
2·63	34	6·9169	235·1746	89·42
2·88	115	8·2944	953·8560	331·20
3·13	175	9·7969	1714·4575	547·75
3·38	281	11·4244	3210·2564	949·78
3·63	261	13·1769	3439·1709	947·43
3·88	212	15·0544	3191·5328	822·56
4·13	94	17·0569	1603·3486	388·22
4·38	47	19·1844	901·6668	205·86
4·63	14	21·4369	300·1166	64·82
4·88	6	23·8144	142·8864	29·28
5·13	2	26·3169	52·6338	10·26
	1260 (Σf)		15840·822* (Σfx^2)	4429·05 (Σfx)

* Eight digits accuracy.

$$S = \sqrt{\frac{\Sigma fx^2 - (\Sigma fx)^2/\Sigma f}{\Sigma f - 1}}$$

$$= \sqrt{\frac{15840\cdot822 - (4429\cdot05)^2/1260}{1259}}$$

$$= 0\cdot4650$$

frequencies (f) observed in each class, and the sum of their values (Σf) is the total sample size. Column 3 contains the square of each x value and column 4 gives each of these x^2 values multiplied by its frequency f. The sum of this column is Σfx^2. Column 5 gives each observed value multiplied by its frequency giving the sum Σfx. Σf, Σfx and Σfx^2 are then substituted into Eqn. A.4 to give the standard deviation. Again the original values, x, can if necessary be rescaled to make the calculations more manageable on a pocket calculator.

A.3 The χ^2 test for independent 2 × 2 tables

An alternative to the usual χ^2 formula in 2 × 2 tables (Eqn. 7.16)

$$\chi^2 = \Sigma\frac{(O - E)^2}{E}$$

Table A.4. Short-cut χ^2 formula for independent 2×2 tables

a	b	r_1	
c	d	r_2	$\chi^2 = \dfrac{(ad - bc)^2 n}{r_1 r_2 s_1 s_2}$ on 1 degree of freedom
s_1	s_2	n	

which is computationally simpler, is often used. It has the disadvantage, however, that the expected values (E) are not computed so that there is no direct check on whether all of these are greater than 5, as required in the usual assumptions for the use of the test.

Table A.4 shows the layout of a general 2×2 contingency table. a, b, c and d are the four observed quantities, r_1 and r_2 are the row totals and s_1 and s_2 are the column totals, n is the sample size. With this notation,

$$\chi^2 = \frac{(ad - bc)^2 n}{r_1 r_2 s_1 s_2}. \tag{A.5}$$

When using a pocket calculator, the numerator of this expression may exceed the capacity of the display. This can be avoided by first calculating $(ad - bc)^2$, then dividing by r_1 and r_2, multiplying by n and finally dividing by s_1 and s_2.

A.4 Regression and correlation

The formulae for both the regression and correlation coefficients (Eqns. 9.4 and 9.7) involve the expression

$$\Sigma(x - \bar{x})(y - \bar{y})$$

while the formula for the standard error of the estimate (Eqn. 9.12) requires the calculation of

$$\Sigma(y - \hat{y})^2$$

where the ys are the observed values of the dependent variable and the $\hat{y}$s are the predicted or expected values on the basis of the regression equation. As they stand, both these expressions are computationally awkward and alternatives are available. Firstly

$$\Sigma(x - \bar{x})(y - \bar{y}) = \Sigma xy - \frac{(\Sigma x)(\Sigma y)}{n} \tag{A.6}$$

where n is the number of pairs on which the regression equation or correlation coefficient is being calculated. This expression involves calculating the product of each pair of x and y variables and summing to obtain Σxy. The Σx and Σy terms are the sums of the x and y variables separately.

Table A.5 shows the original data for the regression of left ventricular ejection fraction (LVEF) on the QRS score discussed in Chapter 9.* Columns 1 and 2 give the QRS values (x), and the corresponding LVEF values (y), which summed give Σx and Σy. Column 3 gives the xy values obtained by multiplying each x value by its y value, and the sum of these is Σxy. Columns 4 and 5 give the squares of the x and y values and their sums. These are the basic quantities required for regression

Table A.5. Computation of basic quantities required for simple regression calculations (data from Fig. 9.6)

1 QRS score x	2 LVEF y	3 xy	4 x^2	5 y^2
0	51	0	0	2601
0	57	0	0	3249
0	58	0	0	3364
0	60	0	0	3600
0	66	0	0	4356
0	71	0	0	5041
1	58	58	1	3364
1	60	60	1	3600
1	65	65	1	4225
2	57	114	4	3249
3	52	156	9	2704
4	51	204	16	2601
5	44	220	25	1936
5	46	230	25	2116
6	32	192	36	1024
6	40	240	36	1600
6	42	252	36	1764
6	48	288	36	2304
7	37	259	49	1369
8	28	224	64	784
8	38	304	64	1444
9	28	252	81	784
9	31	279	81	961
9	43	387	81	1849
11	21	231	121	441
11	22	242	121	484
11	24	264	121	576
13	18	234	169	324
142 (Σx)	1248 (Σy)	4755 (Σxy)	1178 (Σx^2)	61714 (Σy^2)

* These data are based on the published diagram (Palmeri *et al.* 1982) and the resulting calculations differ slightly from those appearing in the publication.

Table A.6. Regression calculations for LVEF/QRS data

Quantity	Computational formula	Value	
$\Sigma(x - \bar{x})(y - \bar{y})$	$\Sigma xy - (\Sigma x)(\Sigma y)/n$	$4755 - (142)(1248)/28$	$-1574 \cdot 1429$
$\Sigma(x - \bar{x})^2$	$\Sigma x^2 - (\Sigma x)^2/n$	$1178 - (142)^2/28$	$457 \cdot 85714$
$\Sigma(y - \bar{y})^2$	$\Sigma y^2 - (\Sigma y)^2/n$	$61714 - (1248)^2/28$	$6088 \cdot 8572$
$\bar{x}$	$\Sigma x/n$	$142/28$	$5 \cdot 0714$
$\bar{y}$	$\Sigma y/n$	$1248/28$	$44 \cdot 5714$
Regression coefficient b (Eqn. 9.4)	$\Sigma(x - \bar{x})(y - \bar{y})/\Sigma(x - \bar{x})^2$	$-1574 \cdot 1429/457 \cdot 85714$	$-3 \cdot 4381$
Regression coefficient a (Eqn. 9.6)	$\bar{y} - b\bar{x}$	$44 \cdot 5714 + 3 \cdot 4381(5 \cdot 0714)$	$62 \cdot 0074$
Correlation coefficient r (Eqn. 9.7)	$\dfrac{\Sigma(x - \bar{x})(y - \bar{y})}{\sqrt{\Sigma(x - \bar{x})^2 \; \Sigma(y - \bar{y})^2}}$	$\dfrac{-1574 \cdot 1429}{\sqrt{457 \cdot 85714 \times 6088 \cdot 8572}}$	$-0 \cdot 9428$

and correlation calculations. The number of pairs, n, is 28. Table A.6 shows, explicitly, the calculations for the regression coefficients (Eqns. 9.4 and 9.6) and the correlation coefficient (Eqn. 9.7) for the LVEF data.

The computational expression for $\Sigma(y - \hat{y})^2$ is given by

$$\Sigma(y - \bar{y})^2 - \frac{[\Sigma(x - \bar{x})(y - \bar{y})]^2}{\Sigma(x - \bar{x})^2}. \tag{A.7}$$

All these quantities have already been calculated and Table A.7 shows the final computations for $S_{y.x}$ using Eqn. 9.12.

Table A.7. Calculation of $S_{y.x}$ for the LVEF/QRS data

$$\Sigma(y - \hat{y})^2 = \Sigma(y - \bar{y})^2 - \frac{[\Sigma(x - \bar{x})(y - \bar{y})]^2}{\Sigma(x - \bar{x})^2}$$

$$= 6088 \cdot 8572 - \frac{(-1574 \cdot 1429)^2}{457 \cdot 85714}$$

$$= 676 \cdot 8501$$

$$S_{y.x} = \sqrt{\frac{\Sigma(y - \hat{y})^2}{n - 2}}$$

$$= \sqrt{\frac{676 \cdot 8501}{26}}$$

$$= 5 \cdot 1022$$

A.5. Sums of squares in ANOVA

Underlying all calculations in the analysis of variance are the quantities referred to as 'sums of squares' (see Section 8.4). The formulae for these, as presented, are tedious to compute and a more convenient approach is described below.

$$\text{Total SSq} = \Sigma_i \Sigma_j \, (x_{ij} - \bar{x})^2$$

$$\text{Within-group SSq} = \Sigma_i \Sigma_j \, (x_{ij} - \bar{x}_i)^2$$

$$\text{Between-group SSq} = \Sigma_i \Sigma_j \, (\bar{x}_i - \bar{x})^2$$

where Σ_i means summation over the number of groups being compared (k) and Σ_j means summation over the n_i values in a group (see Eqn. 8.9).

The easiest way to compute these quantities is to first calculate the total SSq using the methods of Section A.1 (Eqn. A.1). Letting T be the sum of all the observations, and S be the sum of all the observations after squaring,[*]

$$T = \Sigma_i \Sigma_j x_{ij} \quad \text{and} \quad S = \Sigma_i \Sigma_j x_{ij}^2,$$

it is easy to see that

$$\text{Total SSq} = S - \frac{T^2}{N} \tag{A.8}$$

where N is the total sample size in all k groups.

The within-group SSq for a single group — group i — is

$$\Sigma_j \, (x_{ij} - \bar{x}_i)^2 = S_i - \frac{T_i^2}{n_i}$$

where T_i and S_i denote the sums of the observations and the squared observations in group i, and n_i is the sample size in that group. The within-group SSq for all the groups is then

$$\text{Within-group SSq} = \Sigma_i S_i - \Sigma_i (T_i^2/n_i)$$
$$= S - \Sigma_i \, (T_i^2/n_i). \tag{A.9}$$

The between-group SSq can be obtained, after the total and within-group SSqs have been calculated with Eqns. A.8 and A.9, by using Eqn. 8.10:

$$\text{Between-group SSq} = \text{Total SSq} - \text{Within-group SSq}. \tag{A.10}$$

These calculations are illustrated in Table A.8 on the data from Section 8.3 (Table 8.2).

---

[*] *S in this section* refers to the sum of the squared observations and should not be confused with the standard deviation which, elsewhere in this text, is also denoted S.

Table A.8. Illustration of sums of squares calculations on the data of Table 8.2

Group i	Smokers (1)	Ex-smokers (2)	Non-smokers (3)	$k = 3$
Systolic blood	125	115	95	
pressures	135	125	100	
	140	135	105	
	145		120	
	155			
n_i	5	3	4	$N = 12$
T_i	700	375	420	$T = 1495$
T_i^2	490000	140625	176400	
T_i^2/n_i	98000	46875	44100	$\Sigma_i\,(T_i^2/n_i) = 188975$

S (obtained directly) $= 190025$

Total SSq $\quad = S - (T^2/N)$
$\qquad\quad = 190025 - (1495)^2/12$
$\qquad\quad = 3772.9$

Within-group SSq $\quad = S - \Sigma_i\,(T_i^2/n_i)$
$\qquad\qquad\quad = 190025 - 188975$
$\qquad\qquad\quad = 1050$

Between-group SSq $= 3772.9 - 1050$
$\qquad\qquad\qquad = 2722.9$

B

Statistical Tables

B.1 Introduction

This appendix gives the statistical (and other) tables necessary in the calculation of significance levels and confidence intervals for the methods described in this book. For ease of use, an attempt has been made to employ a uniform layout for these tables and the upper and lower critical values for a range of one- and two-sided significance levels are presented. Consequently, some of the tables may have a different appearance from those that are more customary, but hopefully they will prove easier to employ in practice. Note also that the tables relate to the critical values of the test statistic as described in this text, which may have a slightly different formulation (especially for the non-parametric tests) from that given in other sources. Most of the tables have been reproduced or adapted from the *Geigy Scientific Tables* (Lentner, 1982), which is a very useful reference work, but Tables B.11, B.12 and B.13 have been produced directly using algorithms written for the SAS statistical software (SAS User's Guide: Basics, 1985).

Sometimes the sample size may be too large for use of the statistical tables for the non-parametric tests. In such cases, if a non-parametric test must be used, the *Geigy Scientific Tables* give formulae for approximate large sample-size significance levels. The non-parametric tests, however, tend to be used more often with small sample sizes, so this should not be a major problem in most practical applications. Note, too, that in many of the non-parametric tests, the significance levels given in the tables are not exact, due to the discrete nature of the particular distributions. The actual probability or p value associated with a given critical value may, in fact, be slightly less than that presented. The tables included in the appendix are:

B.2 Tables

Table B.I. Table of random numbers. Abbreviated from *Geigy Scientific Tables* Vol. 2, 8th edn. with permission

20557	43375	50914	83628	73935	72502	48174	62551	96122	22375	96488
83936	45842	78222	88481	44933	12839	20750	47116	58973	99018	22769
36077	82577	16210	76092	87730	90049	02115	37096	20505	91937	69776
78267	31568	58297	88922	50436	86135	42726	54307	29170	13045	65527
00232	98059	07255	90786	95246	15280	61692	45137	17539	31799	64780
65869	64355	91271	49295	98354	28005	69792	01480	51557	70726	35862
35454	51623	98381	11055	32951	28363	16451	67912	66404	76254	75495
99542	44247	12762	54488	74321	36224	95619	16238	25374	13653	25345
36087	32326	52225	72447	77804	57045	27552	72387	34001	83792	66764
64899	62390	68375	42921	28545	33167	85710	11035	40171	04840	69848
11994	97820	06653	27477	61364	22681	02280	53815	47479	44017	37563
02915	81553	92012	50435	73814	96290	86827	81430	45597	82296	28947
62895	09202	48494	95974	33534	94657	71126	71770	16092	03942	90111
39202	82110	82254	03669	03281	11613	36336	98297	48100	71594	52667
53252	18175	09457	83810	46392	02705	85591	33192	65127	80852	42030
17820	50756	80608	35695	72641	26306	76298	32532	22644	96853	18610
85245	12710	60264	74650	92126	08152	32147	17457	56298	48964	64733
85822	44424	88508	66190	74060	93206	92840	44833	81146	64060	62975
24804	24720	66501	74157	42246	41688	72835	87258	89384	11251	34329
31942	85419	93017	28087	78323	77109	56832	78400	24190	37978	85863
72838	10933	99964	13468	17211	48046	51122	92668	96750	11139	06275
38546	49559	71671	53603	24491	57570	90789	32932	67449	05115	45941
38051	39391	92039	71664	40219	97707	93975	66981	19556	24605	52169
28101	38543	54214	48928	32818	51963	87353	15094	29529	87305	01361
70476	44242	54227	28598	64422	29361	20359	48577	05971	92373	22765
64999	11468	74149	81386	94127	67342	38010	92522	57728	39432	27914
73641	52165	54336	89196	40042	37889	06003	58033	59082	94988	62152
67421	83093	77038	55399	67893	89597	85630	08059	35757	49479	63531
30976	66455	90708	08450	50120	17795	55604	51222	17900	55553	02980
29660	30790	65154	19582	20942	81439	83917	90452	64753	99645	19799
82747	97297	74420	18783	93471	89055	56413	77817	10655	52915	68198
46978	87390	53319	90155	03154	20301	47831	86786	11284	49160	79852
19783	82215	35810	39852	43795	21530	96315	55657	76473	08217	46810
12249	35844	63265	26451	06986	08707	99251	06260	74779	96285	31998
58785	53473	06308	56778	30474	57277	23425	27092	47759	18422	56074
69373	73674	97914	77989	47280	71804	74587	70563	77813	50242	60398
95662	83923	90790	49474	11901	30322	80254	99608	17019	17892	76813
97758	08206	54199	41327	01170	21745	71318	07978	35440	26128	10545
72154	86385	39490	57482	32921	33795	43155	30432	48384	85430	51828
25583	74101	87573	01556	89183	64830	16779	35724	82103	61658	20296

Table B.2. The z test: critical values for the standard normal distribution. Abbreviated and adapted from *Geigy Scientific Tables* Vol. 2, 8th edn. with permission

	Area in two tails (two-sided significance level)	0·10	0·05	0·02	0·01
	Area in one tail (one-sided significance level)	0·05	0·025	0·01	0·005
Critical value z_c		1·645	1·960	2·326	2·576

Significant result if $z \geqslant z_c$ or $z \leqslant -z_c$

Table B.3. The *t* test: critical values for the Student's *t* distribution. Abbreviated and adapted from *Geigy Scientific Tables* Vol. 2, 8th edn. with permission

	Area in two tails (two-sided significance level)	0·10	0·05	0·02	0·01
	Area in one tail (one-sided significance level)	0·05	0·025	0·01	0·005
d.f.		Critical value t_c			
1		6·314	12·706	31·821	63·657
2		2·920	4·303	6·965	9·925
3		2·353	3·182	4·541	5·841
4		2·132	2·776	3·747	4·604
5		2·015	2·571	3·365	4·032
6		1·943	2·447	3·143	3·707
7		1·895	2·365	2·998	3·499
8		1·860	2·306	2·896	3·355
9		1·833	2·262	2·821	3·250
10		1·812	2·228	2·764	3·169
11		1·796	2·201	2·718	3·106
12		1·782	2·179	2·681	3·055
13		1·771	2·160	2·650	3·012
14		1·761	2·145	2·624	2·977
15		1·753	2·131	2·602	2·947
16		1·746	2·120	2·583	2·921
17		1·740	2·110	2·567	2·898
18		1·734	2·101	2·552	2·878
19		1·729	2·093	2·539	2·861
20		1·725	2·086	2·528	2·845
21		1·721	2·080	2·518	2·831
22		1·717	2·074	2·508	2·819
23		1·714	2·069	2·500	2·807
24		1·711	2·064	2·492	2·797
25		1·708	2·060	2·485	2·787
30		1·697	2·042	2·457	2·750
40		1·684	2·021	2·423	2·704
60		1·671	2·000	2·390	2·660
80		1·664	1·990	2·374	2·639
100		1·660	1·984	2·364	2·626
∞		1·645	1·960	2·326	2·576

Significant result if $t \geq t_c$ or $t \leq -t_c$

Table B.4. The χ^2 test: critical values for the chi-square distribution. Abbreviated and adapted from *Geigy Scientific Tables* Vol. 2, 8th edn. with permission

Two-sided significance level	0·10	0·05	0·02	0·01
One-sided significance level	0·05	0·025	0·01	0·005
d.f.	Critical value χ^2_c			
1	2·706	3·841	5·412	6·635
2	4·605	5·991	7·824	9·210
3	6·251	7·815	9·837	11·345
4	7·779	9·488	11·668	13·277
5	9·236	11·070	13·388	15·086
6	10·645	12·592	15·033	16·812
7	12·017	14·067	16·622	18·475
8	13·362	15·507	18·168	20·090
9	14·684	16·919	19·679	21·666
10	15·987	18·307	21·161	23·209
11	17·275	19·675	22·618	24·725
12	18·549	21·026	24·054	26·217
13	19·812	22·362	25·472	27·688
14	21·064	23·685	26·873	29·141
15	22·307	24·996	28·259	30·578
16	23·542	26·296	29·633	32·000
17	24·769	27·587	30·995	33·409
18	25·989	28·869	32·346	34·805
19	27·204	30·144	33·687	36·191
20	28·412	31·410	35·020	37·566
21	29·615	32·671	36·343	38·932
22	30·813	33·924	37·659	40·289
23	32·007	35·172	38·968	41·638
24	33·196	36·415	40·270	42·980
25	34·382	37·652	41·566	44·314
26	35·563	38·885	42·856	45·642
27	36·741	40·113	44·140	46·963
28	37·916	41·337	45·419	48·278
29	39·087	42·557	46·693	49·588
30	40·256	43·773	47·962	50·892

Significant result if $\chi^2 \geqslant \chi^2_c$

Table B.5(a). The Wilcoxon two-sample rank sum test for sample sizes $n_1 = 1$ to 9, $n_2 = 1$ to 35. Critical lower (T_l) and upper (T_u) values for the sum of ranks T_1 from sample sized n_1. Abbreviated and adapted from *Geigy Scientific Tables* Vol. 2, 8th edn. with permission

Two-sided significance level: 0·10
One-sided significance level: 0·05

n_1	1	2	3	4	5	6	7	8	9
n_2	$T_l\ T_u$	$T_l\ T_u$	$T_l\ T_u$	$T_l\ T_u$	$T_l\ T_u$	$T_l\ T_u$	$T_l\ T_u$	$T_l\ T_u$	$T_l\ T_u$
1	—	—	—	—	—	—	—	—	—
2	—	—	—	—	15 – 25	21 – 33	28 – 42	37 – 51	46 – 62
3	—	—	6 – 15	10 – 22	16 – 29	23 – 37	30 – 47	39 – 57	49 – 68
4	—	—	6 – 18	11 – 25	17 – 33	24 – 42	32 – 52	41 – 63	51 – 75
5	—	3 – 13	7 – 20	12 – 28	19 – 36	26 – 46	34 – 57	44 – 68	54 – 81
6	—	3 – 15	8 – 22	13 – 31	20 – 40	28 – 50	36 – 62	46 – 74	57 – 87
7	—	3 – 17	8 – 25	14 – 34	21 – 44	29 – 55	39 – 66	49 – 79	60 – 93
8	—	4 – 18	9 – 27	15 – 37	23 – 47	31 – 59	41 – 71	51 – 85	63 – 99
9	—	4 – 20	10 – 29	16 – 40	24 – 51	33 – 63	43 – 76	54 – 90	66 – 105
10	—	4 – 22	10 – 32	17 – 43	26 – 54	35 – 67	45 – 81	56 – 96	69 – 111
11	—	4 – 24	11 – 34	18 – 46	27 – 58	37 – 71	47 – 86	59 – 101	72 – 117
12	—	5 – 25	11 – 37	19 – 49	28 – 62	38 – 76	49 – 91	62 – 106	75 – 123
13	—	5 – 27	12 – 39	20 – 52	30 – 65	40 – 80	52 – 95	64 – 112	78 – 129
14	—	6 – 28	13 – 41	21 – 55	31 – 69	42 – 84	54 – 100	67 – 117	81 – 135
15	—	6 – 30	13 – 44	22 – 58	33 – 72	44 – 88	56 – 105	69 – 123	84 – 141
16	—	6 – 32	14 – 46	24 – 60	34 – 76	46 – 92	58 – 110	72 – 128	87 – 147
17	—	6 – 34	15 – 48	25 – 63	35 – 80	47 – 97	61 – 114	75 – 133	90 – 153
18	—	7 – 35	15 – 51	26 – 66	37 – 83	49 – 101	63 – 119	77 – 139	93 – 159
19	1 – 20	7 – 37	16 – 53	27 – 69	38 – 87	51 – 105	65 – 124	80 – 144	96 – 165
20	1 – 21	7 – 39	17 – 55	28 – 72	40 – 90	53 – 109	67 – 129	83 – 149	99 – 171
21	1 – 22	8 – 40	17 – 58	29 – 75	41 – 94	55 – 113	69 – 134	85 – 155	102 – 177
22	1 – 23	8 – 42	18 – 60	30 – 78	43 – 97	57 – 117	72 – 138	88 – 160	105 – 183
23	1 – 24	8 – 44	19 – 62	31 – 81	44 – 101	58 – 122	74 – 143	90 – 166	108 – 189
24	1 – 25	9 – 45	19 – 62	32 – 84	45 – 105	60 – 126	76 – 148	93 – 171	111 – 195
25	1 – 26	9 – 47	20 – 67	33 – 87	47 – 108	62 – 130	78 – 153	96 – 176	114 – 201
26	1 – 27	9 – 49	21 – 69	34 – 90	48 – 112	64 – 134	81 – 157	98 – 182	117 – 207
27	1 – 28	10 – 50	21 – 72	35 – 93	50 – 115	66 – 138	83 – 162	101 – 187	120 – 213
28	1 – 29	10 – 52	22 – 74	36 – 96	51 – 119	67 – 143	85 – 167	104 – 192	123 – 219
29	1 – 30	10 – 54	23 – 76	37 – 99	53 – 122	69 – 147	87 – 172	106 – 198	127 – 224
30	1 – 31	10 – 56	23 – 79	38 – 102	54 – 126	71 – 151	89 – 177	109 – 203	130 – 230
31	1 – 32	11 – 57	24 – 81	39 – 105	55 – 130	73 – 155	92 – 181	112 – 208	133 – 236
32	1 – 33	11 – 59	25 – 83	40 – 108	57 – 133	75 – 159	94 – 186	114 – 214	136 – 242
33	1 – 34	11 – 61	25 – 86	41 – 111	58 – 137	77 – 163	96 – 191	117 – 219	139 – 248
34	1 – 35	12 – 62	26 – 88	42 – 114	60 – 140	78 – 168	98 – 196	120 – 224	142 – 254
35	1 – 36	12 – 64	27 – 90	43 – 117	61 – 144	80 – 172	101 – 200	122 – 230	145 – 260

Significant result if $T_1 \geqslant T_u$ or $T_1 \leqslant T_l$

Table B.5(a). (*Continued*)

Two-sided significance level: 0·05
One-sided significance level: 0·025

n_1	1	2	3	4	5	6	7	8	9
n_2	$T_l\ T_u$	$T_l\ T_u$	$T_l\ T_u$	$T_l\ T_u$	$T_l\ T_u$	$T_l\ T_u$	$T_l\ T_u$	$T_l\ T_u$	$T_l\ T_u$
1	—	—	—	—	—	—	—	—	—
2	—	—	—	—	—	—	—	36 − 52	45 − 63
3	—	—	—	—	15 − 30	22 − 38	29 − 48	38 − 58	47 − 70
4	—	—	—	10 − 26	16 − 34	23 − 43	31 − 53	40 − 64	49 − 77
5	—	—	6 − 21	11 − 29	17 − 38	24 − 48	33 − 58	42 − 70	52 − 83
6	—	—	7 − 23	12 − 32	18 − 42	26 − 52	34 − 64	44 − 76	55 − 89
7	—	—	7 − 26	13 − 35	20 − 45	27 − 57	36 − 69	46 − 82	57 − 96
8	—	3 − 19	8 − 28	14 − 38	21 − 49	29 − 61	38 − 74	49 − 87	60 − 102
9	—	3 − 21	8 − 31	14 − 42	22 − 53	31 − 65	40 − 79	51 − 93	62 − 109
10	—	3 − 23	9 − 33	15 − 45	23 − 57	32 − 70	42 − 84	53 − 99	65 − 115
11	—	3 − 25	9 − 36	16 − 48	24 − 61	34 − 74	44 − 89	55 − 105	68 − 121
12	—	4 − 26	10 − 38	17 − 51	26 − 64	35 − 79	46 − 94	58 − 110	71 − 127
13	—	4 − 28	10 − 41	18 − 54	27 − 68	37 − 83	48 − 99	60 − 116	73 − 134
14	—	4 − 30	11 − 43	19 − 57	28 − 72	38 − 88	50 − 104	62 − 122	76 − 140
15	—	4 − 32	11 − 46	20 − 60	29 − 76	40 − 92	52 − 109	65 − 127	79 − 146
16	—	4 − 34	12 − 48	21 − 63	30 − 80	42 − 96	54 − 114	67 − 133	82 − 152
17	—	5 − 35	12 − 51	21 − 67	32 − 83	43 − 101	56 − 119	70 − 138	84 − 159
18	—	5 − 37	13 − 53	22 − 70	33 − 87	45 − 105	58 − 124	72 − 144	87 − 165
19	—	5 − 39	13 − 56	23 − 73	34 − 91	46 − 110	60 − 129	74 − 150	90 − 171
20	—	5 − 41	14 − 58	24 − 76	35 − 95	48 − 114	62 − 134	77 − 155	93 − 177
21	—	6 − 42	14 − 61	25 − 79	37 − 98	50 − 118	64 − 139	79 − 161	95 − 184
22	—	6 − 44	15 − 63	26 − 82	38 − 102	51 − 123	66 − 144	81 − 167	98 − 190
23	—	6 − 46	15 − 66	27 − 85	39 − 106	53 − 127	68 − 149	84 − 172	101 − 196
24	—	6 − 48	16 − 68	27 − 89	40 − 110	54 − 132	70 − 154	86 − 178	104 − 202
25	—	6 − 50	16 − 71	28 − 92	42 − 113	56 − 136	72 − 159	89 − 183	107 − 208
26	—	7 − 51	17 − 73	29 − 95	43 − 117	58 − 140	74 − 164	91 − 189	109 − 215
27	—	7 − 53	17 − 76	30 − 98	44 − 121	59 − 145	76 − 169	93 − 195	112 − 221
28	—	7 − 55	18 − 78	31 − 101	45 − 125	61 − 149	78 − 174	96 − 200	115 − 227
29	—	7 − 57	19 − 80	32 − 104	47 − 128	63 − 153	80 − 179	98 − 206	118 − 233
30	—	8 − 58	19 − 83	33 − 107	48 − 132	64 − 158	82 − 184	101 − 211	121 − 239
31	—	8 − 60	20 − 85	34 − 110	49 − 136	66 − 162	84 − 189	103 − 217	123 − 246
32	—	8 − 62	20 − 88	34 − 114	50 − 140	67 − 167	86 − 194	105 − 223	126 − 252
33	—	8 − 64	21 − 90	35 − 117	52 − 143	69 − 171	88 − 199	108 − 228	129 − 258
34	—	8 − 66	21 − 93	36 − 120	53 − 147	71 − 175	90 − 204	110 − 234	132 − 264
35	—	9 − 67	22 − 95	37 − 123	54 − 151	72 − 180	92 − 209	113 − 239	134 − 271

Significant result if $T_1 \geqslant T_u$ or $T_1 \leqslant T_l$ *Continued*

Table B.5(a). (*Continued*) The Wilcoxon two-sample rank sum test for sample sizes $n_1 = 1$ to 9, $n_2 = 1$ to 35. Critical lower (T_l) and upper (T_u) values for the sum of ranks T_1 from sample sized n_1

Two-sided significance level: 0·02
One-sided significance level: 0·01

n_1	1	2	3	4	5	6	7	8	9
n_2	$T_l\ T_u$	$T_l\ T_u$	$T_l\ T_u$	$T_l\ T_u$	$T_l\ T_u$	$T_l\ T_u$	$T_l\ T_u$	$T_l\ T_u$	$T_l\ T_u$
1	—	—	—	—	—	—	—	—	—
2	—	—	—	—	—	—	—	—	—
3	—	—	—	—	—	—	28 − 49	36 − 60	46 − 71
4	—	—	—	—	15 − 35	22 − 44	29 − 55	38 − 66	48 − 78
5	—	—	—	10 − 30	16 − 39	23 − 49	31 − 60	40 − 72	50 − 85
6	—	—	—	11 − 33	17 − 43	24 − 54	32 − 66	42 − 78	52 − 92
7	—	—	6 − 27	11 − 37	18 − 47	25 − 59	34 − 71	43 − 85	54 − 99
8	—	—	6 − 30	12 − 40	19 − 51	27 − 63	35 − 77	45 − 91	56 − 106
9	—	—	7 − 32	13 − 43	20 − 55	28 − 68	37 − 82	47 − 97	59 − 112
10	—	—	7 − 35	13 − 47	21 − 59	29 − 73	39 − 87	49 − 103	61 − 119
11	—	—	7 − 38	14 − 50	22 − 63	30 − 78	40 − 93	51 − 109	63 − 126
12	—	—	8 − 40	15 − 53	23 − 67	32 − 82	42 − 98	53 − 115	66 − 132
13	—	3 − 29	8 − 43	15 − 57	24 − 71	33 − 87	44 − 103	56 − 120	68 − 139
14	—	3 − 31	8 − 46	16 − 60	25 − 75	34 − 92	45 − 109	58 − 126	71 − 145
15	—	3 − 33	9 − 48	17 − 63	26 − 79	36 − 96	47 − 114	60 − 132	73 − 152
16	—	3 − 35	9 − 51	17 − 67	27 − 83	37 − 101	49 − 119	62 − 138	76 − 158
17	—	3 − 37	10 − 53	18 − 70	28 − 87	39 − 105	51 − 124	64 − 144	78 − 165
18	—	3 − 39	10 − 56	19 − 73	29 − 91	40 − 110	52 − 130	66 − 150	81 − 171
19	—	4 − 40	10 − 59	19 − 77	30 − 95	41 − 115	54 − 135	68 − 156	83 − 178
20	—	4 − 42	11 − 61	20 − 80	31 − 99	43 − 119	56 − 140	70 − 162	85 − 185
21	—	4 − 44	11 − 64	21 − 83	32 − 103	44 − 124	58 − 145	72 − 168	88 − 191
22	—	4 − 46	12 − 66	21 − 87	33 − 107	45 − 129	59 − 151	74 − 174	90 − 198
23	—	4 − 48	12 − 69	22 − 90	34 − 111	47 − 133	61 − 156	76 − 180	93 − 204
24	—	4 − 50	12 − 72	23 − 93	35 − 115	48 − 138	63 − 161	78 − 186	95 − 211
25	—	4 − 52	13 − 74	23 − 97	36 − 119	50 − 142	64 − 167	81 − 191	98 − 217
26	—	4 − 54	13 − 77	24 − 100	37 − 123	51 − 147	66 − 172	83 − 197	100 − 224
27	—	5 − 55	13 − 80	25 − 103	38 − 127	52 − 152	68 − 177	85 − 203	103 − 230
28	—	5 − 57	14 − 82	26 − 106	39 − 131	54 − 156	70 − 182	87 − 209	105 − 237
29	—	5 − 59	14 − 85	26 − 110	40 − 135	55 − 161	71 − 188	89 − 215	108 − 243
30	—	5 − 61	15 − 87	27 − 113	41 − 139	56 − 166	73 − 193	91 − 221	110 − 250
31	—	5 − 63	15 − 90	28 − 116	42 − 143	58 − 170	75 − 198	93 − 227	113 − 256
32	—	5 − 65	15 − 93	28 − 120	43 − 147	59 − 175	77 − 203	95 − 233	115 − 263
33	—	·5 − 67	16 − 95	29 − 123	44 − 151	61 − 179	78 − 209	97 − 239	118 − 269
34	—	6 − 68	16 − 98	30 − 126	45 − 155	62 − 184	80 − 214	100 − 244	120 − 276
35	—	6 − 70	17 − 100	30 − 130	46 − 159	63 − 189	82 − 219	102 − 250	123 − 282

Significant result if $T_1 \geq T_u$ or $T_1 \leq T_l$

Table B.5(a). (*Continued*)

Two-sided significance level: 0·01
One-sided significance level: 0·005

n_1	1	2	3	4	5	6	7	8	9
n_2	$T_l\ T_u$	$T_l\ T_u$	$T_l\ T_u$	$T_l\ T_u$	$T_l\ T_u$	$T_l\ T_u$	$T_l\ T_u$	$T_l\ T_u$	$T_l\ T_u$
1	—	—	—	—	—	—	—	—	—
2	—	—	—	—	—	—	—	—	—
3	—	—	—	—	—	—	—	—	45 − 72
4	—	—	—	—	—	21 − 45	28 − 56	37 − 67	46 − 80
5	—	—	—	—	15 − 40	22 − 50	29 − 62	38 − 74	48 − 87
6	—	—	—	10 − 34	16 − 44	23 − 55	31 − 67	40 − 80	50 − 94
7	—	—	—	10 − 38	16 − 49	24 − 60	32 − 73	42 − 86	52 − 101
8	—	—	—	11 − 41	17 − 53	25 − 65	34 − 78	43 − 93	54 − 108
9	—	—	6 − 33	11 − 45	18 − 57	26 − 70	35 − 84	45 − 99	56 − 115
10	—	—	6 − 36	12 − 48	19 − 61	27 − 75	37 − 89	47 − 105	58 − 122
11	—	—	6 − 39	12 − 52	20 − 65	28 − 80	38 − 95	49 − 111	61 − 128
12	—	—	7 − 41	13 − 55	21 − 69	30 − 84	40 − 100	51 − 117	63 − 135
13	—	—	7 − 44	13 − 59	22 − 73	31 − 89	41 − 106	53 − 123	65 − 142
14	—	—	7 − 47	14 − 62	22 − 78	32 − 94	43 − 111	54 − 130	67 − 149
15	—	—	8 − 49	15 − 65	23 − 82	33 − 99	44 − 117	56 − 136	69 − 156
16	—	—	8 − 52	15 − 69	24 − 86	34 − 104	46 − 122	58 − 142	72 − 162
17	—	—	8 − 55	16 − 72	25 − 90	36 − 108	47 − 128	60 − 148	74 − 169
18	—	—	8 − 58	16 − 76	26 − 94	37 − 113	49 − 133	62 − 154	76 − 176
19	—	3 − 41	9 − 60	17 − 79	27 − 98	38 − 118	50 − 139	64 − 160	78 − 183
20	—	3 − 43	9 − 63	18 − 82	28 − 102	39 − 123	52 − 144	66 − 166	81 − 189
21	—	3 − 45	9 − 66	18 − 86	29 − 106	40 − 128	53 − 150	68 − 172	83 − 196
22	—	3 − 47	10 − 68	19 − 89	29 − 111	42 − 132	55 − 155	70 − 178	85 − 203
23	—	3 − 49	10 − 71	19 − 93	30 − 115	43 − 137	57 − 160	71 − 185	88 − 209
24	—	3 − 51	10 − 74	20 − 96	31 − 119	44 − 142	58 − 166	73 − 191	90 − 216
25	—	3 − 53	11 − 76	20 − 100	32 − 123	45 − 147	60 − 171	75 − 197	92 − 223
26	—	3 − 55	11 − 79	21 − 103	33 − 127	46 − 152	61 − 177	77 − 203	94 − 230
27	—	4 − 56	11 − 82	22 − 106	34 − 131	48 − 156	63 − 182	79 − 209	97 − 236
28	—	4 − 58	11 − 85	22 − 110	35 − 135	49 − 161	64 − 188	81 − 215	99 − 243
29	—	4 − 60	12 − 87	23 − 113	36 − 139	50 − 166	66 − 193	83 − 221	101 − 250
30	—	4 − 62	12 − 90	23 − 117	37 − 143	51 − 171	68 − 198	85 − 227	103 − 257
31	—	4 − 64	12 − 93	24 − 120	37 − 148	53 − 175	69 − 204	87 − 233	106 − 263
32	—	4 − 66	13 − 95	24 − 124	38 − 152	54 − 180	71 − 209	89 − 239	108 − 270
33	—	4 − 68	13 − 98	25 − 127	39 − 156	55 − 185	72 − 215	91 − 245	110 − 277
34	—	4 − 70	13 − 101	26 − 130	40 − 160	56 − 190	74 − 220	93 − 251	113 − 283
35	—	4 − 72	14 − 103	26 − 134	41 − 164	58 − 194	75 − 226	95 − 257	115 − 290

Significant result if $T_1 \geqslant T_u$ or $T_1 \geqslant T_l$

Appendix B: Statistical Tables

Table B.5(b). The Wilcoxon two-sample rank sum test for sample sizes $n_1 = 10$ to 17, $n_2 = 1$ to 35. Critical lower (T_l) and upper (T_u) values for the sum of ranks T_1 from sample sized n_1. Abbreviated and adapted from *Geigy Scientific Tables* Vol. 2, 8th edn. with permission

Two-sided significance level: 0·10
One-sided significance level: 0·05

n_1	10	11	12	13	14	15	16	17
n_2	T_l T_u	T_l T_u	T_l T_u	T_l T_u	T_l T_u	T_l T_u	T_l T_u	T_l T_u
1	—	—	—	—	—	—	—	—
2	56 – 74	67 – 87	80 – 100	93 – 115	108 – 130	123 – 147	139 – 165	156 – 184
3	59 – 81	71 – 94	83 – 109	97 – 124	112 – 140	127 – 158	144 – 176	162 – 195
4	62 – 88	74 – 102	87 – 117	101 – 133	116 – 150	132 – 168	150 – 186	168 – 206
5	66 – 94	78 – 109	91 – 125	106 – 141	121 – 159	138 – 177	155 – 197	173 – 218
6	69 – 101	82 – 116	95 – 133	110 – 150	126 – 168	143 – 187	161 – 207	179 – 229
7	72 – 108	85 – 124	99 – 141	115 – 158	131 – 177	148 – 197	166 – 218	186 – 239
8	75 – 115	89 – 131	104 – 148	119 – 167	136 – 186	153 – 207	172 – 228	192 – 250
9	79 – 121	93 – 138	108 – 156	124 – 175	141 – 195	159 – 216	178 – 238	198 – 261
10	82 – 128	97 – 145	112 – 164	128 – 184	146 – 204	164 – 226	184 – 248	204 – 272
11	86 – 134	100 – 153	116 – 172	133 – 192	151 – 213	170 – 235	190 – 258	210 – 283
12	89 – 141	104 – 160	120 – 180	138 – 200	156 – 222	175 – 245	196 – 268	217 – 293
13	92 – 148	108 – 167	125 – 187	142 – 209	161 – 231	181 – 254	201 – 279	223 – 304
14	96 – 154	112 – 174	129 – 195	147 – 217	166 – 240	186 – 264	207 – 289	230 – 314
15	99 – 161	116 – 181	133 – 203	152 – 225	171 – 249	192 – 273	213 – 299	236 – 325
16	103 – 167	120 – 188	138 – 210	156 – 234	176 – 258	197 – 283	219 – 309	242 – 336
17	106 – 174	123 – 196	142 – 218	161 – 242	182 – 266	203 – 292	225 – 319	249 – 346
18	110 – 180	127 – 203	146 – 226	166 – 250	187 – 275	208 – 302	231 – 329	255 – 357
19	113 – 187	131 – 210	150 – 234	171 – 258	192 – 284	214 – 311	237 – 339	262 – 367
20	117 – 193	135 – 217	155 – 241	175 – 267	197 – 293	220 – 320	243 – 349	268 – 378
21	120 – 200	135 – 224	159 – 249	180 – 275	202 – 302	225 – 330	249 – 359	274 – 389
22	123 – 207	143 – 231	163 – 257	185 – 283	207 – 311	231 – 339	255 – 369	281 – 399
23	127 – 213	147 – 238	168 – 264	189 – 292	212 – 320	236 – 349	261 – 379	287 – 410
24	130 – 220	151 – 245	172 – 272	194 – 300	218 – 328	242 – 358	267 – 389	294 – 420
25	134 – 226	155 – 252	176 – 280	199 – 308	223 – 337	248 – 367	273 – 399	300 – 431
26	137 – 233	158 – 260	181 – 287	204 – 316	228 – 346	253 – 377	279 – 409	307 – 441
27	141 – 239	162 – 267	185 – 295	208 – 325	233 – 355	259 – 386	285 – 419	313 – 452
28	144 – 246	166 – 274	189 – 303	213 – 333	238 – 364	264 – 396	292 – 428	320 – 462
29	148 – 252	170 – 281	194 – 310	218 – 341	243 – 373	270 – 405	298 – 438	326 – 473
30	151 – 259	174 – 288	198 – 318	223 – 349	249 – 381	276 – 414	304 – 448	333 – 483
31	155 – 265	178 – 295	202 – 326	227 – 358	254 – 390	281 – 424	310 – 458	339 – 494
32	158 – 272	182 – 302	206 – 334	232 – 366	259 – 399	287 – 433	316 – 468	346 – 504
33	162 – 278	186 – 309	211 – 341	237 – 374	264 – 408	292 – 443	322 – 478	352 – 515
34	165 – 285	190 – 316	215 – 349	242 – 382	269 – 417	298 – 452	328 – 488	359 – 525
35	169 – 291	194 – 323	219 – 357	247 – 390	275 – 425	304 – 461	334 – 498	365 – 536

Significant result if $T_1 \geqslant T_u$ or $T_1 \leqslant T_l$

Table B.5(b). (*Continued*)

Two-sided significance level: 0·05
One-sided significance level: 0·025

n_1	10	11	12	13	14	15	16	17
n_2	$T_l\ T_u$	$T_l\ T_u$	$T_l\ T_u$	$T_l\ T_u$	$T_l\ T_u$	$T_l\ T_u$	$T_l\ T_u$	$T_l\ T_u$
1	—	—	—	—	—	—	—	—
2	55 − 75	66 − 88	79 − 101	92 − 116	106 − 132	121 − 149	137 − 167	155 − 185
3	58 − 82	69 − 96	82 − 110	95 − 126	110 − 142	125 − 160	142 − 178	159 − 198
4	60 − 90	72 − 104	85 − 119	99 − 135	114 − 152	130 − 170	147 − 189	164 − 210
5	63 − 97	75 − 112	89 − 127	103 − 144	118 − 162	134 − 181	151 − 201	170 − 221
6	66 − 104	79 − 119	92 − 136	107 − 153	122 − 172	139 − 191	157 − 211	175 − 233
7	69 − 111	82 − 127	96 − 144	111 − 162	127 − 181	144 − 201	162 − 222	181 − 244
8	72 − 118	85 − 135	100 − 152	115 − 171	131 − 191	149 − 211	167 − 233	187 − 255
9	75 − 125	89 − 142	104 − 160	119 − 180	136 − 200	154 − 221	173 − 243	192 − 267
10	78 − 132	92 − 150	107 − 169	124 − 188	141 − 209	159 − 231	178 − 254	198 − 278
11	81 − 139	96 − 157	111 − 177	128 − 197	145 − 219	164 − 241	183 − 265	204 − 289
12	84 − 146	99 − 165	115 − 185	132 − 206	150 − 228	169 − 251	189 − 275	210 − 300
13	88 − 152	103 − 172	119 − 193	136 − 215	155 − 237	174 − 261	195 − 285	216 − 311
14	91 − 159	106 − 180	123 − 201	141 − 223	160 − 246	179 − 271	200 − 296	222 − 322
15	94 − 166	110 − 187	127 − 209	145 − 232	164 − 256	184 − 281	206 − 306	228 − 333
16	97 − 173	113 − 195	131 − 217	150 − 240	169 − 265	190 − 290	211 − 317	234 − 344
17	100 − 180	117 − 202	135 − 225	154 − 249	174 − 274	195 − 300	217 − 327	240 − 355
18	103 − 187	121 − 209	139 − 233	158 − 258	179 − 283	200 − 310	222 − 338	246 − 366
19	107 − 193	124 − 217	143 − 241	163 − 266	183 − 293	205 − 320	228 − 348	252 − 377
20	110 − 200	128 − 224	147 − 249	167 − 275	188 − 302	210 − 330	234 − 358	258 − 388
21	113 − 207	131 − 232	151 − 257	171 − 284	193 − 311	216 − 339	239 − 369	264 − 399
22	116 − 214	135 − 239	155 − 265	176 − 292	198 − 320	221 − 349	245 − 379	270 − 410
23	119 − 221	139 − 246	159 − 273	180 − 301	203 − 329	226 − 359	251 − 389	276 − 421
24	122 − 228	142 − 254	163 − 281	185 − 309	207 − 339	231 − 369	256 − 400	282 − 432
25	126 − 234	146 − 261	167 − 289	189 − 318	212 − 348	237 − 378	262 − 410	288 − 443
26	129 − 241	149 − 269	171 − 297	193 − 327	217 − 357	242 − 388	268 − 420	294 − 454
27	132 − 248	153 − 276	175 − 305	198 − 335	222 − 366	247 − 398	273 − 431	300 − 465
28	135 − 255	156 − 284	179 − 313	202 − 344	227 − 375	252 − 408	279 − 441	307 − 475
29	138 − 262	160 − 291	183 − 321	207 − 352	232 − 384	258 − 417	285 − 451	313 − 486
30	142 − 268	164 − 298	187 − 329	211 − 361	236 − 394	263 − 427	290 − 462	319 − 497
31	145 − 275	167 − 306	191 − 337	216 − 369	241 − 403	268 − 437	296 − 472	325 − 508
32	148 − 282	171 − 313	195 − 345	220 − 378	246 − 412	273 − 447	302 − 482	331 − 519
33	151 − 289	174 − 321	199 − 353	224 − 387	251 − 421	279 − 456	307 − 493	337 − 530
34	154 − 296	178 − 328	203 − 361	229 − 395	256 − 430	284 − 466	313 − 503	343 − 541
35	158 − 302	182 − 335	207 − 369	233 − 404	261 − 439	289 − 476	319 − 513	349 − 552

Significant result if $T_1 \geqslant T_u$ or $T_1 \leqslant T_l$

Continued

Table B.5(b). (*Continued*) The Wilcoxon two-sample rank sum test for sample sizes $n_1 = 10$ to 17, $n_2 = 1$ to 35. Critical lower (T_l) and upper (T_u) values for the sum of ranks T_1 from sample sized n_1

Two-sided significance level: 0·02
One-sided significance level: 0·01

n_1	10	11	12	13	14	15	16	17
n_2	$T_l \; T_u$	$T_l \; T_u$	$T_l \; T_u$	$T_l \; T_u$	$T_l \; T_u$	$T_l \; T_u$	$T_l \; T_u$	$T_l \; T_u$
1	–	–	–	–	–	–	–	–
2	–	–	–	91 – 117	105 – 133	120 – 150	136 – 168	153 – 187
3	56 – 84	67 – 98	80 – 112	93 – 128	107 – 145	123 – 162	139 – 181	157 – 200
4	58 – 92	70 – 106	83 – 121	96 – 138	111 – 155	127 – 173	143 – 193	161 – 213
5	61 – 99	73 – 114	86 – 130	100 – 147	115 – 165	131 – 184	148 – 204	166 – 225
6	63 – 107	75 – 123	89 – 139	103 – 157	118 – 176	135 – 195	152 – 216	171 – 237
7	66 – 114	78 – 131	92 – 148	107 – 166	122 – 186	139 – 206	157 – 227	176 – 249
8	68 – 122	81 – 139	95 – 157	111 – 175	127 – 195	144 – 216	162 – 238	181 – 261
9	71 – 129	84 – 147	99 – 165	114 – 185	131 – 205	148 – 227	167 – 249	186 – 273
10	74 – 136	88 – 154	102 – 174	118 – 194	135 – 215	153 – 237	172 – 260	191 – 285
11	77 – 143	91 – 162	106 – 182	122 – 203	139 – 225	157 – 248	177 – 271	197 – 296
12	79 – 151	94 – 170	109 – 191	126 – 212	143 – 235	162 – 258	182 – 282	202 – 308
13	82 – 158	97 – 178	113 – 199	130 – 221	148 – 244	167 – 268	187 – 293	208 – 319
14	85 – 165	100 – 186	116 – 208	134 – 230	152 – 254	171 – 279	192 – 304	213 – 331
15	88 – 172	103 – 194	120 – 216	138 – 239	156 – 264	176 – 289	197 – 315	219 – 342
16	91 – 179	107 – 201	124 – 224	142 – 248	161 – 273	181 – 299	202 – 326	224 – 354
17	93 – 187	110 – 209	127 – 233	146 – 257	165 – 283	186 – 309	207 – 337	230 – 365
18	96 – 194	113 – 217	131 – 241	150 – 266	170 – 292	190 – 320	212 – 348	235 – 377
19	99 – 201	116 – 225	134 – 250	154 – 275	174 – 302	195 – 330	218 – 358	241 – 388
20	102 – 208	119 – 233	138 – 258	158 – 284	178 – 312	200 – 340	223 – 369	246 – 400
21	105 – 215	123 – 240	142 – 266	162 – 293	183 – 321	205 – 350	228 – 380	252 – 411
22	108 – 222	126 – 248	145 – 275	166 – 302	187 – 331	210 – 360	233 – 391	258 – 422
23	110 – 230	129 – 256	149 – 283	170 – 311	192 – 340	214 – 371	238 – 402	263 – 434
24	113 – 237	132 – 264	153 – 291	174 – 320	196 – 350	219 – 381	244 – 412	269 – 445
25	116 – 244	136 – 271	156 – 300	178 – 329	200 – 360	224 – 391	249 – 423	275 – 456
26	119 – 251	139 – 279	160 – 308	182 – 338	205 – 369	229 – 401	254 – 434	280 – 468
27	122 – 258	142 – 287	163 – 317	186 – 347	209 – 379	234 – 411	259 – 445	286 – 479
28	125 – 265	145 – 295	167 – 325	190 – 356	214 – 388	239 – 421	265 – 455	292 – 490
29	128 – 272	149 – 302	171 – 333	194 – 365	218 – 398	243 – 432	270 – 466	297 – 502
30	131 – 279	152 – 310	174 – 342	198 – 374	223 – 407	248 – 442	275 – 477	303 – 513
31	133 – 287	155 – 318	178 – 350	202 – 383	227 – 417	253 – 452	280 – 488	309 – 524
32	136 – 294	158 – 326	182 – 358	206 – 392	232 – 426	258 – 462	286 – 498	314 – 536
33	139 – 301	162 – 333	185 – 367	210 – 401	236 – 436	263 – 472	291 – 509	320 – 547
34	142 – 308	165 – 341	189 – 375	214 – 410	240 – 446	268 – 482	296 – 520	326 – 558
35	145 – 315	168 – 349	193 – 383	218 – 419	245 – 455	273 – 492	301 – 531	331 – 570

Significant result if $T_1 \geqslant T_u$ or $T_1 \leqslant T_l$

Table B.5(b). (*Continued*)

Two-sided significance level: 0·01
One-sided significance level: 0·005

n_1	10	11	12	13	14	15	16	17
n_2	$T_l \ T_u$	$T_l \ T_u$	$T_l \ T_u$	$T_l \ T_u$	$T_l \ T_u$	$T_l \ T_u$	$T_l \ T_u$	$T_l \ T_u$
1	—	—	—	—	—	—	—	—
2	—	—	—	—	—	—	—	—
3	55 – 85	66 – 99	79 – 113	92 – 129	106 – 146	122 – 163	138 – 182	155 – 202
4	57 – 93	68 – 108	81 – 123	94 – 140	109 – 157	125 – 175	141 – 195	159 – 215
5	59 – 101	71 – 116	84 – 132	98 – 149	112 – 168	128 – 187	145 – 207	163 – 228
6	61 – 109	73 – 125	87 – 141	101 – 159	116 – 178	132 – 198	149 – 219	168 – 240
7	64 – 116	76 – 133	90 – 150	104 – 169	120 – 188	136 – 209	154 – 230	172 – 253
8	66 – 124	79 – 141	93 – 159	108 – 178	123 – 199	140 – 220	158 – 242	177 – 265
9	68 – 132	82 – 149	96 – 168	111 – 188	127 – 209	144 – 231	163 – 253	182 – 277
10	71 – 139	84 – 158	99 – 177	115 – 197	131 – 219	149 – 241	167 – 265	187 – 289
11	73 – 147	87 – 166	102 – 186	118 – 207	135 – 229	153 – 252	172 – 276	192 – 301
12	76 – 154	90 – 174	105 – 195	122 – 216	139 – 239	157 – 263	177 – 287	197 – 313
13	79 – 161	93 – 182	109 – 203	125 – 226	143 – 249	162 – 273	181 – 299	202 – 325
14	81 – 169	96 – 190	112 – 212	129 – 235	147 – 259	166 – 284	186 – 310	207 – 337
15	84 – 176	99 – 198	115 – 221	133 – 244	151 – 269	171 – 294	191 – 321	213 – 348
16	86 – 184	102 – 206	119 – 229	136 – 254	155 – 279	175 – 305	196 – 332	218 – 360
17	89 – 191	105 – 214	122 – 238	140 – 263	159 – 289	180 – 315	201 – 343	223 – 372
18	92 – 198	108 – 222	125 – 247	144 – 272	163 – 299	184 – 326	206 – 354	228 – 384
19	94 – 206	111 – 230	129 – 255	148 – 281	168 – 308	189 – 336	210 – 366	234 – 395
20	97 – 213	114 – 238	132 – 264	151 – 291	172 – 318	193 – 347	215 – 377	239 – 407
21	99 – 221	117 – 246	136 – 272	155 – 300	176 – 328	198 – 357	220 – 388	244 – 419
22	102 – 228	120 – 254	139 – 281	159 – 309	180 – 338	202 – 368	225 – 399	249 – 431
23	105 – 235	123 – 262	142 – 290	163 – 318	184 – 348	207 – 378	230 – 410	255 – 442
24	107 – 243	126 – 270	146 – 298	166 – 328	188 – 358	211 – 389	235 – 421	260 – 454
25	110 – 250	129 – 278	149 – 307	170 – 337	192 – 368	216 – 399	240 – 432	265 – 466
26	113 – 257	132 – 286	152 – 316	174 – 346	197 – 377	220 – 410	245 – 443	271 – 477
27	115 – 265	135 – 294	156 – 324	178 – 355	201 – 387	225 – 420	250 – 454	276 – 489
28	118 – 272	138 – 302	159 – 333	182 – 364	205 – 397	229 – 431	255 – 465	281 – 501
29	121 – 279	141 – 310	163 – 341	185 – 374	209 – 407	234 – 441	260 – 476	287 – 512
30	123 – 287	144 – 318	166 – 350	189 – 383	213 – 417	239 – 451	265 – 487	292 – 524
31	126 – 294	147 – 326	170 – 358	193 – 392	218 – 426	243 – 462	270 – 498	298 – 535
32	129 – 301	150 – 334	173 – 367	197 – 401	222 – 436	248 – 472	275 – 509	303 – 547
33	131 – 309	153 – 342	176 – 376	201 – 410	226 – 446	252 – 483	280 – 520	308 – 559
34	134 – 316	156 – 350	180 – 384	204 – 420	230 – 456	257 – 493	285 – 531	314 – 570
35	137 – 323	159 – 358	183 – 393	208 – 429	234 – 466	262 – 503	290 – 542	319 – 582

Significant result if $T_1 \geqslant T_u$ or $T_1 \leqslant T_l$

Table B.5(c). The Wilcoxon two-sample rank sum test for samples sizes $n_1 = 18$ to 25, $n_2 = 1$ to 35. Critical lower (T_l) and upper (T_u) values for the sum of ranks T_1 from sample sized n_1. Abbreviated and adapted from *Geigy Scientific Tables* Vol. 2, 8th edn. with permission

Two-sided significance level: 0·10
One-sided significance level: 0·05

n_1	18	19	20	21	22	23	24	25
n_2	$T_l\ T_u$	$T_l\ T_u$	$T_l\ T_u$	$T_l\ T_u$	$T_l\ T_u$	$T_l\ T_u$	$T_l\ T_u$	$T_l\ T_u$
1	–	190 – 209	210 – 230	231 – 252	253 – 275	276 – 299	300 – 324	325 – 350
2	175 – 203	194 – 224	214 – 246	236 – 268	258 – 292	281 – 317	306 – 342	331 – 369
3	180 – 216	200 – 237	221 – 259	242 – 283	265 – 307	289 – 332	313 – 359	339 – 386
4	187 – 227	207 – 249	228 – 272	250 – 296	273 – 321	297 – 347	322 – 374	348 – 402
5	193 – 239	213 – 262	235 – 285	257 – 310	281 – 335	305 – 362	330 – 390	357 – 418
6	199 – 251	220 – 274	242 – 298	265 – 323	289 – 349	313 – 377	339 – 405	366 – 434
7	206 – 262	227 – 286	249 – 311	272 – 337	297 – 363	322 – 391	348 – 420	375 – 450
8	212 – 274	234 – 298	257 – 323	280 – 350	305 – 377	330 – 406	357 – 435	385 – 465
9	219 – 285	241 – 310	264 – 336	288 – 363	313 – 391	339 – 420	366 – 450	394 – 481
10	226 – 296	248 – 322	272 – 348	296 – 376	321 – 405	348 – 434	375 – 465	404 – 496
11	232 – 308	255 – 334	279 – 361	304 – 389	330 – 418	357 – 448	385 – 479	414 – 511
12	239 – 319	262 – 346	287 – 373	312 – 402	338 – 432	366 – 462	394 – 494	423 – 527
13	246 – 330	270 – 357	294 – 386	320 – 415	347 – 445	374 – 477	403 – 509	433 – 542
14	253 – 341	277 – 369	302 – 398	328 – 428	355 – 459	383 – 491	413 – 523	443 – 557
15	259 – 353	284 – 381	310 – 410	336 – 441	364 – 472	392 – 505	422 – 538	453 – 572
16	266 – 364	291 – 393	317 – 423	344 – 454	372 – 486	401 – 519	431 – 553	462 – 588
17	273 – 375	299 – 404	325 – 435	352 – 467	381 – 499	410 – 533	441 – 567	472 – 603
18	280 – 386	306 – 416	333 – 447	361 – 479	389 – 513	419 – 547	450 – 582	482 – 618
19	287 – 397	313 – 428	340 – 460	369 – 492	398 – 526	428 – 561	460 – 596	492 – 633
20	294 – 408	320 – 440	348 – 472	377 – 505	407 – 539	437 – 575	469 – 611	502 – 648
21	301 – 419	328 – 451	356 – 484	385 – 518	415 – 553	446 – 589	479 – 625	512 – 663
22	307 – 431	335 – 463	364 – 496	393 – 531	424 – 566	455 – 603	488 – 640	522 – 678
23	314 – 442	342 – 475	371 – 509	401 – 544	432 – 580	465 – 616	498 – 654	532 – 693
24	321 – 453	350 – 486	379 – 521	410 – 556	441 – 593	474 – 630	507 – 669	542 – 708
25	328 – 464	357 – 498	387 – 533	418 – 569	450 – 606	483 – 644	517 – 683	552 – 723
26	335 – 475	364 – 510	395 – 545	426 – 582	458 – 620	492 – 658	526 – 698	562 – 738
27	342 – 486	372 – 521	402 – 558	434 – 595	467 – 633	501 – 672	536 – 712	572 – 753
28	349 – 497	379 – 533	410 – 570	443 – 607	476 – 646	510 – 686	545 – 727	582 – 768
29	356 – 508	386 – 545	418 – 582	451 – 620	484 – 660	519 – 700	555 – 741	592 – 783
30	363 – 519	394 – 556	426 – 594	459 – 633	493 – 673	528 – 714	564 – 756	602 – 798
31	370 – 530	401 – 568	434 – 606	467 – 646	502 – 686	537 – 728	574 – 770	612 – 813
32	377 – 541	408 – 580	441 – 619	475 – 659	510 – 700	547 – 741	584 – 784	622 – 828
33	383 – 553	416 – 591	449 – 631	484 – 671	519 – 713	556 – 755	593 – 799	632 – 843
34	390 – 564	423 – 603	457 – 643	492 – 684	528 – 726	565 – 769	603 – 813	642 – 858
35	397 – 575	431 – 614	465 – 655	500 – 697	537 – 739	574 – 783	612 – 828	652 – 873

Significant result if $T_1 \geqslant T_u$ or $T_1 \leqslant T_l$

Table B.5(c). (*Continued*)

Two-sided significance level: 0·05
One-sided significance level: 0·025

n_1	18	19	20	21	22	23	24	25
n_2	$T_l \; T_u$	$T_l \; T_u$	$T_l \; T_u$	$T_l \; T_u$	$T_l \; T_u$	$T_l \; T_u$	$T_l \; T_u$	$T_l \; T_u$
1	–	–	–	–	–	–	–	–
2	173 – 205	192 – 226	212 – 248	234 – 270	256 – 294	279 – 319	303 – 345	328 – 372
3	178 – 218	197 – 240	218 – 262	239 – 286	262 – 310	285 – 336	310 – 362	335 – 390
4	183 – 231	203 – 235	224 – 276	246 – 300	269 – 325	293 – 351	317 – 379	343 – 407
5	189 – 243	209 – 266	230 – 290	253 – 314	276 – 340	300 – 367	325 – 395	352 – 423
6	195 – 255	215 – 279	237 – 303	260 – 328	283 – 355	308 – 382	333 – 411	360 – 440
7	201 – 267	222 – 291	244 – 316	267 – 342	291 – 269	316 – 397	342 – 426	369 – 456
8	207 – 279	228 – 304	251 – 329	274 – 356	298 – 384	324 – 412	350 – 442	378 – 472
9	213 – 291	235 – 316	258 – 342	281 – 370	306 – 398	332 – 427	359 – 457	387 – 488
10	219 – 303	242 – 328	265 – 355	289 – 383	314 – 412	340 – 442	367 – 473	396 – 504
11	226 – 314	248 – 341	272 – 368	296 – 397	322 – 426	349 – 456	376 – 488	405 – 520
12	232 – 326	255 – 353	279 – 381	304 – 410	330 – 440	357 – 471	385 – 503	414 – 536
13	238 – 338	262 – 365	286 – 394	311 – 424	338 – 454	365 – 486	394 – 518	423 – 552
14	245 – 349	268 – 378	293 – 407	319 – 437	346 – 468	374 – 500	402 – 534	432 – 568
15	251 – 361	275 – 390	300 – 420	327 – 450	354 – 482	382 – 515	411 – 549	442 – 583
16	257 – 373	282 – 402	308 – 432	334 – 464	362 – 496	391 – 529	420 – 564	451 – 599
17	264 – 384	289 – 414	315 – 445	342 – 477	370 – 510	399 – 544	429 – 579	460 – 615
18	270 – 396	296 – 426	322 – 458	350 – 490	378 – 524	408 – 558	438 – 594	470 – 630
19	277 – 407	303 – 438	329 – 471	357 – 504	386 – 538	416 – 573	447 – 609	479 – 646
20	283 – 419	309 – 451	337 – 483	365 – 517	394 – 552	425 – 587	456 – 624	488 – 662
21	290 – 430	316 – 463	344 – 496	373 – 530	403 – 656	433 – 602	465 – 639	498 – 677
22	296 – 442	323 – 475	351 – 509	381 – 543	411 – 579	442 – 616	474 – 654	507 – 693
23	303 – 453	330 – 487	359 – 521	388 – 557	419 – 593	451 – 630	483 – 669	517 – 708
24	309 – 465	337 – 499	366 – 534	396 – 707	427 – 607	459 – 645	492 – 684	526 – 724
25	316 – 476	344 – 511	373 – 547	404 – 583	435 – 621	468 – 659	501 – 699	536 – 739
26	322 – 488	351 – 523	381 – 559	412 – 596	444 – 634	476 – 674	510 – 714	545 – 755
27	329 – 499	358 – 535	388 – 572	419 – 610	452 – 648	485 – 688	519 – 729	555 – 770
28	335 – 511	365 – 547	396 – 584	427 – 623	460 – 662	494 – 702	528 – 744	564 – 786
29	342 – 522	372 – 559	403 – 597	435 – 636	468 – 676	502 – 717	538 – 758	574 – 801
30	348 – 534	379 – 571	410 – 610	443 – 649	476 – 690	511 – 731	547 – 773	583 – 817
31	355 – 545	386 – 583	418 – 622	451 – 662	485 – 703	520 – 745	556 – 788	593 – 832
32	361 – 557	393 – 595	425 – 635	458 – 676	493 – 717	528 – 760	565 – 803	602 – 848
33	368 – 568	400 – 607	432 – 648	466 – 689	501 – 731	537 – 774	574 – 818	612 – 863
34	374 – 580	407 – 619	440 – 660	474 – 702	509 – 745	546 – 788	583 – 833	622 – 878
35	381 – 591	414 – 631	447 – 673	482 – 715	518 – 758	554 – 803	592 – 848	631 – 894

Significant result if $T_1 \geqslant T_u$ or $T_1 \leqslant T_l$

Continued

Table B.5(c). (*Continued*) The Wilcoxon two-sample rank sum test for sample sizes $n_1 = 18$ to 25, $n_2 = 1$ to 35. Critical lower (T_l) and upper (T_u) values for the sum of ranks T_1 from sample sized n_1

Two-sided significance level: 0·02
One-sided significance level: 0·01

n_1	18	19	20	21	22	23	24	25
n_2	T_l T_u	T_l T_u	T_l T_u	T_l T_u	T_l T_u	T_l T_u	T_l T_u	T_l T_u
1	—	—	—	—	—	—	—	—
2	171 − 207	191 − 227	211 − 249	232 − 272	254 − 296	277 − 321	301 − 347	326 − 374
3	175 − 221	194 − 243	215 − 265	236 − 289	259 − 313	282 − 339	306 − 366	332 − 393
4	180 − 234	199 − 257	220 − 280	242 − 304	264 − 330	288 − 356	313 − 383	338 − 412
5	185 − 247	205 − 270	226 − 294	248 − 319	271 − 345	295 − 372	320 − 400	346 − 429
6	190 − 260	210 − 284	232 − 308	254 − 334	277 − 361	302 − 388	327 − 417	354 − 446
7	195 − 273	216 − 297	238 − 322	261 − 348	284 − 376	309 − 404	335 − 433	361 − 464
8	201 − 285	222 − 310	244 − 336	267 − 363	291 − 391	316 − 420	342 − 450	370 − 480
9	207 − 297	228 − 323	250 − 350	274 − 377	298 − 406	324 − 435	350 − 466	378 − 497
10	212 − 310	234 − 336	257 − 363	281 − 391	306 − 420	331 − 451	358 − 482	386 − 514
11	218 − 322	240 − 349	263 − 377	288 − 405	313 − 435	339 − 466	366 − 498	395 − 530
12	224 − 334	246 − 362	270 − 390	295 − 419	320 − 450	347 − 481	375 − 513	403 − 547
13	230 − 346	253 − 374	277 − 403	302 − 433	328 − 464	355 − 496	383 − 529	412 − 563
14	236 − 358	259 − 387	283 − 417	309 − 447	335 − 479	363 − 511	391 − 545	420 − 580
15	241 − 371	265 − 400	290 − 430	316 − 461	343 − 493	370 − 527	399 − 561	429 − 596
16	247 − 383	272 − 412	297 − 443	323 − 475	350 − 508	378 − 542	408 − 576	438 − 612
17	253 − 395	278 − 425	303 − 457	330 − 489	358 − 522	386 − 557	416 − 592	447 − 628
18	259 − 407	284 − 438	310 − 470	337 − 503	365 − 537	394 − 572	424 − 608	455 − 645
19	265 − 419	291 − 450	317 − 483	344 − 517	373 − 551	402 − 587	433 − 623	464 − 661
20	271 − 431	297 − 463	324 − 496	352 − 530	380 − 566	410 − 602	441 − 639	473 − 677
21	277 − 443	303 − 476	331 − 509	359 − 544	388 − 580	418 − 617	450 − 654	482 − 693
22	283 − 455	310 − 488	337 − 523	366 − 558	396 − 594	426 − 632	458 − 670	491 − 709
23	289 − 467	316 − 501	344 − 536	373 − 572	403 − 609	434 − 647	467 − 685	500 − 725
24	295 − 479	323 − 513	351 − 549	381 − 585	411 − 623	443 − 661	475 − 701	509 − 741
25	301 − 491	329 − 526	358 − 562	388 − 599	419 − 637	451 − 676	484 − 716	517 − 758
26	307 − 503	336 − 538	365 − 575	395 − 613	426 − 652	459 − 691	492 − 732	526 − 774
27	313 − 515	342 − 551	372 − 588	402 − 627	434 − 666	467 − 706	501 − 747	535 − 790
28	320 − 526	349 − 563	379 − 601	410 − 640	442 − 680	475 − 721	509 − 763	544 − 806
29	326 − 538	355 − 576	386 − 614	417 − 654	450 − 694	483 − 736	518 − 778	553 − 822
30	332 − 550	362 − 588	392 − 628	424 − 668	457 − 709	491 − 751	526 − 794	562 − 838
31	338 − 562	368 − 601	399 − 641	432 − 681	465 − 723	499 − 766	535 − 809	571 − 854
32	344 − 574	375 − 613	406 − 654	439 − 695	473 − 737	508 − 780	543 − 825	580 − 870
33	350 − 586	381 − 626	413 − 667	446 − 709	481 − 751	516 − 795	552 − 840	589 − 886
34	356 − 598	388 − 638	420 − 680	454 − 722	488 − 766	524 − 810	561 − 855	598 − 902
35	362 − 610	394 − 651	427 − 693	461 − 736	496 − 780	532 − 825	569 − 871	607 − 918

Significant result if $T_1 \geqslant T_u$ or $T_1 \leqslant T_l$

Table B.5(c). (*Continued*)

Two-sided significance level: 0·01
One-sided significance level: 0·005

n_1	18	19	20	21	22	23	24	25
n_2	$T_l\ T_u$	$T_l\ T_u$	$T_l\ T_u$	$T_l\ T_u$	$T_l\ T_u$	$T_l\ T_u$	$T_l\ T_u$	$T_l\ T_u$
1	–	–	–	–	–	–	–	–
2	–	190 – 228	210 – 250	231 – 273	253 – 297	276 – 322	300 – 348	325 – 375
3	173 – 223	193 – 244	213 – 267	234 – 291	257 – 315	280 – 341	304 – 368	330 – 395
4	177 – 237	197 – 259	218 – 282	239 – 307	262 – 332	285 – 359	310 – 386	335 – 415
5	182 – 250	202 – 273	223 – 297	245 – 322	267 – 349	291 – 376	316 – 404	342 – 433
6	187 – 263	207 – 287	228 – 312	250 – 338	274 – 364	298 – 392	323 – 421	349 – 451
7	192 – 276	212 – 301	234 – 326	256 – 353	280 – 380	305 – 408	330 – 438	357 – 468
8	197 – 289	218 – 314	240 – 340	263 – 367	287 – 395	311 – 425	337 – 455	364 – 486
9	202 – 302	223 – 328	246 – 354	269 – 382	293 – 411	319 – 440	345 – 471	372 – 503
10	208 – 314	229 – 341	252 – 368	275 – 397	300 – 426	326 – 456	352 – 488	380 – 520
11	213 – 327	235 – 354	258 – 382	282 – 411	307 – 441	333 – 472	360 – 504	388 – 537
12	218 – 340	241 – 367	264 – 396	289 – 425	314 – 456	340 – 488	368 – 520	396 – 554
13	224 – 352	247 – 380	270 – 410	295 – 440	321 – 471	348 – 503	375 – 537	404 – 571
14	229 – 365	253 – 393	277 – 423	302 – 454	328 – 486	355 – 519	383 – 553	412 – 588
15	235 – 377	259 – 406	283 – 437	309 – 468	335 – 501	363 – 534	391 – 569	421 – 604
16	241 – 389	264 – 420	289 – 451	315 – 483	342 – 516	370 – 550	399 – 585	429 – 621
17	246 – 402	271 – 432	296 – 464	322 – 497	349 – 531	378 – 565	407 – 601	437 – 638
18	252 – 414	277 – 445	302 – 478	329 – 511	357 – 545	385 – 581	415 – 617	446 – 654
19	258 – 426	283 – 458	309 – 491	336 – 525	364 – 560	393 – 596	423 – 633	454 – 671
20	263 – 439	289 – 471	315 – 505	343 – 539	371 – 575	401 – 611	431 – 649	463 – 687
21	269 – 451	295 – 484	322 – 518	349 – 554	378 – 590	408 – 627	439 – 665	471 – 704
22	275 – 463	301 – 497	328 – 532	356 – 568	386 – 604	416 – 642	447 – 681	480 – 720
23	280 – 476	307 – 510	335 – 545	363 – 582	393 – 619	424 – 657	455 – 697	488 – 737
24	286 – 488	313 – 523	341 – 559	370 – 596	400 – 634	431 – 673	464 – 712	497 – 753
25	292 – 500	319 – 536	348 – 572	377 – 610	408 – 648	439 – 688	472 – 728	505 – 770
26	298 – 512	325 – 549	354 – 586	384 – 624	415 – 663	447 – 703	480 – 744	514 – 786
27	303 – 525	332 – 561	361 – 599	391 – 638	422 – 678	455 – 718	488 – 760	522 – 803
28	309 – 537	338 – 574	367 – 613	398 – 652	430 – 692	462 – 734	496 – 776	531 – 819
29	315 – 549	344 – 587	374 – 626	405 – 666	437 – 707	470 – 749	504 – 792	540 – 835
30	321 – 561	350 – 600	380 – 640	412 – 680	444 – 722	478 – 764	513 – 807	548 – 852
31	326 – 574	356 – 613	387 – 653	419 – 694	452 – 736	486 – 779	521 – 823	557 – 868
32	332 – 586	362 – 626	394 – 666	426 – 708	459 – 751	494 – 794	529 – 839	565 – 885
33	338 – 598	369 – 638	400 – 680	433 – 722	467 – 765	501 – 810	537 – 855	574 – 901
34	344 – 610	375 – 651	407 – 693	440 – 736	474 – 780	509 – 825	545 – 871	583 – 917
35	350 – 622	381 – 664	413 – 707	447 – 750	482 – 794	517 – 840	554 – 886	591 – 934

Significant result if $T_1 \geq T_u$ or $T_1 \leq T_l$

Table B.6. (a) The sign test (paired data). Critical lower (S_l) and upper (S_u) values for the number of positive differences n_+ from a sample with n non-zero differences.
(b) The exact test for correlated proportions. Critical values for the number of untied pairs 'c' in favour of one of the 'treatments' with n untied pairs altogether. Abbreviated and adapted from *Geigy Scientific Tables* Vol. 2, 8th edn. with permission

Two-sided significance level	0·10	0·05	0·02	0·01
One-sided significance level	0·05	0·025	0·01	0·005
n	$S_l\ S_u$	$S_l\ S_u$	$S_l\ S_u$	$S_l\ S_u$
5	0 − 5	—	—	—
6	0 − 6	0 − 6	—	—
7	0 − 7	0 − 7	0 − 7	—
8	1 − 7	0 − 8	0 − 8	0 − 8
9	1 − 8	1 − 8	0 − 9	0 − 9
10	1 − 9	1 − 9	0 − 10	0 − 10
11	2 − 9	1 − 10	1 − 10	0 − 11
12	2 − 10	2 − 10	1 − 11	1 − 11
13	3 − 10	2 − 11	1 − 12	1 − 12
14	3 − 11	2 − 12	2 − 12	1 − 13
15	3 − 12	3 − 12	2 − 13	2 − 13
16	4 − 12	3 − 13	2 − 14	2 − 14
17	4 − 13	4 − 13	3 − 14	2 − 15
18	5 − 13	4 − 14	3 − 15	3 − 15
19	5 − 14	4 − 15	4 − 15	3 − 16
20	5 − 15	5 − 15	4 − 16	3 − 17
21	6 − 15	5 − 16	4 − 17	4 − 17
22	6 − 16	5 − 17	5 − 17	4 − 18
23	7 − 16	6 − 17	5 − 18	4 − 19
24	7 − 17	6 − 18	6 − 19	5 − 20
25	7 − 18	7 − 18	6 − 19	5 − 20
26	8 − 18	7 − 19	6 − 20	6 − 20
27	8 − 19	7 − 20	7 − 20	6 − 21
28	9 − 19	8 − 20	7 − 21	6 − 22
29	9 − 20	8 − 21	7 − 22	7 − 22
30	10 − 20	9 − 21	8 − 22	7 − 23
31	10 − 21	9 − 22	8 − 23	7 − 24
32	10 − 22	9 − 23	8 − 24	8 − 24
33	11 − 22	10 − 23	9 − 24	8 − 25
34	11 − 23	10 − 24	9 − 25	9 − 25
35	12 − 23	11 − 24	10 − 25	9 − 26

Significant result if (a) $n_+ \geqslant S_u$ or $n_+ \leqslant S_l$
(b) $c \geqslant S_u$ or $c \leqslant S_l$

Table B.6. (*Continued*)

Two-sided significance level	0·10	0·05	0·02	0·01
One-sided significance level	0·05	0·025	0·01	0·005
n	S_l S_u	S_l S_u	S_l S_u	S_l S_u
36	12 − 24	11 − 25	10 − 26	9 − 27
37	13 − 24	12 − 25	10 − 27	10 − 27
38	13 − 25	12 − 26	11 − 27	10 − 28
39	13 − 26	12 − 57	11 − 28	11 − 28
40	14 − 26	13 − 27	12 − 28	11 − 29
41	14 − 27	13 − 28	12 − 29	11 − 30
42	15 − 27	14 − 28	13 − 29	12 − 30
43	15 − 28	14 − 29	13 − 30	12 − 31
44	16 − 28	15 − 29	13 − 31	13 − 31
45	16 − 29	15 − 30	14 − 31	13 − 32
46	16 − 30	15 − 31	14 − 32	13 − 33
47	17 − 30	16 − 31	15 − 32	14 − 33
48	17 − 31	16 − 32	15 − 33	14 − 34
49	18 − 31	17 − 32	15 − 34	15 − 34
50	18 − 32	17 − 33	16 − 34	15 − 35
51	19 − 32	18 − 33	16 − 35	15 − 36
52	19 − 33	18 − 34	17 − 35	16 − 36
53	20 − 33	18 − 35	17 − 36	16 − 37
54	20 − 34	19 − 35	18 − 36	17 − 37
55	20 − 35	19 − 36	18 − 37	17 − 38
56	21 − 35	20 − 36	18 − 38	17 − 39
57	21 − 36	20 − 37	19 − 38	18 − 39
58	22 − 36	21 − 37	19 − 39	18 − 40
59	22 − 37	21 − 38	20 − 39	19 − 40
60	23 − 37	21 − 39	20 − 40	19 − 41
61	23 − 38	22 − 39	20 − 41	20 − 41
62	24 − 38	22 − 40	21 − 41	20 − 42
63	24 − 39	23 − 40	21 − 42	20 − 43
64	24 − 40	23 − 41	22 − 42	21 − 43
65	25 − 40	24 − 41	22 − 43	21 − 44
66	25 − 41	24 − 42	23 − 43	22 − 44
67	26 − 41	25 − 42	23 − 44	22 − 45
68	26 − 42	25 − 43	23 − 45	22 − 46
69	27 − 42	25 − 44	24 − 45	23 − 46
70	27 − 43	26 − 44	24 − 46	23 − 47

Significant result if (a) $n_+ \geqslant S_u$ or $n_+ \leqslant S_l$

(b) $c \geqslant S_u$ or $c \leqslant S_l$

Continued

Table B.6. (*Continued*) (a) The sign test (paired data). Critical lower (S_l) and upper (S_u) values for the number of positive differences n_+ from a sample with n non-zero differences.
(b) The exact test for correlated proportions. Critical values for the number of untied pairs 'c' in favour of one of the 'treatments' with n untied pairs altogether

Two-sided significance level	0·10	0·05	0·02	0·01
One-sided significance level	0·05	0·025	0·01	0·005
n	S_l S_u	S_l S_u	S_l S_u	S_l S_u
71	28 – 43	26 – 45	25 – 46	24 – 47
72	28 – 44	27 – 45	25 – 47	24 – 48
73	28 – 45	27 – 46	26 – 47	25 – 48
74	29 – 45	28 – 46	26 – 48	25 – 49
75	29 – 46	28 – 47	26 – 49	25 – 50
76	30 – 46	28 – 48	27 – 49	26 – 50
77	30 – 47	29 – 48	27 – 50	26 – 51
78	31 – 47	29 – 40	28 – 50	27 – 51
79	31 – 48	30 – 49	28 – 51	27 – 52
80	32 – 48	30 – 50	29 – 51	28 – 52
81	32 – 49	31 – 50	29 – 52	28 – 53
82	33 – 49	31 – 51	30 – 52	28 – 54
83	33 – 50	32 – 51	30 – 53	29 – 54
84	33 – 51	31 – 52	30 – 54	29 – 55
85	34 – 51	32 – 53	31 – 54	30 – 55
86	34 – 52	33 – 53	31 – 55	30 – 56
87	35 – 52	33 – 54	32 – 55	31 – 56
88	35 – 53	34 – 54	32 – 56	31 – 57
89	36 – 53	34 – 55	33 – 56	31 – 58
90	36 – 54	35 – 55	33 – 57	32 – 58
91	37 – 54	35 – 56	33 – 58	32 – 59
92	37 – 55	36 – 56	34 – 58	33 – 59
93	38 – 55	36 – 57	34 – 59	33 – 60
94	38 – 56	37 – 57	35 – 59	34 – 60
95	38 – 57	37 – 58	35 – 60	34 – 61
96	39 – 57	37 – 59	36 – 60	34 – 62
97	39 – 58	38 – 59	36 – 61	35 – 62
98	40 – 58	38 – 60	37 – 61	35 – 63
99	40 – 59	39 – 60	37 – 62	36 – 63
100	41 – 59	38 – 61	37 – 63	36 – 64

Significant result if (a) $n_+ \geq S_u$ or $n_+ \leq S_l$
                (b) $c \geq S_u$ or $c \leq S_l$

Table B.7. The Wilcoxon signed rank test (paired data). Critical lower (T_l) and upper (T_u) values for the sum of the positive ranks (T_+) from a study with n non-zero differences. Abbreviated and adapted from *Geigy Scientific Tables* Vol. 2, 8th edn. with permission

Two-sided significance level	0·10	0·05	0·02	0·01
One-sided significance level	0·05	0·025	0·01	0·005
n	$T_l\ T_u$	$T_l\ T_u$	$T_l\ T_u$	$T_l\ T_u$
5	0 – 15	—	—	—
6	2 – 19	0 – 21	—	—
7	3 – 25	2 – 26	0 – 28	—
8	5 – 31	3 – 33	1 – 35	0 – 36
9	8 – 37	5 – 40	3 – 42	1 – 44
10	10 – 45	8 – 47	5 – 50	3 – 52
11	13 – 53	10 – 56	7 – 59	5 – 61
12	17 – 61	13 – 65	9 – 69	7 – 71
13	21 – 70	17 – 74	12 – 79	9 – 82
14	25 – 80	21 – 84	15 – 90	12 – 93
15	30 – 90	25 – 95	19 – 101	15 – 105
16	35 – 101	29 – 107	23 – 113	19 – 117
17	41 – 112	34 – 119	28 – 125	23 – 130
18	47 – 124	40 – 131	32 – 139	27 – 144
19	53 – 137	46 – 144	37 – 153	32 – 158
20	60 – 150	52 – 158	43 – 167	37 – 173
21	67 – 164	58 – 173	49 – 182	42 – 189
22	75 – 178	66 – 187	55 – 198	48 – 205
23	83 – 193	73 – 203	62 – 214	54 – 222
24	91 – 209	81 – 219	69 – 231	61 – 239
25	100 – 225	89 – 236	76 – 249	68 – 257

Significant result if $T_+ \geq T_u$ or $T_+ \leq T_l$

Table B.8. Logs of the factorials of $n = 0$ to 99. Abbreviated from *Geigy Scientific Tables* Vol. 2, 8th edn. with permission

n	0	1	2	3	4	5	6	7	8	9
0	0·00000	0·00000	0·30103	0·77815	1·38021	2·07918	2·85733	3·70243	4·60552	5·55976
10	6·55976	7·60116	8·68034	9·79428	10·94041	12·11650	13·32062	14·55107	15·80634	17·08509
20	18·38612	19·70834	21·05077	22·41249	23·79271	25·19065	26·60562	28·03698	29·48414	30·94654
30	32·42366	33·91502	35·42017	36·93869	38·47016	40·01423	41·57054	43·13874	44·71852	46·30959
40	47·91165	49·52443	51·14768	52·78115	54·42460	56·07781	57·74057	59·41267	61·09391	62·78410
50	64·48307	66·19064	67·90665	69·63092	71·36332	73·10368	74·85187	76·60774	78·37117	80·14202
60	81·92017	83·70550	85·49790	87·29724	89·10342	90·91633	92·73587	94·56195	96·39446	98·23331
70	100·07841	101·92966	103·78700	105·65032	107·51955	109·39461	111·27543	113·16192	115·05401	116·95164
80	118·85473	120·76321	122·67703	124·59610	126·52038	128·44980	130·38430	132·32382	134·26830	136·21769
90	138·17194	140·13098	142·09476	144·06325	146·03638	148·01410	149·99637	151·98314	153·97437	155·97000

Table B.9. Antilogarithm table. Reprinted from *Geigy Scientific Tables*, Vol. 2, 8th edn. with permission

$\log_{10}x$	0	1	2	3	4	5	6	7	8	9	1	2	3	4	5	6	7	8	9
				x										Proportional parts					
0·00	1000	1002	1005	1007	1009	1012	1014	1016	1019	1021	0	0	1	1	1	1	2	2	2
0·01	1023	1026	1028	1030	1033	1035	1038	1040	1042	1045	0	0	1	1	1	1	2	2	2
0·02	1047	1050	1052	1054	1057	1059	1062	1064	1067	1069	0	0	1	1	1	1	2	2	2
0·03	1072	1074	1076	1079	1081	1084	1086	1089	1091	1094	0	0	1	1	1	1	2	2	2
0·04	1096	1099	1102	1104	1107	1109	1112	1114	1117	1119	0	1	1	1	1	2	2	2	2
0·05	1122	1125	1127	1130	1132	1135	1138	1140	1143	1146	0	1	1	1	1	2	2	2	2
0·06	1148	1151	1153	1156	1159	1161	1164	1167	1169	1172	0	1	1	1	1	2	2	2	2
0·07	1175	1178	1180	1183	1186	1189	1191	1194	1197	1199	0	1	1	1	1	2	2	2	2
0·08	1202	1205	1208	1211	1213	1216	1219	1222	1225	1227	0	1	1	1	1	2	2	2	3
0·09	1230	1233	1236	1239	1242	1245	1247	1250	1253	1256	0	1	1	1	1	2	2	2	3
0·10	1259	1262	1265	1268	1271	1274	1276	1279	1282	1285	0	1	1	1	1	2	2	2	3
0·11	1288	1291	1294	1297	1300	1303	1306	1309	1312	1315	0	1	1	1	2	2	2	2	3
0·12	1318	1321	1324	1327	1330	1334	1337	1340	1343	1346	0	1	1	1	2	2	2	2	3
0·13	1349	1352	1355	1358	1361	1365	1368	1371	1374	1377	0	1	1	1	2	2	2	3	3
0·14	1380	1384	1387	1390	1393	1396	1400	1403	1406	1409	0	1	1	1	2	2	2	3	3
0·15	1413	1416	1419	1422	1426	1429	1432	1435	1439	1442	0	1	1	1	2	2	2	3	3
0·16	1445	1449	1452	1455	1459	1462	1466	1469	1472	1476	0	1	1	1	2	2	2	3	3
0·17	1479	1483	1486	1489	1493	1496	1500	1503	1507	1510	0	1	1	1	2	2	2	3	3
0·18	1514	1517	1521	1524	1528	1531	1535	1538	1542	1545	0	1	1	1	2	2	2	3	3
0·19	1549	1552	1556	1560	1563	1567	1570	1574	1578	1581	0	1	1	1	2	2	3	3	3
0·20	1585	1589	1592	1596	1600	1603	1607	1611	1614	1618	0	1	1	1	2	2	3	3	3
0·21	1622	1626	1629	1633	1637	1641	1644	1648	1652	1656	0	1	1	2	2	2	3	3	3
0·22	1660	1663	1667	1671	1675	1679	1683	1687	1690	1694	0	1	1	2	2	2	3	3	3
0·23	1698	1702	1706	1710	1714	1718	1722	1726	1730	1734	0	1	1	2	2	2	3	3	4
0·24	1738	1742	1746	1750	1754	1758	1762	1766	1770	1774	0	1	1	2	2	2	3	3	4

Continued

Table B.9. (*Continued*) Antilogarithm table

$\log_{10}x$	0	1	2	3	4	5	6	7	8	9	1	2	3	4	5	6	7	8	9
					x									Proportional parts					
0·25	1778	1782	1786	1791	1795	1799	1803	1807	1811	1816	0	1	1	2	2	2	3	3	4
0·26	1820	1824	1828	1832	1837	1841	1845	1849	1854	1858	0	1	1	2	2	3	3	3	4
0·27	1862	1866	1871	1875	1879	1884	1888	1892	1897	1901	0	1	1	2	2	3	3	3	4
0·28	1905	1910	1914	1919	1923	1928	1932	1936	1941	1945	0	1	1	2	2	3	3	3	4
0·29	1950	1954	1959	1963	1968	1972	1977	1982	1986	1991	0	1	1	2	2	3	3	4	4
0·30	1995	2000	2004	2009	2014	2018	2023	2028	2032	2037	0	1	1	2	2	3	3	4	4
0·31	2042	2046	2051	2056	2061	2065	2070	2075	2080	2084	0	1	1	2	2	3	3	4	4
0·32	2089	2094	2099	2104	2109	2113	2118	2123	2128	2133	0	1	1	2	2	3	3	4	4
0·33	2138	2143	2148	2153	2158	2163	2168	2173	2178	2183	0	1	1	2	2	3	3	4	4
0·34	2188	2193	2198	2203	2208	2213	2218	2223	2228	2234	1	1	2	2	3	3	4	4	5
0·35	2239	2244	2249	2254	2259	2265	2270	2275	2280	2286	1	1	2	2	3	3	4	4	5
0·36	2291	2296	2301	2307	2312	2317	2323	2328	2333	2339	1	1	2	2	3	3	4	4	5
0·37	2344	2350	2355	2360	2366	2371	2377	2382	2388	2393	1	1	2	2	3	3	4	4	5
0·38	2399	2404	2410	2415	2421	2427	2432	2438	2443	2449	1	1	2	2	3	3	4	4	5
0·39	2455	2460	2466	2472	2477	2483	2489	2495	2500	2506	1	1	2	2	3	3	4	5	5
0·40	2512	2518	2523	2529	2535	2541	2547	2553	2559	2564	1	1	2	2	3	4	4	5	5
0·41	2570	2576	2582	2588	2594	2600	2606	2612	2618	2624	1	1	2	2	3	4	4	5	5
0·42	2630	2636	2642	2649	2655	2661	2667	2673	2679	2685	1	1	2	2	3	4	4	5	6
0·43	2692	2698	2704	2710	2716	2723	2729	2735	2742	2748	1	1	2	3	3	4	4	5	6
0·44	2754	2761	2767	2773	2780	2786	2793	2799	2805	2812	1	1	2	3	3	4	4	5	6
0·45	2818	2825	2831	2838	2844	2851	2858	2864	2871	2877	1	1	2	3	3	4	5	5	6
0·46	2884	2891	2897	2904	2911	2917	2924	2931	2938	2944	1	1	2	3	3	4	5	5	6
0·47	2951	2958	2965	2972	2979	2985	2992	2999	3006	3013	1	1	2	3	3	4	5	5	6
0·48	3020	3027	3034	3041	3048	3055	3062	3069	3076	3083	1	1	2	3	4	4	5	6	6
0·49	3090	3097	3105	3112	3119	3126	3133	3141	3148	3155	1	1	2	3	4	4	5	6	6

	0	1	2	3	4	5	6	7	8	9	1	2	3	4	5	6	7	8	9
0·50	3162	3170	3177	3184	3192	3199	3206	3214	3221	3228	1	1	2	3	4	4	5	6	7
0·51	3236	3243	3251	3258	3266	3273	3281	3289	3296	3304	1	2	2	3	4	5	5	6	7
0·52	3311	3319	3327	3334	3342	3350	3357	3365	3373	3381	1	2	2	3	4	5	5	6	7
0·53	3388	3396	3404	3412	3420	3428	3436	3443	3451	3459	1	2	2	3	4	5	6	6	7
0·54	3467	3475	3483	3491	3499	3508	3516	3524	3532	3540	1	2	2	3	4	5	6	6	7
0·55	3548	3556	3565	3573	3581	3589	3597	3606	3614	3622	1	2	2	3	4	5	6	7	7
0·56	3631	3639	3648	3656	3664	3673	3681	3690	3698	3707	1	2	3	3	4	5	6	7	8
0·57	3715	3724	3733	3741	3750	3758	3767	3776	3784	3793	1	2	3	3	4	5	6	7	8
0·58	3802	3811	3819	3828	3837	3846	3855	3864	3873	3882	1	2	3	4	4	5	6	7	8
0·59	3890	3899	3908	3917	3926	3936	3945	3954	3963	3972	1	2	3	4	5	5	6	7	8
0·60	3981	3990	3999	4009	4018	4027	4036	4046	4055	4064	1	2	3	4	5	6	6	7	8
0·61	4074	4083	4093	4102	4111	4121	4130	4140	4150	4159	1	2	3	4	5	6	7	8	9
0·62	4169	4178	4188	4198	4207	4217	4227	4236	4246	4256	1	2	3	4	5	6	7	8	9
0·63	4266	4276	4285	4295	4305	4315	4325	4335	4345	4355	1	2	3	4	5	6	7	8	9
0·64	4365	4375	4385	4395	4406	4416	4426	4436	4446	4457	1	2	3	4	5	6	7	8	9
0·65	4467	4477	4487	4498	4508	4519	4529	4539	4550	4560	1	2	3	4	5	6	7	8	9
0·66	4571	4581	4592	4603	4613	4624	4634	4645	4656	4667	1	2	3	4	5	6	7	9	10
0·67	4677	4688	4699	4710	4721	4732	4742	4753	4764	4775	1	2	3	4	5	6	8	9	10
0·68	4786	4797	4808	4819	4831	4842	4853	4864	4875	4887	1	2	4	5	6	7	8	9	10
0·69	4898	4909	4920	4932	4943	4955	4966	4977	4989	5000	1	2	4	5	6	7	8	9	10
0·70	5012	5023	5035	5047	5058	5070	5082	5093	5105	5117	1	2	4	5	6	7	8	9	11
0·71	5129	5140	5152	5164	5176	5188	5200	5212	5224	5236	1	2	4	5	6	7	8	10	11
0·72	5248	5260	5272	5284	5297	5309	5321	5333	5346	5358	1	2	4	5	6	7	9	10	11
0·73	5370	5383	5395	5408	5420	5433	5445	5458	5470	5483	1	3	4	5	6	8	9	10	11
0·74	5495	5508	5521	5534	5546	5559	5572	5585	5598	5610	1	3	4	5	6	8	9	10	12
0·75	5623	5636	5649	5662	5675	5689	5702	5715	5728	5741	1	3	4	5	7	8	9	10	12
0·76	5754	5768	5781	5794	5808	5821	5834	5848	5861	5875	1	3	4	5	7	8	9	11	12
0·77	5888	5902	5916	5929	5943	5957	5970	5984	5998	6012	1	3	4	5	7	8	10	11	12
0·78	6026	6039	6053	6067	6081	6095	6109	6124	6138	6152	1	3	4	6	7	8	10	11	13
0·79	6166	6180	6194	6209	6223	6237	6252	6266	6281	6295	1	3	4	6	7	9	10	11	13

Continued

Table B.9. (*Continued*) Antilogarithm table

$\log_{10}x$	0	1	2	3	4	5	6	7	8	9	1	2	3	4	5	6	7	8	9
						x							Proportional parts						
0·80	6310	6324	6339	6353	6368	6383	6397	6412	6427	6442	1	3	4	6	7	9	10	12	13
0·81	6457	6471	6486	6501	6516	6531	6546	6561	6577	6592	2	3	5	6	8	9	11	12	14
0·82	6607	6622	6637	6653	6668	6683	6699	6714	6730	6745	2	3	5	6	8	9	11	12	14
0·83	6761	6776	6792	6808	6823	6839	6855	6871	6887	6902	2	3	5	6	8	9	11	13	14
0·84	6918	6934	6950	6966	6982	6998	7015	7031	7047	7063	2	3	5	6	8	10	11	13	15
0·85	7079	7096	7112	7129	7145	7161	7178	7194	7211	7228	2	3	5	7	8	10	12	13	15
0·86	7244	7261	7278	7295	7311	7328	7345	7362	7379	7396	2	3	5	7	8	10	12	13	15
0·87	7413	7430	7447	7464	7482	7499	7516	7534	7551	7568	2	3	5	7	9	10	12	14	16
0·88	7586	7603	7621	7638	7656	7674	7691	7709	7727	7745	2	4	5	7	9	11	12	14	16
0·89	7762	7780	7798	7816	7834	7852	7870	7889	7907	7925	2	4	5	7	9	11	13	14	16
0·90	7943	7962	7980	7998	8017	8035	8054	8072	8091	8110	2	4	6	7	9	11	13	15	17
0·91	8128	8147	8166	8185	8204	8222	8241	8260	8279	8299	2	4	6	8	9	11	13	15	17
0·92	8318	8337	8356	8375	8395	8414	8433	8453	8472	8492	2	4	6	8	10	12	14	15	17
0·93	8511	8531	8551	8570	8590	8610	8630	8650	8670	8690	2	4	6	8	10	12	14	16	18
0·94	8710	8730	8750	8770	8790	8810	8831	8851	8872	8892	2	4	6	8	10	12	14	16	18
0·95	8913	8933	8954	8974	8995	9016	9036	9057	9078	9099	2	4	6	8	10	12	15	17	19
0·96	9120	9141	9162	9183	9204	9226	9247	9268	9290	9311	2	4	6	8	11	13	15	17	19
0·97	9333	9354	9376	9397	9419	9441	9462	9484	9506	9528	2	4	7	9	11	13	15	17	20
0·98	9550	9572	9594	9616	9638	9661	9683	9705	9727	9750	2	4	7	9	11	13	16	18	20
0·99	9772	9795	9817	9840	9863	9886	9908	9931	9954	9977	2	5	7	9	11	14	16	18	20

Table B.10. Spearman's rank correlation coefficient: critical values for the correlation coefficient r_S calculated on n pairs of observations. Abbreviated from *Geigy Scientific Tables*, Vol. 2, 8th edn. with permission

Two-sided significance level	0·10	0·05	0·02	0·01
One-sided significance level	0·05	0·025	0·01	0·005
n	Critical values r_c			
4	0·9999	—	—	—
5	0·9000	0·9999	0·9999	—
6	0·8286	0·8857	0·9429	0·9999
7	0·7143	0·7857	0·8929	0·9286
8	0·6429	0·7381	0·8333	0·8810
9	0·6000	0·6833	0·7833	0·8333
10	0·5636	0·6485	0·7333	0·7939
11	0·5364	0·6182	0·7000	0·7545
12	0·5035	0·5874	0·6783	0·7343
13	0·4835	0·5604	0·6484	0·7033
14	0·4637	0·5385	0·6264	0·6791
15	0·4464	0·5214	0·6036	0·6571
16	0·4294	0·5029	0·5853	0·6353
17	0·4142	0·4877	0·5662	0·6176
18	0·4014	0·4737	0·5501	0·5996
19	0·3912	0·4596	0·5351	0·5842
20	0·3805	0·4466	0·5218	0·5699
21	0·3701	0·4364	0·5091	0·5558
22	0·3608	0·4252	0·4975	0·5438
23	0·3528	0·4160	0·4862	0·5316
24	0·3443	0·4070	0·4757	0·5209
25	0·3369	0·3985	0·4662	0·5108
26	0·3306	0·3901	0·4571	0·5009
27	0·3242	0·3828	0·4487	0·4921
28	0·3180	0·3755	0·4406	0·4833
29	0·3118	0·3690	0·4325	0·4749
30	0·3063	0·3624	0·4256	0·4670

Significant result if $r_S \geq r_c$ or $r_S \leq -r_c$

Table B.11. Exact confidence limits for a binomial proportion: x events are observed in a sample sized n. $p = x/n$ is the observed proportion. p_l and p_u are the lower and upper confidence limits for the population proportion

Confidence level

n	x	p	95% p_l	95% p_u	99% p_l	99% p_u
2	0	0.0000	0.0000	0.8419	0.0000	0.9293
	1	0.5000	0.0126	0.9874	0.0025	0.9975
	2	1.0000	0.1581	1.0000	0.0707	1.0000
3	0	0.0000	0.0000	0.7076	0.0000	0.8290
	1	0.3333	0.0084	0.9057	0.0017	0.9586
	2	0.6667	0.0943	0.9916	0.0414	0.9983
	3	1.0000	0.2924	1.0000	0.1710	1.0000
4	0	0.0000	0.0000	0.6024	0.0000	0.7341
	1	0.2500	0.0063	0.8059	0.0013	0.8891
	2	0.5000	0.0676	0.9324	0.0294	0.9706
	3	0.7500	0.1941	0.9937	0.1109	0.9987
	4	1.0000	0.3976	1.0000	0.2659	1.0000
5	0	0.0000	0.0000	0.5218	0.0000	0.6534
	1	0.2000	0.0051	0.7164	0.0010	0.8149
	2	0.4000	0.0527	0.8534	0.0229	0.9172
	3	0.6000	0.1466	0.9473	0.0828	0.9771
	4	0.8000	0.2836	0.9949	0.1851	0.9990
	5	1.0000	0.4782	1.0000	0.3466	1.0000
6	0	0.0000	0.0000	0.4593	0.0000	0.5865
	1	0.1667	0.0042	0.6412	0.0008	0.7460
	2	0.3333	0.0433	0.7772	0.0187	0.8564
	3	0.5000	0.1181	0.8819	0.0663	0.9337
	4	0.6667	0.2228	0.9567	0.1436	0.9813
	5	0.8333	0.3588	0.9958	0.2540	0.9992
	6	1.0000	0.5407	1.0000	0.4135	1.0000
7	0	0.0000	0.0000	0.4096	0.0000	0.5309
	1	0.1429	0.0036	0.5787	0.0007	0.6849
	2	0.2857	0.0367	0.7096	0.0158	0.7970
	3	0.4286	0.0990	0.8159	0.0553	0.8823
	4	0.5714	0.1841	0.9010	0.1177	0.9447
	5	0.7143	0.2904	0.9633	0.2030	0.9842
	6	0.8571	0.4213	0.9964	0.3151	0.9993
	7	1.0000	0.5904	1.0000	0.4691	1.0000

Confidence level

n	x	p	95% p_l	95% p_u	99% p_l	99% p_u
12	0	0.0000	0.0000	0.2646	0.0000	0.3569
	1	0.0833	0.0021	0.3848	0.0004	0.4770
	2	0.1667	0.0209	0.4841	0.0090	0.5729
	3	0.2500	0.0549	0.5719	0.0303	0.6552
	4	0.3333	0.0992	0.6511	0.0624	0.7275
	5	0.4167	0.1517	0.7233	0.1034	0.7915
	6	0.5000	0.2109	0.7891	0.1522	0.8478
	7	0.5833	0.2767	0.8483	0.2085	0.8966
	8	0.6667	0.3489	0.9008	0.2725	0.9376
	9	0.7500	0.4281	0.9451	0.3448	0.9697
	10	0.8333	0.5159	0.9791	0.4271	0.9910
	11	0.9167	0.6152	0.9979	0.5230	0.9996
	12	1.0000	0.7354	1.0000	0.6431	1.0000
13	0	0.0000	0.0000	0.2471	0.0000	0.3347
	1	0.0769	0.0019	0.3603	0.0004	0.4490
	2	0.1538	0.0192	0.4545	0.0083	0.5410
	3	0.2308	0.0504	0.5381	0.0278	0.6206
	4	0.3077	0.0909	0.6143	0.0571	0.6913
	5	0.3846	0.1386	0.6842	0.0942	0.7546
	6	0.4615	0.1922	0.7487	0.1383	0.8113
	7	0.5385	0.2513	0.8078	0.1887	0.8617
	8	0.6154	0.3158	0.8614	0.2454	0.9058
	9	0.6923	0.3857	0.9091	0.3087	0.9429
	10	0.7692	0.4619	0.9496	0.3794	0.9722
	11	0.8462	0.5455	0.9808	0.4590	0.9917
	12	0.9231	0.6397	0.9981	0.5510	0.9996
	13	1.0000	0.7529	1.0000	0.6653	1.0000
14	0	0.0000	0.0000	0.2316	0.0000	0.3151
	1	0.0714	0.0018	0.3387	0.0004	0.4240
	2	0.1429	0.0178	0.4281	0.0076	0.5123
	3	0.2143	0.0466	0.5080	0.0257	0.5892
	4	0.2857	0.0839	0.5810	0.0526	0.6579
	5	0.3571	0.1276	0.6486	0.0866	0.7201
	6	0.4286	0.1766	0.7114	0.1267	0.7766

8	**0**	0.0000	0.0000	0.3694	0.0000	0.4843
	1	0.1250	0.0032	0.5265	0.0006	0.6315
	2	0.2500	0.0319	0.6509	0.0137	0.7422
	3	0.3750	0.0852	0.7551	0.0475	0.8303
	4	0.5000	0.1570	0.8430	0.0999	0.9001
	5	0.6250	0.2449	0.9148	0.1697	0.9525
	6	0.7500	0.3491	0.9681	0.2578	0.9863
	7	0.8750	0.4735	0.9968	0.3685	0.9994
	8	1.0000	0.6306	1.0000	0.5157	1.0000
9	**0**	0.0000	0.0000	0.3363	0.0000	0.4450
	1	0.1111	0.0028	0.4825	0.0006	0.5850
	2	0.2222	0.0281	0.6001	0.0121	0.6926
	3	0.3333	0.0749	0.7007	0.0416	0.7809
	4	0.4444	0.1370	0.7880	0.0868	0.8539
	5	0.5556	0.2120	0.8630	0.1461	0.9132
	6	0.6667	0.2993	0.9251	0.2191	0.9584
	7	0.7778	0.3999	0.9719	0.3074	0.9879
	8	0.8889	0.5175	0.9972	0.4150	0.9994
	9	1.0000	0.6637	1.0000	0.5550	1.0000
10	**0**	0.0000	0.0000	0.3085	0.0000	0.4113
	1	0.1000	0.0025	0.4450	0.0005	0.5443
	2	0.2000	0.0252	0.5561	0.0109	0.6482
	3	0.3000	0.0667	0.6525	0.0370	0.7351
	4	0.4000	0.1216	0.7376	0.0768	0.8091
	5	0.5000	0.1871	0.8129	0.1283	0.8717
	6	0.6000	0.2624	0.8784	0.1909	0.9232
	7	0.7000	0.3475	0.9333	0.2649	0.9630
	8	0.8000	0.4439	0.9748	0.3518	0.9891
	9	0.9000	0.5550	0.9975	0.4557	0.9995
	10	1.0000	0.6915	1.0000	0.5887	1.0000
11	**0**	0.0000	0.0000	0.2849	0.0000	0.3822
	1	0.0909	0.0023	0.4128	0.0005	0.5086
	2	0.1818	0.0228	0.5178	0.0098	0.6085
	3	0.2727	0.0602	0.6097	0.0333	0.6933
	4	0.3636	0.1093	0.6921	0.0688	0.7668
	5	0.4545	0.1675	0.7662	0.1145	0.8307
	6	0.5455	0.2338	0.8325	0.1693	0.8855
	7	0.6364	0.3079	0.8907	0.2332	0.9312
	8	0.7273	0.3903	0.9398	0.3067	0.9667
	9	0.8182	0.4822	0.9772	0.3915	0.9902
	10	0.9091	0.5872	0.9977	0.4914	0.9995
	11	1.0000	0.7151	1.0000	0.6178	1.0000
14	7	0.5000	0.2304	0.7696	0.1724	0.8276
	8	0.5714	0.2886	0.8234	0.2234	0.8733
	9	0.6429	0.3514	0.8724	0.2799	0.9134
	10	0.7143	0.4190	0.9161	0.3421	0.9474
	11	0.7857	0.4920	0.9534	0.4108	0.9743
	12	0.8571	0.5719	0.9822	0.4877	0.9924
	13	0.9286	0.6613	0.9982	0.5760	0.9996
	14	1.0000	0.7684	1.0000	0.6849	1.0000
15	**0**	0.0000	0.0000	0.2180	0.0000	0.2976
	1	0.0667	0.0017	0.3195	0.0003	0.4016
	2	0.1333	0.0166	0.4046	0.0071	0.4863
	3	0.2000	0.0433	0.4809	0.0239	0.5605
	4	0.2667	0.0779	0.5510	0.0488	0.6273
	5	0.3333	0.1182	0.6162	0.0801	0.6882
	6	0.4000	0.1634	0.6771	0.1170	0.7439
	7	0.4667	0.2127	0.7341	0.1587	0.7949
	8	0.5333	0.2659	0.7873	0.2051	0.8413
	9	0.6000	0.3229	0.8366	0.2561	0.8830
	10	0.6667	0.3838	0.8818	0.3118	0.9199
	11	0.7333	0.4490	0.9221	0.3727	0.9512
	12	0.8000	0.5191	0.9567	0.4395	0.9761
	13	0.8667	0.5954	0.9834	0.5137	0.9929
	14	0.9333	0.6805	0.9983	0.5984	0.9997
	15	1.0000	0.7820	1.0000	0.7024	1.0000
16	**0**	0.0000	0.0000	0.2059	0.0000	0.2819
	1	0.0625	0.0016	0.3023	0.0003	0.3814
	2	0.1250	0.0155	0.3835	0.0067	0.4628
	3	0.1875	0.0405	0.4565	0.0223	0.5344
	4	0.2500	0.0727	0.5238	0.0455	0.5991
	5	0.3125	0.1102	0.5866	0.0745	0.6585
	6	0.3750	0.1520	0.6457	0.1086	0.7132
	7	0.4375	0.1975	0.7012	0.1471	0.7638
	8	0.5000	0.2465	0.7535	0.1897	0.8103
	9	0.5625	0.2988	0.8025	0.2362	0.8529
	10	0.6250	0.3543	0.8480	0.2868	0.8914
	11	0.6875	0.4134	0.8898	0.3415	0.9255
	12	0.7500	0.4762	0.9273	0.4009	0.9545
	13	0.8125	0.5435	0.9595	0.4656	0.9777
	14	0.8750	0.6165	0.9845	0.5372	0.9933
	15	0.9375	0.6977	0.9984	0.6186	0.9997
	16	1.0000	0.7941	1.0000	0.7181	1.0000

Continued

Table B.11. Exact confidence limits for a binomial proportion: x events are observed in a sample sized n. $p = x/n$ is the observed proportion. p_l and p_u are the lower and upper confidence limits for the population proportion

Confidence level

n	x	p	95% p_l	95% p_u	99% p_l	99% p_u
17	0	0.0000	0.0000	0.1951	0.0000	0.2678
	1	0.0588	0.0015	0.2869	0.0003	0.3630
	2	0.1176	0.0146	0.3644	0.0063	0.4413
	3	0.1765	0.0380	0.4343	0.0209	0.5104
	4	0.2353	0.0681	0.4990	0.0426	0.5732
	5	0.2941	0.1031	0.5596	0.0697	0.6310
	6	0.3529	0.1421	0.6167	0.1014	0.6846
	7	0.4118	0.1844	0.6708	0.1371	0.7344
	8	0.4706	0.2298	0.7219	0.1764	0.7807
	9	0.5294	0.2781	0.7702	0.2193	0.8236
	10	0.5882	0.3292	0.8156	0.2656	0.8629
	11	0.6471	0.3833	0.8579	0.3154	0.8986
	12	0.7059	0.4404	0.8969	0.3690	0.9303
	13	0.7647	0.5010	0.9319	0.4268	0.9574
	14	0.8235	0.5657	0.9620	0.4896	0.9791
	15	0.8824	0.6356	0.9854	0.5587	0.9937
	16	0.9412	0.7131	0.9985	0.6370	0.9997
	17	1.0000	0.8049	1.0000	0.7322	1.0000
18	0	0.0000	0.0000	0.1853	0.0000	0.2550
	1	0.0556	0.0014	0.2729	0.0003	0.3463
	2	0.1111	0.0138	0.3471	0.0059	0.4217
	3	0.1667	0.0358	0.4142	0.0197	0.4884
	4	0.2222	0.0641	0.4764	0.0400	0.5492
	5	0.2778	0.0969	0.5348	0.0654	0.6055
	6	0.3333	0.1334	0.5901	0.0951	0.6579
	7	0.3889	0.1730	0.6425	0.1284	0.7068
	8	0.4444	0.2153	0.6924	0.1649	0.7526
	9	0.5000	0.2602	0.7398	0.2047	0.7953
	10	0.5556	0.3076	0.7847	0.2474	0.8351
	11	0.6111	0.3575	0.8270	0.2932	0.8716
	12	0.6667	0.4099	0.8666	0.3421	0.9049
	13	0.7222	0.4652	0.9031	0.3945	0.9346
	14	0.7778	0.5236	0.9359	0.4508	0.9600
	15	0.8333	0.5858	0.9642	0.5116	0.9803
	16	0.8889	0.6529	0.9862	0.5783	0.9941

Confidence level

n	x	p	95% p_l	95% p_u	99% p_l	99% p_u
20	19	0.9500	0.7513	0.9987	0.6829	0.9997
	20	1.0000	0.8316	1.0000	0.7673	1.0000
21	0	0.0000	0.0000	0.1611	0.0000	0.2230
	1	0.0476	0.0012	0.2382	0.0002	0.3043
	2	0.0952	0.0117	0.3038	0.0050	0.3718
	3	0.1429	0.0305	0.3634	0.0168	0.4322
	4	0.1905	0.0545	0.4191	0.0339	0.4876
	5	0.2381	0.0822	0.4717	0.0553	0.5392
	6	0.2857	0.1128	0.5218	0.0801	0.5878
	7	0.3333	0.1459	0.5697	0.1078	0.6337
	8	0.3810	0.1811	0.6156	0.1381	0.6772
	9	0.4286	0.2182	0.6598	0.1707	0.7185
	10	0.4762	0.2571	0.7022	0.2055	0.7576
	11	0.5238	0.2978	0.7429	0.2424	0.7945
	12	0.5714	0.3402	0.7818	0.2815	0.8293
	13	0.6190	0.3844	0.8189	0.3228	0.8619
	14	0.6667	0.4303	0.8541	0.3663	0.8922
	15	0.7143	0.4782	0.8872	0.4122	0.9199
	16	0.7619	0.5283	0.9178	0.4608	0.9447
	17	0.8095	0.5809	0.9455	0.5124	0.9661
	18	0.8571	0.6366	0.9695	0.5678	0.9832
	19	0.9048	0.6962	0.9883	0.6282	0.9950
	20	0.9524	0.7618	0.9988	0.6957	0.9998
	21	1.0000	0.8389	1.0000	0.7770	1.0000
22	0	0.0000	0.0000	0.1544	0.0000	0.2140
	1	0.0455	0.0012	0.2284	0.0002	0.2924
	2	0.0909	0.0112	0.2916	0.0048	0.3577
	3	0.1364	0.0291	0.3491	0.0160	0.4161
	4	0.1818	0.0519	0.4028	0.0323	0.4699
	5	0.2273	0.0782	0.4537	0.0526	0.5201
	6	0.2727	0.1073	0.5022	0.0761	0.5674
	7	0.3182	0.1386	0.5487	0.1024	0.6123
	8	0.3636	0.1720	0.5934	0.1310	0.6549
	9	0.4091	0.2071	0.6365	0.1618	0.6954
	10	0.4545	0.2439	0.6779	0.1946	0.7340

n	k					
18	17	0.9444	0.7271	0.9986	0.6537	0.9997
	18	1.0000	0.8147	1.0000	0.7450	1.0000
19	0	0.0000	0.0000	0.1765	0.0000	0.2434
	1	0.0526	0.0013	0.2603	0.0003	0.3311
	2	0.1053	0.0130	0.3314	0.0056	0.4037
	3	0.1579	0.0338	0.3958	0.0186	0.4682
	4	0.2105	0.0605	0.4557	0.0378	0.5271
	5	0.2632	0.0915	0.5120	0.0617	0.5818
	6	0.3158	0.1258	0.5655	0.0895	0.6329
	7	0.3684	0.1629	0.6164	0.1207	0.6809
	8	0.4211	0.2025	0.6650	0.1549	0.7260
	9	0.4737	0.2445	0.7114	0.1919	0.7684
	10	0.5263	0.2886	0.7555	0.2316	0.8081
	11	0.5789	0.3350	0.7975	0.2740	0.8451
	12	0.6316	0.3836	0.8371	0.3191	0.8793
	13	0.6842	0.4345	0.8742	0.3671	0.9105
	14	0.7368	0.4880	0.9085	0.4182	0.9383
	15	0.7895	0.5443	0.9395	0.4729	0.9622
	16	0.8421	0.6042	0.9662	0.5318	0.9814
	17	0.8947	0.6686	0.9870	0.5963	0.9944
	18	0.9474	0.7397	0.9987	0.6689	0.9997
	19	1.0000	0.8235	1.0000	0.7566	1.0000
20	0	0.0000	0.0000	0.1684	0.0000	0.2327
	1	0.0500	0.0013	0.2487	0.0003	0.3171
	2	0.1000	0.0123	0.3170	0.0053	0.3871
	3	0.1500	0.0321	0.3789	0.0176	0.4495
	4	0.2000	0.0573	0.4366	0.0358	0.5066
	5	0.2500	0.0866	0.4910	0.0583	0.5598
	6	0.3000	0.1189	0.5428	0.0846	0.6096
	7	0.3500	0.1539	0.5922	0.1139	0.6566
	8	0.4000	0.1912	0.6395	0.1460	0.7009
	9	0.4500	0.2306	0.6847	0.1806	0.7428
	10	0.5000	0.2720	0.7280	0.2177	0.7823
	11	0.5500	0.3153	0.7694	0.2572	0.8194
	12	0.6000	0.3605	0.8088	0.2991	0.8540
	13	0.6500	0.4078	0.8461	0.3434	0.8861
	14	0.7000	0.4572	0.8811	0.3904	0.9154
	15	0.7500	0.5090	0.9134	0.4402	0.9417
	16	0.8000	0.5634	0.9427	0.4934	0.9642
	17	0.8500	0.6211	0.9679	0.5505	0.9824
	18	0.9000	0.6830	0.9877	0.6129	0.9947

n	k					
22	11	0.7707	0.2293	0.7178	0.2822	0.5000
	12	0.8054	0.2660	0.7561	0.3221	0.5455
	13	0.8382	0.3046	0.7929	0.3635	0.5909
	14	0.8690	0.3451	0.8280	0.4066	0.6364
	15	0.8976	0.3877	0.8614	0.4513	0.6818
	16	0.9239	0.4326	0.8927	0.4978	0.7273
	17	0.9474	0.4799	0.9218	0.5463	0.7727
	18	0.9677	0.5301	0.9481	0.5972	0.8182
	19	0.9840	0.5839	0.9709	0.6509	0.8636
	20	0.9952	0.6423	0.9888	0.7084	0.9091
	21	0.9998	0.7076	0.9988	0.7716	0.9545
	22	1.0000	0.7860	1.0000	0.8456	1.0000
23	0	0.2058	0.0000	0.1482	0.0000	0.0000
	1	0.2814	0.0002	0.2195	0.0011	0.0435
	2	0.3446	0.0046	0.2804	0.0107	0.0870
	3	0.4012	0.0153	0.3359	0.0278	0.1304
	4	0.4534	0.0308	0.3878	0.0495	0.1739
	5	0.5022	0.0502	0.4370	0.0746	0.2174
	6	0.5483	0.0725	0.4841	0.1023	0.2609
	7	0.5921	0.0974	0.5292	0.1321	0.3043
	8	0.6338	0.1246	0.5727	0.1638	0.3478
	9	0.6736	0.1537	0.6146	0.1971	0.3913
	10	0.7116	0.1848	0.6551	0.2319	0.4348
	11	0.7479	0.2176	0.6941	0.2682	0.4783
	12	0.7824	0.2521	0.7318	0.3059	0.5217
	13	0.8152	0.2884	0.7681	0.3449	0.5652
	14	0.8463	0.3264	0.8029	0.3854	0.6087
	15	0.8754	0.3662	0.8362	0.4273	0.6522
	16	0.9026	0.4079	0.8679	0.4708	0.6957
	17	0.9275	0.4517	0.8977	0.5159	0.7391
	18	0.9498	0.4978	0.9254	0.5630	0.7826
	19	0.9692	0.5466	0.9505	0.6122	0.8261
	20	0.9847	0.5988	0.9722	0.6641	0.8696
	21	0.9954	0.6554	0.9893	0.7196	0.9130
	22	0.9998	0.7186	0.9989	0.7805	0.9565
	23	1.0000	0.7942	1.0000	0.8518	1.0000
24	0	0.1981	0.0000	0.1425	0.0000	0.0000
	1	0.2713	0.0002	0.2112	0.0011	0.0417
	2	0.3324	0.0044	0.2700	0.0103	0.0833
	3	0.3873	0.0146	0.3236	0.0266	0.1250
	4	0.4379	0.0295	0.3738	0.0474	0.1667

Continued

Table B.11. Exact confidence limits for a binomial proportion: x events are observed in a sample sized n. $p = x/n$ is the observed proportion. p_l and p_u are the lower and upper confidence limits for the population proportion

Confidence level

n	x	p	95% p_l	95% p_u	99% p_l	99% p_u
24	5	0.2083	0.0713	0.4215	0.0479	0.4855
	6	0.2500	0.0977	0.4671	0.0692	0.5304
	7	0.2917	0.1262	0.5109	0.0930	0.5732
	8	0.3333	0.1563	0.5532	0.1188	0.6140
	9	0.3750	0.1880	0.5941	0.1465	0.6530
	10	0.4167	0.2211	0.6336	0.1759	0.6904
	11	0.4583	0.2555	0.6718	0.2070	0.7262
	12	0.5000	0.2912	0.7088	0.2396	0.7604
	13	0.5417	0.3282	0.7445	0.2738	0.7930
	14	0.5833	0.3664	0.7789	0.3096	0.8241
	15	0.6250	0.4059	0.8120	0.3470	0.8535
	16	0.6667	0.4468	0.8437	0.3860	0.8812
	17	0.7083	0.4891	0.8738	0.4268	0.9070
	18	0.7500	0.5329	0.9023	0.4696	0.9308
	19	0.7917	0.5785	0.9287	0.5145	0.9521
	20	0.8333	0.6262	0.9526	0.5621	0.9705
	21	0.8750	0.6764	0.9734	0.6127	0.9854
	22	0.9167	0.7300	0.9897	0.6676	0.9956
	23	0.9583	0.7888	0.9989	0.7287	0.9998
	24	1.0000	0.8575	1.0000	0.8019	1.0000
25	0	0.0000	0.0000	0.1372	0.0000	0.1910
	1	0.0400	0.0010	0.2035	0.0002	0.2618
	2	0.0800	0.0098	0.2603	0.0042	0.3210
	3	0.1200	0.0255	0.3122	0.0140	0.3743
	4	0.1600	0.0454	0.3608	0.0282	0.4235
	5	0.2000	0.0683	0.4070	0.0459	0.4698
	6	0.2400	0.0936	0.4513	0.0663	0.5136
	7	0.2800	0.1207	0.4939	0.0889	0.5553
	8	0.3200	0.1495	0.5350	0.1135	0.5952
	9	0.3600	0.1797	0.5748	0.1399	0.6335
	10	0.4000	0.2113	0.6133	0.1679	0.6702
	11	0.4400	0.2440	0.6507	0.1974	0.7054
	12	0.4800	0.2780	0.6869	0.2283	0.7393
	13	0.5200	0.3131	0.7220	0.2607	0.7717
	14	0.5600	0.3493	0.7560	0.2946	0.8026
	15	0.6000	0.3867	0.7887	0.3298	0.8321

Confidence level

n	x	p	95% p_l	95% p_u	99% p_l	99% p_u
27	5	0.1852	0.0630	0.3808	0.0423	0.4411
	6	0.2222	0.0862	0.4226	0.0610	0.4828
	7	0.2593	0.1111	0.4628	0.0817	0.5226
	8	0.2963	0.1375	0.5018	0.1042	0.5608
	9	0.3333	0.1652	0.5396	0.1283	0.5975
	10	0.3704	0.1940	0.5763	0.1538	0.6328
	11	0.4074	0.2239	0.6120	0.1807	0.6669
	12	0.4444	0.2548	0.6467	0.2088	0.6998
	13	0.4815	0.2867	0.6805	0.2381	0.7314
	14	0.5185	0.3195	0.7133	0.2686	0.7619
	15	0.5556	0.3533	0.7452	0.3002	0.7912
	16	0.5926	0.3880	0.7761	0.3331	0.8193
	17	0.6296	0.4237	0.8060	0.3672	0.8462
	18	0.6667	0.4604	0.8348	0.4025	0.8717
	19	0.7037	0.4982	0.8625	0.4392	0.8958
	20	0.7407	0.5372	0.8889	0.4774	0.9183
	21	0.7778	0.5774	0.9138	0.5172	0.9390
	22	0.8148	0.6192	0.9370	0.5589	0.9577
	23	0.8519	0.6627	0.9581	0.6027	0.9740
	24	0.8889	0.7084	0.9765	0.6493	0.9871
	25	0.9259	0.7571	0.9909	0.6996	0.9961
	26	0.9630	0.8103	0.9991	0.7554	0.9998
	27	1.0000	0.8723	1.0000	0.8218	1.0000
28	0	0.0000	0.0000	0.1234	0.0000	0.1724
	1	0.0357	0.0009	0.1835	0.0002	0.2369
	2	0.0714	0.0088	0.2350	0.0038	0.2911
	3	0.1071	0.0227	0.2823	0.0124	0.3399
	4	0.1429	0.0403	0.3267	0.0251	0.3853
	5	0.1786	0.0606	0.3689	0.0407	0.4280
	6	0.2143	0.0830	0.4095	0.0586	0.4687
	7	0.2500	0.1069	0.4487	0.0786	0.5076
	8	0.2857	0.1322	0.4867	0.1002	0.5449
	9	0.3214	0.1588	0.5235	0.1232	0.5808
	10	0.3571	0.1864	0.5593	0.1477	0.6155
	11	0.3929	0.2150	0.5942	0.1733	0.6490
	12	0.4286	0.2446	0.6282	0.2002	0.6814

n = 28

k					
13	0.4643	0.2751	0.6613	0.2282	0.7126
14	0.5000	0.3065	0.6935	0.2572	0.7428
15	0.5357	0.3387	0.7249	0.2874	0.7718
16	0.5714	0.3718	0.7554	0.3186	0.7998
17	0.6071	0.4058	0.7850	0.3510	0.8267
18	0.6429	0.4407	0.8136	0.3845	0.8523
19	0.6786	0.4765	0.8412	0.4192	0.8768
20	0.7143	0.5133	0.8678	0.4551	0.8998
21	0.7500	0.5513	0.8931	0.4924	0.9214
22	0.7857	0.5905	0.9170	0.5313	0.9414
23	0.8214	0.6311	0.9394	0.5720	0.9593
24	0.8571	0.6733	0.9597	0.6147	0.9749
25	0.8929	0.7177	0.9773	0.6601	0.9876
26	0.9286	0.7650	0.9912	0.7089	0.9962
27	0.9643	0.8165	0.9991	0.7631	0.9998
28	1.0000	0.8766	1.0000	0.8276	1.0000

n = 29

k					
0	0.0000	0.0000	0.1194	0.0000	0.1670
1	0.0345	0.0009	0.1776	0.0002	0.2296
2	0.0690	0.0085	0.2277	0.0036	0.2823
3	0.1034	0.0219	0.2735	0.0120	0.3298
4	0.1379	0.0389	0.3166	0.0242	0.3740
5	0.1724	0.0585	0.3577	0.0392	0.4157
6	0.2069	0.0799	0.3972	0.0565	0.4554
7	0.2414	0.1030	0.4354	0.0756	0.4933
8	0.2759	0.1273	0.4724	0.0964	0.5299
9	0.3103	0.1528	0.5083	0.1185	0.5651
10	0.3448	0.1794	0.5433	0.1420	0.5991
11	0.3793	0.2069	0.5774	0.1666	0.6320
12	0.4138	0.2352	0.6106	0.1923	0.6638
13	0.4483	0.2645	0.6431	0.2191	0.6946
14	0.4828	0.2945	0.6747	0.2469	0.7243
15	0.5172	0.3253	0.7055	0.2757	0.7531
16	0.5517	0.3569	0.7355	0.3054	0.7809
17	0.5862	0.3894	0.7648	0.3362	0.8077
18	0.6207	0.4226	0.7931	0.3680	0.8334
19	0.6552	0.4567	0.8206	0.4009	0.8580
20	0.6897	0.4917	0.8472	0.4349	0.8815
21	0.7241	0.5276	0.8727	0.4701	0.9036
22	0.7586	0.5646	0.8970	0.5067	0.9244
23	0.7931	0.6028	0.9201	0.5446	0.9435
24	0.8276	0.6423	0.9415	0.5843	0.9608
25	0.8621	0.6834	0.9611	0.6260	0.9758

n = 25

k					
16	0.6400	0.4252	0.8203	0.3665	0.8601
17	0.6800	0.4650	0.8505	0.4048	0.8865
18	0.7200	0.5061	0.8793	0.4447	0.9111
19	0.7600	0.5487	0.9064	0.4864	0.9337
20	0.8000	0.5930	0.9317	0.5302	0.9541
21	0.8400	0.6392	0.9546	0.5765	0.9718
22	0.8800	0.6878	0.9745	0.6257	0.9860
23	0.9200	0.7397	0.9902	0.6790	0.9958
24	0.9600	0.7965	0.9990	0.7382	0.9998
25	1.0000	0.8628	1.0000	0.8090	1.0000

n = 26

k					
0	0.0000	0.0000	0.1323	0.0000	0.1844
1	0.0385	0.0010	0.1964	0.0002	0.2529
2	0.0769	0.0095	0.2513	0.0041	0.3104
3	0.1154	0.0245	0.3015	0.0134	0.3621
4	0.1538	0.0436	0.3487	0.0271	0.4100
5	0.1923	0.0655	0.3935	0.0440	0.4550
6	0.2308	0.0897	0.4365	0.0635	0.4977
7	0.2692	0.1157	0.4779	0.0852	0.5385
8	0.3077	0.1433	0.5179	0.1087	0.5775
9	0.3462	0.1721	0.5567	0.1338	0.6150
10	0.3846	0.2023	0.5943	0.1605	0.6510
11	0.4231	0.2335	0.6308	0.1886	0.6857
12	0.4615	0.2659	0.6663	0.2181	0.7191
13	0.5000	0.2993	0.7007	0.2489	0.7511
14	0.5385	0.3337	0.7341	0.2809	0.7819
15	0.5769	0.3692	0.7665	0.3143	0.8114
16	0.6154	0.4057	0.7977	0.3490	0.8395
17	0.6538	0.4433	0.8279	0.3850	0.8662
18	0.6923	0.4821	0.8567	0.4225	0.8913
19	0.7308	0.5221	0.8843	0.4615	0.9148
20	0.7692	0.5635	0.9103	0.5023	0.9365
21	0.8077	0.6065	0.9345	0.5450	0.9560
22	0.8462	0.6513	0.9564	0.5900	0.9729
23	0.8846	0.6985	0.9755	0.6379	0.9866
24	0.9231	0.7487	0.9905	0.6896	0.9959
25	0.9615	0.8036	0.9990	0.7471	0.9998
26	1.0000	0.8677	1.0000	0.8156	1.0000

n = 27

k					
0	0.0000	0.0000	0.1277	0.0000	0.1782
1	0.0370	0.0009	0.1897	0.0002	0.2446
2	0.0741	0.0091	0.2429	0.0039	0.3004
3	0.1111	0.0235	0.2916	0.0129	0.3507
4	0.1481	0.0419	0.3373	0.0260	0.3973

Continued

Table B.11. Exact confidence limits for a binomial proportion: x events are observed in a sample sized n. $p = x/n$ is the observed proportion. p_l and p_u are the lower and upper confidence limits for the population proportion

Confidence level

n	x	p	95% p_l	95% p_u	99% p_l	99% p_u
29	26	0.8966	0.7265	0.9781	0.6702	0.9880
	27	0.9310	0.7723	0.9915	0.7177	0.9964
	28	0.9655	0.8224	0.9991	0.7704	0.9998
	29	1.0000	0.8806	1.0000	0.8330	1.0000
30	0	0.0000	0.0000	0.1157	0.0000	0.1619
	1	0.0333	0.0008	0.1722	0.0002	0.2228
	2	0.0667	0.0082	0.2207	0.0035	0.2740
	3	0.1000	0.0211	0.2653	0.0116	0.3203
	4	0.1333	0.0376	0.3072	0.0233	0.3634
	5	0.1667	0.0564	0.3472	0.0378	0.4040
	6	0.2000	0.0771	0.3857	0.0545	0.4428
	7	0.2333	0.0993	0.4228	0.0729	0.4799
	8	0.2667	0.1228	0.4589	0.0929	0.5156
	9	0.3000	0.1473	0.4940	0.1142	0.5501
	10	0.3333	0.1729	0.5281	0.1367	0.5834
	11	0.3667	0.1993	0.5614	0.1604	0.6157
	12	0.4000	0.2266	0.5940	0.1850	0.6470
	13	0.4333	0.2546	0.6257	0.2107	0.6773
	14	0.4667	0.2834	0.6567	0.2373	0.7067
	15	0.5000	0.3130	0.6870	0.2648	0.7352
	16	0.5333	0.3433	0.7166	0.2933	0.7627
	17	0.5667	0.3743	0.7454	0.3227	0.7893
	18	0.6000	0.4060	0.7734	0.3530	0.8150
	19	0.6333	0.4386	0.8007	0.3843	0.8396
	20	0.6667	0.4719	0.8271	0.4166	0.8633
	21	0.7000	0.5060	0.8527	0.4499	0.8858
	22	0.7333	0.5411	0.8772	0.4844	0.9071
	23	0.7667	0.5772	0.9007	0.5201	0.9271
	24	0.8000	0.6143	0.9229	0.5572	0.9455
	25	0.8333	0.6528	0.9436	0.5960	0.9622
	26	0.8667	0.6928	0.9624	0.6366	0.9767
	27	0.9000	0.7347	0.9789	0.6797	0.9884
	28	0.9333	0.7793	0.9918	0.7260	0.9965
	29	0.9667	0.8278	0.9992	0.7772	0.9998
	30	1.0000	0.8843	1.0000	0.8381	1.0000
32	11	0.3438	0.1857	0.5319	0.1492	0.5854
	12	0.3750	0.2110	0.5631	0.1720	0.6156
	13	0.4063	0.2370	0.5936	0.1957	0.6450
	14	0.4375	0.2636	0.6234	0.2203	0.6735
	15	0.4688	0.2909	0.6526	0.2456	0.7013
	16	0.5000	0.3189	0.6811	0.2718	0.7282
	17	0.5313	0.3474	0.7091	0.2987	0.7544
	18	0.5625	0.3766	0.7364	0.3265	0.7797
	19	0.5938	0.4064	0.7630	0.3550	0.8043
	20	0.6250	0.4369	0.7890	0.3844	0.8280
	21	0.6563	0.4681	0.8143	0.4146	0.8508
	22	0.6875	0.4999	0.8388	0.4457	0.8727
	23	0.7188	0.5325	0.8625	0.4777	0.8936
	24	0.7500	0.5660	0.8854	0.5108	0.9134
	25	0.7813	0.6003	0.9072	0.5450	0.9320
	26	0.8125	0.6356	0.9279	0.5805	0.9491
	27	0.8438	0.6721	0.9472	0.6175	0.9647
	28	0.8750	0.7101	0.9649	0.6562	0.9782
	29	0.9063	0.7498	0.9802	0.6972	0.9892
	30	0.9375	0.7919	0.9923	0.7412	0.9967
	31	0.9688	0.8378	0.9992	0.7898	0.9998
	32	1.0000	0.8911	1.0000	0.8474	1.0000
33	0	0.0000	0.0000	0.1058	0.0000	0.1483
	1	0.0303	0.0008	0.1576	0.0002	0.2044
	2	0.0606	0.0074	0.2023	0.0032	0.2518
	3	0.0909	0.0192	0.2433	0.0105	0.2947
	4	0.1212	0.0340	0.2820	0.0211	0.3347
	5	0.1515	0.0511	0.3190	0.0342	0.3726
	6	0.1818	0.0698	0.3546	0.0492	0.4087
	7	0.2121	0.0898	0.3891	0.0658	0.4434
	8	0.2424	0.1109	0.4226	0.0838	0.4769
	9	0.2727	0.1330	0.4552	0.1029	0.5093
	10	0.3030	0.1559	0.4871	0.1231	0.5408
	11	0.3333	0.1796	0.5183	0.1442	0.5713
	12	0.3636	0.2040	0.5488	0.1662	0.6010

31

0	0.0000	0.0000	0.1122	0.0000	0.1571
1	0.0323	0.0008	0.1670	0.0002	0.2163
2	0.0645	0.0079	0.2142	0.0034	0.2662
3	0.0968	0.0204	0.2575	0.0112	0.3113
4	0.1290	0.0363	0.2983	0.0225	0.3533
5	0.1613	0.0545	0.3373	0.0365	0.3930
6	0.1935	0.0745	0.3747	0.0526	0.4308
7	0.2258	0.0959	0.4110	0.0704	0.4671
8	0.2581	0.1186	0.4461	0.0896	0.5021
9	0.2903	0.1422	0.4804	0.1102	0.5358
10	0.3226	0.1668	0.5137	0.1318	0.5685
11	0.3548	0.1923	0.5463	0.1546	0.6002
12	0.3871	0.2185	0.5781	0.1783	0.6309
13	0.4194	0.2455	0.6092	0.2029	0.6608
14	0.4516	0.2732	0.6397	0.2285	0.6898
15	0.4839	0.3015	0.6694	0.2549	0.7179
16	0.5161	0.3306	0.6985	0.2821	0.7451
17	0.5484	0.3603	0.7268	0.3102	0.7715
18	0.5806	0.3908	0.7545	0.3392	0.7971
19	0.6129	0.4219	0.7815	0.3691	0.8217
20	0.6452	0.4537	0.8077	0.3998	0.8454
21	0.6774	0.4863	0.8332	0.4315	0.8682
22	0.7097	0.5196	0.8578	0.4642	0.8898
23	0.7419	0.5539	0.8814	0.4979	0.9104
24	0.7742	0.5890	0.9041	0.5329	0.9296
25	0.8065	0.6253	0.9255	0.5692	0.9474
26	0.8387	0.6627	0.9455	0.6070	0.9635
27	0.8710	0.7017	0.9637	0.6467	0.9775
28	0.9032	0.7425	0.9796	0.6887	0.9888
29	0.9355	0.7858	0.9921	0.7338	0.9966
30	0.9677	0.8330	0.9992	0.7837	0.9998
31	1.0000	0.8878	1.0000	0.8429	1.0000

32

0	0.0000	0.0000	0.1089	0.0000	0.1526
1	0.0313	0.0008	0.1622	0.0002	0.2102
2	0.0625	0.0077	0.2081	0.0033	0.2588
3	0.0938	0.0198	0.2502	0.0108	0.3028
4	0.1250	0.0351	0.2899	0.0218	0.3438
5	0.1563	0.0528	0.3279	0.0353	0.3825
6	0.1875	0.0721	0.3644	0.0509	0.4195
7	0.2188	0.0928	0.3997	0.0680	0.4550
8	0.2500	0.1146	0.4340	0.0866	0.4892
9	0.2813	0.1375	0.4675	0.1064	0.5223
10	0.3125	0.1612	0.5001	0.1273	0.5543

33

13	0.3939	0.2291	0.5786	0.1890	0.6298
14	0.4242	0.2548	0.6078	0.2127	0.6579
15	0.4545	0.2811	0.6365	0.2371	0.6853
16	0.4848	0.3080	0.6646	0.2622	0.7119
17	0.5152	0.3354	0.6920	0.2881	0.7378
18	0.5455	0.3635	0.7189	0.3147	0.7629
19	0.5758	0.3922	0.7452	0.3421	0.7873
20	0.6061	0.4214	0.7709	0.3702	0.8110
21	0.6364	0.4512	0.7960	0.3990	0.8338
22	0.6667	0.4817	0.8204	0.4287	0.8558
23	0.6970	0.5129	0.8441	0.4592	0.8769
24	0.7273	0.5448	0.8670	0.4907	0.8971
25	0.7576	0.5774	0.8891	0.5231	0.9162
26	0.7879	0.6109	0.9102	0.5566	0.9342
27	0.8182	0.6454	0.9302	0.5913	0.9508
28	0.8485	0.6810	0.9489	0.6274	0.9658
29	0.8788	0.7180	0.9660	0.6653	0.9789
30	0.9091	0.7567	0.9808	0.7053	0.9895
31	0.9394	0.7977	0.9926	0.7482	0.9968
32	0.9697	0.8424	0.9992	0.7956	0.9998
33	1.0000	0.8942	1.0000	0.8517	1.0000

34

0	0.0000	0.0000	0.1028	0.0000	0.1443
1	0.0294	0.0007	0.1533	0.0001	0.1990
2	0.0588	0.0072	0.1968	0.0031	0.2452
3	0.0882	0.0186	0.2368	0.0102	0.2871
4	0.1176	0.0330	0.2745	0.0205	0.3262
5	0.1471	0.0495	0.3106	0.0332	0.3631
6	0.1765	0.0676	0.3453	0.0477	0.3985
7	0.2059	0.0870	0.3790	0.0638	0.4324
8	0.2353	0.1075	0.4117	0.0811	0.4652
9	0.2647	0.1288	0.4436	0.0996	0.4970
10	0.2941	0.1510	0.4748	0.1191	0.5278
11	0.3235	0.1739	0.5053	0.1395	0.5578
12	0.3529	0.1975	0.5351	0.1607	0.5869
13	0.3824	0.2217	0.5644	0.1828	0.6153
14	0.4118	0.2465	0.5930	0.2056	0.6430
15	0.4412	0.2719	0.6211	0.2291	0.6700
16	0.4706	0.2978	0.6487	0.2533	0.6962
17	0.5000	0.3243	0.6757	0.2782	0.7218
18	0.5294	0.3513	0.7022	0.3038	0.7467
19	0.5588	0.3789	0.7281	0.3300	0.7709
20	0.5882	0.4070	0.7535	0.3570	0.7944
21	0.6176	0.4356	0.7783	0.3847	0.8172

Continued

Table B.11. Exact confidence limits for a binomial proportion: x events are observed in a sample sized n. $p = x/n$ is the observed proportion. p_l and p_u are the lower and upper confidence limits for the population proportion

Confidence level

n	x	p	95% p_l	95% p_u	99% p_l	99% p_u
36	29	0.8056	0.6398	0.9181	0.5880	0.9400
	30	0.8333	0.6719	0.9363	0.6206	0.9551
	31	0.8611	0.7050	0.9533	0.6544	0.9688
	32	0.8889	0.7394	0.9689	0.6898	0.9807
	33	0.9167	0.7753	0.9825	0.7271	0.9904
	34	0.9444	0.8134	0.9932	0.7670	0.9971
	35	0.9722	0.8547	0.9993	0.8111	0.9999
	36	1.0000	0.9026	1.0000	0.8631	1.0000
37	0	0.0000	0.0000	0.0949	0.0000	0.1334
	1	0.0270	0.0007	0.1416	0.0001	0.1842
	2	0.0541	0.0066	0.1819	0.0028	0.2273
	3	0.0811	0.0170	0.2191	0.0093	0.2663
	4	0.1081	0.0303	0.2542	0.0188	0.3028
	5	0.1351	0.0454	0.2877	0.0304	0.3375
	6	0.1622	0.0619	0.3201	0.0436	0.3706
	7	0.1892	0.0796	0.3516	0.0583	0.4025
	8	0.2162	0.0983	0.3821	0.0741	0.4333
	9	0.2432	0.1177	0.4120	0.0909	0.4633
	10	0.2703	0.1379	0.4412	0.1086	0.4924
	11	0.2973	0.1587	0.4698	0.1271	0.5207
	12	0.3243	0.1801	0.4979	0.1464	0.5483
	13	0.3514	0.2021	0.5254	0.1663	0.5753
	14	0.3784	0.2246	0.5524	0.1869	0.6017
	15	0.4054	0.2475	0.5790	0.2081	0.6275
	16	0.4324	0.2710	0.6051	0.2299	0.6526
	17	0.4595	0.2949	0.6308	0.2522	0.6773
	18	0.4865	0.3192	0.6560	0.2752	0.7013
	19	0.5135	0.3440	0.6808	0.2987	0.7248
	20	0.5405	0.3692	0.7051	0.3227	0.7478
	21	0.5676	0.3949	0.7290	0.3474	0.7701
	22	0.5946	0.4210	0.7525	0.3725	0.7919
	23	0.6216	0.4476	0.7754	0.3983	0.8131
	24	0.6486	0.4746	0.7979	0.4247	0.8337
	25	0.6757	0.5021	0.8199	0.4517	0.8536
	26	0.7027	0.5302	0.8413	0.4793	0.8729

Confidence level

n	x	p	95% p_l	95% p_u	99% p_l	99% p_u
34	22	0.6471	0.4649	0.8025	0.4131	0.8393
	23	0.6765	0.4947	0.8261	0.4422	0.8605
	24	0.7059	0.5252	0.8490	0.4722	0.8809
	25	0.7353	0.5564	0.8712	0.5030	0.9004
	26	0.7647	0.5883	0.8925	0.5348	0.9189
	27	0.7941	0.6210	0.9130	0.5676	0.9362
	28	0.8235	0.6547	0.9324	0.6015	0.9523
	29	0.8529	0.6894	0.9505	0.6369	0.9668
	30	0.8824	0.7255	0.9670	0.6738	0.9795
	31	0.9118	0.7632	0.9814	0.7129	0.9898
	32	0.9412	0.8032	0.9928	0.7548	0.9969
	33	0.9706	0.8467	0.9993	0.8010	0.9999
	34	1.0000	0.8972	1.0000	0.8557	1.0000
35	0	0.0000	0.0000	0.1000	0.0000	0.1405
	1	0.0286	0.0007	0.1492	0.0001	0.1938
	2	0.0571	0.0070	0.1916	0.0030	0.2389
	3	0.0857	0.0180	0.2306	0.0099	0.2798
	4	0.1143	0.0320	0.2674	0.0199	0.3180
	5	0.1429	0.0481	0.3026	0.0322	0.3542
	6	0.1714	0.0656	0.3365	0.0463	0.3887
	7	0.2000	0.0844	0.3694	0.0618	0.4220
	8	0.2286	0.1042	0.4014	0.0786	0.4541
	9	0.2571	0.1249	0.4326	0.0965	0.4852
	10	0.2857	0.1464	0.4630	0.1154	0.5155
	11	0.3143	0.1685	0.4929	0.1351	0.5449
	12	0.3429	0.1913	0.5221	0.1556	0.5735
	13	0.3714	0.2147	0.5508	0.1769	0.6014
	14	0.4000	0.2387	0.5789	0.1989	0.6287
	15	0.4286	0.2632	0.6065	0.2216	0.6552
	16	0.4571	0.2883	0.6335	0.2450	0.6811
	17	0.4857	0.3138	0.6601	0.2690	0.7064
	18	0.5143	0.3399	0.6862	0.2936	0.7310
	19	0.5429	0.3665	0.7117	0.3189	0.7550
	20	0.5714	0.3935	0.7368	0.3448	0.7784
	21	0.6000	0.4211	0.7613	0.3713	0.8011

35

22	0.6286	0.4492	0.7853	0.3986	0.8231
23	0.6571	0.4779	0.8087	0.4265	0.8444
24	0.6857	0.5071	0.8315	0.4551	0.8649
25	0.7143	0.5370	0.8536	0.4845	0.8846
26	0.7429	0.5674	0.8751	0.5148	0.9035
27	0.7714	0.5986	0.8958	0.5459	0.9214
28	0.8000	0.6306	0.9156	0.5780	0.9382
29	0.8286	0.6635	0.9344	0.6113	0.9537
30	0.8571	0.6974	0.9519	0.6458	0.9678
31	0.8857	0.7326	0.9680	0.6820	0.9801
32	0.9143	0.7694	0.9820	0.7202	0.9901
33	0.9429	0.8084	0.9930	0.7611	0.9970
34	0.9714	0.8508	0.9993	0.8062	0.9999
35	1.0000	0.9000	1.0000	0.8595	1.0000

36

0	0.0000	0.0000	0.0974	0.0000	0.1369
1	0.0278	0.0007	0.1453	0.0001	0.1889
2	0.0556	0.0068	0.1866	0.0029	0.2330
3	0.0833	0.0175	0.2247	0.0096	0.2729
4	0.1111	0.0311	0.2606	0.0193	0.3102
5	0.1389	0.0467	0.2950	0.0312	0.3456
6	0.1667	0.0637	0.3281	0.0449	0.3794
7	0.1944	0.0819	0.3602	0.0600	0.4120
8	0.2222	0.1012	0.3915	0.0763	0.4435
9	0.2500	0.1212	0.4220	0.0936	0.4740
10	0.2778	0.1420	0.4519	0.1119	0.5037
11	0.3056	0.1635	0.4811	0.1310	0.5325
12	0.3333	0.1856	0.5097	0.1509	0.5607
13	0.3611	0.2082	0.5378	0.1714	0.5881
14	0.3889	0.2314	0.5654	0.1927	0.6149
15	0.4167	0.2551	0.5924	0.2146	0.6411
16	0.4444	0.2794	0.6190	0.2372	0.6666
17	0.4722	0.3041	0.6451	0.2603	0.6916
18	0.5000	0.3292	0.6708	0.2841	0.7159
19	0.5278	0.3549	0.6959	0.3084	0.7397
20	0.5556	0.3810	0.7206	0.3334	0.7628
21	0.5833	0.4076	0.7449	0.3589	0.7854
22	0.6111	0.4346	0.7686	0.3851	0.8073
23	0.6389	0.4622	0.7918	0.4119	0.8286
24	0.6667	0.4903	0.8144	0.4393	0.8491
25	0.6944	0.5189	0.8365	0.4675	0.8690
26	0.7222	0.5481	0.8580	0.4963	0.8881
27	0.7500	0.5780	0.8788	0.5260	0.9064
28	0.7778	0.6085	0.8988	0.5565	0.9237

37

27	0.7297	0.5588	0.8621	0.5076	0.8914
28	0.7568	0.5880	0.8823	0.5367	0.9091
29	0.7838	0.6179	0.9017	0.5667	0.9259
30	0.8108	0.6484	0.9204	0.5975	0.9417
31	0.8378	0.6799	0.9381	0.6294	0.9564
32	0.8649	0.7123	0.9546	0.6625	0.9696
33	0.8919	0.7458	0.9697	0.6972	0.9812
34	0.9189	0.7809	0.9830	0.7337	0.9907
35	0.9459	0.8181	0.9934	0.7727	0.9972
36	0.9730	0.8584	0.9993	0.8158	0.9999
37	1.0000	0.9051	1.0000	0.8666	1.0000

38

0	0.0000	0.0000	0.0925	0.0000	0.1301
1	0.0263	0.0007	0.1381	0.0001	0.1798
2	0.0526	0.0064	0.1775	0.0028	0.2219
3	0.0789	0.0166	0.2138	0.0091	0.2601
4	0.1053	0.0294	0.2480	0.0183	0.2958
5	0.1316	0.0441	0.2809	0.0295	0.3297
6	0.1579	0.0602	0.3125	0.0424	0.3621
7	0.1842	0.0774	0.3433	0.0567	0.3934
8	0.2105	0.0955	0.3732	0.0720	0.4236
9	0.2368	0.1144	0.4024	0.0883	0.4530
10	0.2632	0.1340	0.4310	0.1055	0.4815
11	0.2895	0.1542	0.4590	0.1235	0.5094
12	0.3158	0.1750	0.4865	0.1421	0.5365
13	0.3421	0.1963	0.5135	0.1614	0.5631
14	0.3684	0.2181	0.5401	0.1814	0.5890
15	0.3947	0.2404	0.5661	0.2019	0.6144
16	0.4211	0.2631	0.5918	0.2230	0.6392
17	0.4474	0.2862	0.6170	0.2447	0.6635
18	0.4737	0.3098	0.6418	0.2668	0.6872
19	0.5000	0.3338	0.6662	0.2895	0.7105
20	0.5263	0.3582	0.6902	0.3128	0.7332
21	0.5526	0.3830	0.7138	0.3365	0.7553
22	0.5789	0.4082	0.7369	0.3608	0.7770
23	0.6053	0.4339	0.7596	0.3856	0.7981
24	0.6316	0.4599	0.7819	0.4110	0.8186
25	0.6579	0.4865	0.8037	0.4369	0.8386
26	0.6842	0.5135	0.8250	0.4635	0.8579
27	0.7105	0.5410	0.8458	0.4906	0.8765
28	0.7368	0.5690	0.8660	0.5185	0.8945
29	0.7632	0.5976	0.8856	0.5470	0.9117
30	0.7895	0.6268	0.9045	0.5764	0.9280
31	0.8158	0.6567	0.9226	0.6066	0.9433

Continued

Table B.11. Exact confidence limits for a binomial proportion: x events are observed in a sample sized n. $p = x/n$ is the observed proportion. p_l and p_u are the lower and upper confidence limits for the population proportion

Confidence level			95%		99%	
n	x	p	p_l	p_u	p_l	p_u
38	32	0.8421	0.6875	0.9398	0.6379	0.9576
	33	0.8684	0.7191	0.9559	0.6703	0.9705
	34	0.8947	0.7520	0.9706	0.7042	0.9817
	35	0.9211	0.7862	0.9834	0.7399	0.9909
	36	0.9474	0.8225	0.9936	0.7781	0.9972
	37	0.9737	0.8619	0.9993	0.8202	0.9999
	38	1.0000	0.9075	1.0000	0.8699	1.0000
39	0	0.0000	0.0000	0.0903	0.0000	0.1270
	1	0.0256	0.0006	0.1348	0.0001	0.1756
	2	0.0513	0.0063	0.1732	0.0027	0.2167
	3	0.0769	0.0162	0.2087	0.0089	0.2541
	4	0.1026	0.0287	0.2422	0.0178	0.2891
	5	0.1282	0.0430	0.2743	0.0287	0.3222
	6	0.1538	0.0586	0.3053	0.0413	0.3540
	7	0.1795	0.0754	0.3353	0.0551	0.3847
	8	0.2051	0.0930	0.3646	0.0700	0.4143
	9	0.2308	0.1113	0.3933	0.0859	0.4431
	10	0.2564	0.1304	0.4213	0.1026	0.4712
	11	0.2821	0.1500	0.4487	0.1200	0.4985
	12	0.3077	0.1702	0.4757	0.1381	0.5252
	13	0.3333	0.1909	0.5022	0.1569	0.5513
	14	0.3590	0.2120	0.5282	0.1762	0.5768
	15	0.3846	0.2336	0.5538	0.1961	0.6018
	16	0.4103	0.2557	0.5790	0.2166	0.6262
	17	0.4359	0.2781	0.6038	0.2375	0.6502
	18	0.4615	0.3009	0.6282	0.2590	0.6736
	19	0.4872	0.3242	0.6522	0.2810	0.6966
	20	0.5128	0.3478	0.6758	0.3034	0.7190
	21	0.5385	0.3718	0.6991	0.3264	0.7410
	22	0.5641	0.3962	0.7219	0.3498	0.7625
	23	0.5897	0.4210	0.7443	0.3738	0.7834
	24	0.6154	0.4462	0.7664	0.3982	0.8039
	25	0.6410	0.4718	0.7880	0.4232	0.8238
	26	0.6667	0.4978	0.8091	0.4487	0.8431
	27	0.6923	0.5243	0.8298	0.4748	0.8619
	28	0.7179	0.5513	0.8500	0.5015	0.8800

Confidence level			95%		99%	
n	x	p	p_l	p_u	p_l	p_u
40	32	0.8000	0.6435	0.9095	0.5946	0.9318
	33	0.8250	0.6722	0.9266	0.6237	0.9463
	34	0.8500	0.7016	0.9429	0.6537	0.9598
	35	0.8750	0.7320	0.9581	0.6849	0.9720
	36	0.9000	0.7634	0.9721	0.7174	0.9827
	37	0.9250	0.7961	0.9843	0.7516	0.9914
	38	0.9500	0.8308	0.9939	0.7882	0.9974
	39	0.9750	0.8684	0.9994	0.8285	0.9999
	40	1.0000	0.9119	1.0000	0.8759	1.0000
41	0	0.0000	0.0000	0.0860	0.0000	0.1212
	1	0.0244	0.0006	0.1286	0.0001	0.1677
	2	0.0488	0.0060	0.1653	0.0026	0.2071
	3	0.0732	0.0154	0.1992	0.0084	0.2429
	4	0.0976	0.0272	0.2313	0.0169	0.2764
	5	0.1220	0.0408	0.2620	0.0273	0.3083
	6	0.1463	0.0557	0.2917	0.0392	0.3389
	7	0.1707	0.0715	0.3206	0.0523	0.3683
	8	0.1951	0.0882	0.3487	0.0664	0.3969
	9	0.2195	0.1056	0.3761	0.0814	0.4246
	10	0.2439	0.1236	0.4030	0.0972	0.4517
	11	0.2683	0.1422	0.4294	0.1137	0.4781
	12	0.2927	0.1613	0.4554	0.1308	0.5038
	13	0.3171	0.1808	0.4809	0.1485	0.5291
	14	0.3415	0.2008	0.5059	0.1667	0.5538
	15	0.3659	0.2212	0.5306	0.1855	0.5780
	16	0.3902	0.2420	0.5550	0.2047	0.6017
	17	0.4146	0.2632	0.5789	0.2244	0.6250
	18	0.4390	0.2847	0.6025	0.2446	0.6478
	19	0.4634	0.3066	0.6258	0.2652	0.6702
	20	0.4878	0.3288	0.6487	0.2863	0.6922
	21	0.5122	0.3513	0.6712	0.3078	0.7137
	22	0.5366	0.3742	0.6934	0.3298	0.7348
	23	0.5610	0.3975	0.7153	0.3522	0.7554
	24	0.5854	0.4211	0.7368	0.3750	0.7756
	25	0.6098	0.4450	0.7580	0.3983	0.7953
	26	0.6341	0.4694	0.7788	0.4220	0.8145

39				
29	0.7436	0.5787	0.8696	0.8974
30	0.7692	0.6067	0.8887	0.9141
31	0.7949	0.6354	0.9070	0.9300
32	0.8205	0.6647	0.9246	0.9449
33	0.8462	0.6947	0.9414	0.9587
34	0.8718	0.7257	0.9570	0.9713
35	0.8974	0.7578	0.9713	0.9822
36	0.9231	0.7913	0.9838	0.9911
37	0.9487	0.8268	0.9937	0.9973
38	0.9744	0.8652	0.9994	0.9999
39	1.0000	0.9097	1.0000	1.0000
40				
0	0.0000	0.0000	0.0881	0.1241
1	0.0250	0.0006	0.1316	0.1715
2	0.0500	0.0061	0.1692	0.2118
3	0.0750	0.0157	0.2039	0.2484
4	0.1000	0.0279	0.2366	0.2826
5	0.1250	0.0419	0.2680	0.3151
6	0.1500	0.0571	0.2984	0.3463
7	0.1750	0.0734	0.3278	0.3763
8	0.2000	0.0905	0.3565	0.4054
9	0.2250	0.1084	0.3845	0.4337
10	0.2500	0.1269	0.4120	0.4612
11	0.2750	0.1460	0.4389	0.4881
12	0.3000	0.1656	0.4653	0.5143
13	0.3250	0.1857	0.4913	0.5400
14	0.3500	0.2063	0.5168	0.5651
15	0.3750	0.2273	0.5420	0.5897
16	0.4000	0.2486	0.5667	0.6138
17	0.4250	0.2704	0.5911	0.6374
18	0.4500	0.2926	0.6151	0.6605
19	0.4750	0.3151	0.6387	0.6832
20	0.5000	0.3380	0.6620	0.7054
21	0.5250	0.3613	0.6849	0.7271
22	0.5500	0.3849	0.7074	0.7484
23	0.5750	0.4089	0.7296	0.7692
24	0.6000	0.4333	0.7514	0.7895
25	0.6250	0.4580	0.7727	0.8094
26	0.6500	0.4832	0.7937	0.8287
27	0.6750	0.5087	0.8143	0.8474
28	0.7000	0.5347	0.8344	0.8656
29	0.7250	0.5611	0.8540	0.8832
30	0.7500	0.5880	0.8731	0.9002
31	0.7750	0.6155	0.8916	0.9164

41					
27	0.6585	0.4941	0.7992	0.4462	0.8333
28	0.6829	0.5191	0.8192	0.4709	0.8515
29	0.7073	0.5446	0.8387	0.4962	0.8692
30	0.7317	0.5706	0.8578	0.5219	0.8863
31	0.7561	0.5970	0.8764	0.5483	0.9028
32	0.7805	0.6239	0.8944	0.5754	0.9186
33	0.8049	0.6513	0.9118	0.6031	0.9336
34	0.8293	0.6794	0.9285	0.6317	0.9477
35	0.8537	0.7083	0.9443	0.6611	0.9608
36	0.8780	0.7380	0.9592	0.6917	0.9727
37	0.9024	0.7687	0.9728	0.7236	0.9831
38	0.9268	0.8008	0.9846	0.7571	0.9916
39	0.9512	0.8347	0.9940	0.7929	0.9974
40	0.9756	0.8714	0.9994	0.8323	0.9999
41	1.0000	0.9140	1.0000	0.8788	1.0000
42					
0	0.0000	0.0000	0.0841	0.0000	0.1185
1	0.0238	0.0006	0.1257	0.0001	0.1640
2	0.0476	0.0058	0.1616	0.0025	0.2026
3	0.0714	0.0150	0.1948	0.0082	0.2377
4	0.0952	0.0266	0.2262	0.0165	0.2705
5	0.1190	0.0398	0.2563	0.0266	0.3018
6	0.1429	0.0543	0.2854	0.0382	0.3318
7	0.1667	0.0697	0.3136	0.0510	0.3607
8	0.1905	0.0860	0.3412	0.0647	0.3887
9	0.2143	0.1030	0.3681	0.0794	0.4159
10	0.2381	0.1205	0.3945	0.0947	0.4425
11	0.2619	0.1386	0.4204	0.1108	0.4684
12	0.2857	0.1572	0.4458	0.1274	0.4938
13	0.3095	0.1762	0.4709	0.1446	0.5186
14	0.3333	0.1957	0.4955	0.1623	0.5429
15	0.3571	0.2155	0.5197	0.1806	0.5668
16	0.3810	0.2357	0.5436	0.1993	0.5902
17	0.4048	0.2563	0.5672	0.2184	0.6131
18	0.4286	0.2772	0.5904	0.2380	0.6356
19	0.4524	0.2985	0.6133	0.2580	0.6577
20	0.4762	0.3200	0.6358	0.2785	0.6794
21	0.5000	0.3419	0.6581	0.2993	0.7007
22	0.5238	0.3642	0.6800	0.3206	0.7215
23	0.5476	0.3867	0.7015	0.3423	0.7420
24	0.5714	0.4096	0.7228	0.3644	0.7620
25	0.5952	0.4328	0.7437	0.3869	0.7816
26	0.6190	0.4564	0.7643	0.4098	0.8007
27	0.6429	0.4803	0.7845	0.4332	0.8194

Continued

Table B.11. Exact confidence limits for a binomial proportion: x events are observed in a sample sized n. $p = x/n$ is the observed proportion. p_l and p_u are the lower and upper confidence limits for the population proportion

| | | | Confidence level | | | |
| | | | 95% | | 99% | |
n	x	p	p_l	p_u	p_l	p_u
42	28	0.6667	0.5045	0.8043	0.4571	0.8377
	29	0.6905	0.5291	0.8238	0.4814	0.8554
	30	0.7143	0.5542	0.8428	0.5062	0.8726
	31	0.7381	0.5796	0.8614	0.5316	0.8892
	32	0.7619	0.6055	0.8795	0.5575	0.9053
	33	0.7857	0.6319	0.8970	0.5841	0.9206
	34	0.8095	0.6588	0.9140	0.6113	0.9353
	35	0.8333	0.6864	0.9303	0.6393	0.9490
	36	0.8571	0.7146	0.9457	0.6682	0.9618
	37	0.8810	0.7437	0.9602	0.6982	0.9734
	38	0.9048	0.7738	0.9734	0.7295	0.9835
	39	0.9286	0.8052	0.9850	0.7623	0.9918
	40	0.9524	0.8384	0.9942	0.7974	0.9975
	41	0.9762	0.8743	0.9994	0.8360	0.9999
	42	1.0000	0.9159	1.0000	0.8815	1.0000
43	**0**	0.0000	0.0000	0.0822	0.0000	0.1159
	1	0.0233	0.0006	0.1229	0.0001	0.1604
	2	0.0465	0.0057	0.1581	0.0024	0.1982
	3	0.0698	0.0146	0.1906	0.0080	0.2327
	4	0.0930	0.0259	0.2214	0.0161	0.2649
	5	0.1163	0.0389	0.2508	0.0260	0.2955
	6	0.1395	0.0530	0.2793	0.0373	0.3249
	7	0.1628	0.0681	0.3070	0.0497	0.3533
	8	0.1860	0.0839	0.3340	0.0632	0.3808
	9	0.2093	0.1004	0.3604	0.0774	0.4076
	10	0.2326	0.1176	0.3863	0.0924	0.4337
	11	0.2558	0.1352	0.4117	0.1080	0.4592
	12	0.2791	0.1533	0.4367	0.1242	0.4841
	13	0.3023	0.1718	0.4613	0.1409	0.5085
	14	0.3256	0.1908	0.4854	0.1582	0.5325
	15	0.3488	0.2101	0.5093	0.1759	0.5559
	16	0.3721	0.2298	0.5327	0.1941	0.5790
	17	0.3953	0.2498	0.5559	0.2127	0.6016
	18	0.4186	0.2701	0.5787	0.2318	0.6238
	19	0.4419	0.2908	0.6012	0.2512	0.6456
	20	0.4651	0.3118	0.6235	0.2711	0.6670

| | | | Confidence level | | | |
| | | | 95% | | 99% | |
n	x	p	p_l	p_u	p_l	p_u
44	**20**	0.4545	0.3039	0.6115	0.2641	0.6551
	21	0.4773	0.3246	0.6331	0.2837	0.6758
	22	0.5000	0.3456	0.6544	0.3038	0.6962
	23	0.5227	0.3669	0.6754	0.3242	0.7163
	24	0.5455	0.3885	0.6961	0.3449	0.7359
	25	0.5682	0.4103	0.7165	0.3661	0.7552
	26	0.5909	0.4325	0.7366	0.3876	0.7741
	27	0.6136	0.4550	0.7564	0.4095	0.7927
	28	0.6364	0.4777	0.7759	0.4318	0.8108
	29	0.6591	0.5008	0.7951	0.4545	0.8285
	30	0.6818	0.5242	0.8139	0.4776	0.8457
	31	0.7045	0.5480	0.8324	0.5012	0.8626
	32	0.7273	0.5721	0.8504	0.5252	0.8789
	33	0.7500	0.5966	0.8681	0.5497	0.8947
	34	0.7727	0.6216	0.8853	0.5748	0.9099
	35	0.7955	0.6470	0.9020	0.6004	0.9245
	36	0.8182	0.6729	0.9181	0.6267	0.9384
	37	0.8409	0.6993	0.9336	0.6537	0.9515
	38	0.8636	0.7265	0.9483	0.6816	0.9636
	39	0.8864	0.7544	0.9621	0.7105	0.9746
	40	0.9091	0.7833	0.9747	0.7405	0.9843
	41	0.9318	0.8134	0.9857	0.7721	0.9922
	42	0.9545	0.8453	0.9944	0.8059	0.9976
	43	0.9773	0.8798	0.9994	0.8430	0.9999
	44	1.0000	0.9196	1.0000	0.8866	1.0000
45	**0**	0.0000	0.0000	0.0787	0.0000	0.1111
	1	0.0222	0.0006	0.1177	0.0001	0.1538
	2	0.0444	0.0054	0.1515	0.0023	0.1901
	3	0.0667	0.0140	0.1827	0.0077	0.2232
	4	0.0889	0.0248	0.2122	0.0153	0.2543
	5	0.1111	0.0371	0.2405	0.0248	0.2838
	6	0.1333	0.0505	0.2679	0.0356	0.3121
	7	0.1556	0.0649	0.2946	0.0474	0.3395
	8	0.1778	0.0800	0.3205	0.0602	0.3660
	9	0.2000	0.0958	0.3460	0.0737	0.3918
	10	0.2222	0.1120	0.3709	0.0880	0.4171

45	11	0.4417	0.1028	0.3954	0.1288	0.2444
	12	0.4658	0.1182	0.4194	0.1460	0.2667
	13	0.4895	0.1341	0.4431	0.1637	0.2889
	14	0.5127	0.1505	0.4665	0.1817	0.3111
	15	0.5354	0.1673	0.4895	0.2000	0.3333
	16	0.5578	0.1846	0.5122	0.2187	0.3556
	17	0.5798	0.2022	0.5346	0.2377	0.3778
	18	0.6014	0.2202	0.5567	0.2570	0.4000
	19	0.6226	0.2386	0.5785	0.2766	0.4222
	20	0.6435	0.2574	0.6000	0.2964	0.4444
	21	0.6640	0.2765	0.6213	0.3166	0.4667
	22	0.6842	0.2960	0.6423	0.3370	0.4889
	23	0.7040	0.3158	0.6630	0.3577	0.5111
	24	0.7235	0.3360	0.6834	0.3787	0.5333
	25	0.7426	0.3565	0.7036	0.4000	0.5556
	26	0.7614	0.3774	0.7234	0.4215	0.5778
	27	0.7798	0.3986	0.7430	0.4433	0.6000
	28	0.7978	0.4202	0.7623	0.4654	0.6222
	29	0.8154	0.4422	0.7813	0.4878	0.6444
	30	0.8327	0.4646	0.8000	0.5105	0.6667
	31	0.8495	0.4873	0.8183	0.5335	0.6889
	32	0.8659	0.5105	0.8363	0.5569	0.7111
	33	0.8818	0.5342	0.8540	0.5806	0.7333
	34	0.8972	0.5583	0.8712	0.6046	0.7556
	35	0.9120	0.5829	0.8880	0.6291	0.7778
	36	0.9263	0.6082	0.9042	0.6540	0.8000
	37	0.9398	0.6340	0.9200	0.6795	0.8222
	38	0.9526	0.6605	0.9351	0.7054	0.8444
	39	0.9644	0.6879	0.9495	0.7321	0.8667
	40	0.9752	0.7162	0.9629	0.7595	0.8889
	41	0.9847	0.7457	0.9752	0.7878	0.9111
	42	0.9923	0.7768	0.9860	0.8173	0.9333
	43	0.9977	0.8099	0.9946	0.8485	0.9556
	44	0.9999	0.8462	0.9994	0.8823	0.9778
	45	1.0000	0.8889	1.0000	0.9213	1.0000
46	0	0.1088	0.0000	0.0771	0.0000	0.0000
	1	0.1507	0.0001	0.1153	0.0006	0.0217
	2	0.1863	0.0023	0.1484	0.0053	0.0435
	3	0.2188	0.0075	0.1790	0.0137	0.0652
	4	0.2493	0.0150	0.2079	0.0242	0.0870
	5	0.2782	0.0242	0.2357	0.0362	0.1087
	6	0.3060	0.0347	0.2626	0.0494	0.1304
	7	0.3329	0.0463	0.2887	0.0634	0.1522

43	21	0.6880	0.2913	0.6454	0.3331	0.4884
	22	0.7087	0.3120	0.6669	0.3546	0.5116
	23	0.7289	0.3330	0.6882	0.3765	0.5349
	24	0.7488	0.3544	0.7092	0.3988	0.5581
	25	0.7682	0.3762	0.7299	0.4213	0.5814
	26	0.7873	0.3984	0.7502	0.4441	0.6047
	27	0.8059	0.4210	0.7702	0.4673	0.6279
	28	0.8241	0.4441	0.7899	0.4907	0.6512
	29	0.8418	0.4675	0.8092	0.5146	0.6744
	30	0.8591	0.4915	0.8282	0.5387	0.6977
	31	0.8758	0.5159	0.8467	0.5633	0.7209
	32	0.8920	0.5408	0.8648	0.5883	0.7442
	33	0.9076	0.5663	0.8824	0.6137	0.7674
	34	0.9226	0.5924	0.8996	0.6396	0.7907
	35	0.9368	0.6192	0.9161	0.6660	0.8140
	36	0.9503	0.6467	0.9319	0.6930	0.8372
	37	0.9627	0.6751	0.9470	0.7207	0.8605
	38	0.9740	0.7045	0.9611	0.7492	0.8837
	39	0.9839	0.7351	0.9741	0.7786	0.9070
	40	0.9920	0.7673	0.9854	0.8094	0.9302
	41	0.9976	0.8018	0.9943	0.8419	0.9535
	42	0.9999	0.8396	0.9994	0.8771	0.9767
	43	1.0000	0.8841	1.0000	0.9178	1.0000
44	0	0.1134	0.0000	0.0804	0.0000	0.0000
	1	0.1570	0.0001	0.1202	0.0006	0.0227
	2	0.1941	0.0024	0.1547	0.0056	0.0455
	3	0.2279	0.0078	0.1866	0.0143	0.0682
	4	0.2595	0.0157	0.2167	0.0253	0.0909
	5	0.2895	0.0254	0.2456	0.0379	0.1136
	6	0.3184	0.0364	0.2735	0.0517	0.1364
	7	0.3463	0.0485	0.3007	0.0664	0.1591
	8	0.3733	0.0616	0.3271	0.0819	0.1818
	9	0.3996	0.0755	0.3530	0.0980	0.2045
	10	0.4252	0.0901	0.3784	0.1147	0.2273
	11	0.4503	0.1053	0.4034	0.1319	0.2500
	12	0.4748	0.1211	0.4279	0.1496	0.2727
	13	0.4988	0.1374	0.4520	0.1676	0.2955
	14	0.5224	0.1543	0.4758	0.1861	0.3182
	15	0.5455	0.1715	0.4992	0.2049	0.3409
	16	0.5682	0.1892	0.5223	0.2241	0.3636
	17	0.5905	0.2073	0.5450	0.2436	0.3864
	18	0.6124	0.2259	0.5675	0.2634	0.4091
	19	0.6339	0.2448	0.5897	0.2835	0.4318

Continued

Table B.11. Exact confidence limits for a binomial proportion: x events are observed in a sample sized n. $p = x/n$ is the observed proportion. p_l and p_u are the lower and upper confidence limits for the population proportion

Confidence level

n	x	p	95% p_l	95% p_u	99% p_l	99% p_u
46	8	0.1739	0.0782	0.3142	0.0588	0.3590
	9	0.1957	0.0936	0.3391	0.0720	0.3844
	10	0.2174	0.1095	0.3636	0.0859	0.4092
	11	0.2391	0.1259	0.3877	0.1004	0.4334
	12	0.2609	0.1427	0.4113	0.1154	0.4572
	13	0.2826	0.1599	0.4346	0.1310	0.4804
	14	0.3043	0.1774	0.4575	0.1469	0.5033
	15	0.3261	0.1953	0.4802	0.1633	0.5257
	16	0.3478	0.2135	0.5025	0.1801	0.5477
	17	0.3696	0.2321	0.5245	0.1973	0.5694
	18	0.3913	0.2509	0.5463	0.2149	0.5907
	19	0.4130	0.2700	0.5677	0.2328	0.6116
	20	0.4348	0.2893	0.5889	0.2511	0.6323
	21	0.4565	0.3090	0.6099	0.2697	0.6525
	22	0.4783	0.3289	0.6305	0.2886	0.6725
	23	0.5000	0.3490	0.6510	0.3079	0.6921
	24	0.5217	0.3695	0.6711	0.3275	0.7114
	25	0.5435	0.3901	0.6910	0.3475	0.7303
	26	0.5652	0.4111	0.7107	0.3677	0.7489
	27	0.5870	0.4323	0.7300	0.3884	0.7672
	28	0.6087	0.4537	0.7491	0.4093	0.7851
	29	0.6304	0.4755	0.7679	0.4306	0.8027
	30	0.6522	0.4975	0.7865	0.4523	0.8199
	31	0.6739	0.5198	0.8047	0.4743	0.8367
	32	0.6957	0.5425	0.8226	0.4967	0.8531
	33	0.7174	0.5654	0.8401	0.5196	0.8690
	34	0.7391	0.5887	0.8573	0.5428	0.8846
	35	0.7609	0.6123	0.8741	0.5666	0.8996
	36	0.7826	0.6364	0.8905	0.5908	0.9141
	37	0.8043	0.6609	0.9064	0.6156	0.9280
	38	0.8261	0.6858	0.9218	0.6410	0.9412
	39	0.8478	0.7113	0.9366	0.6671	0.9537
	40	0.8696	0.7374	0.9506	0.6940	0.9653
	41	0.8913	0.7643	0.9638	0.7218	0.9758
	42	0.9130	0.7921	0.9758	0.7507	0.9850
	43	0.9348	0.8210	0.9863	0.7812	0.9925
	44	0.9565	0.8516	0.9947	0.8137	0.9977

Confidence level

n	x	p	95% p_l	95% p_u	99% p_l	99% p_u
47	42	0.8936	0.7690	0.9645	0.7271	0.9763
	43	0.9149	0.7962	0.9763	0.7556	0.9853
	44	0.9362	0.8246	0.9866	0.7855	0.9927
	45	0.9574	0.8546	0.9948	0.8173	0.9978
	46	0.9787	0.8871	0.9995	0.8523	0.9999
	47	1.0000	0.9245	1.0000	0.8934	1.0000
48	0	0.0000	0.0000	0.0740	0.0000	0.1045
	1	0.0208	0.0005	0.1107	0.0001	0.1448
	2	0.0417	0.0051	0.1425	0.0022	0.1791
	3	0.0625	0.0131	0.1720	0.0072	0.2105
	4	0.0833	0.0232	0.1998	0.0144	0.2398
	5	0.1042	0.0347	0.2266	0.0232	0.2678
	6	0.1250	0.0473	0.2525	0.0332	0.2946
	7	0.1458	0.0607	0.2776	0.0443	0.3206
	8	0.1667	0.0748	0.3022	0.0562	0.3458
	9	0.1875	0.0895	0.3263	0.0689	0.3703
	10	0.2083	0.1047	0.3499	0.0821	0.3943
	11	0.2292	0.1203	0.3731	0.0959	0.4178
	12	0.2500	0.1364	0.3960	0.1103	0.4408
	13	0.2708	0.1528	0.4185	0.1251	0.4633
	14	0.2917	0.1695	0.4406	0.1403	0.4855
	15	0.3125	0.1866	0.4625	0.1559	0.5072
	16	0.3333	0.2040	0.4841	0.1719	0.5286
	17	0.3542	0.2216	0.5054	0.1883	0.5497
	18	0.3750	0.2395	0.5265	0.2050	0.5704
	19	0.3958	0.2577	0.5473	0.2220	0.5908
	20	0.4167	0.2761	0.5679	0.2393	0.6109
	21	0.4375	0.2948	0.5882	0.2570	0.6307
	22	0.4583	0.3137	0.6083	0.2750	0.6501
	23	0.4792	0.3329	0.6281	0.2933	0.6693
	24	0.5000	0.3523	0.6477	0.3118	0.6882
	25	0.5208	0.3719	0.6671	0.3307	0.7067
	26	0.5417	0.3917	0.6863	0.3499	0.7250
	27	0.5625	0.4118	0.7052	0.3693	0.7430
	28	0.5833	0.4321	0.7239	0.3891	0.7607
	29	0.6042	0.4527	0.7423	0.4092	0.7780
	30	0.6250	0.4735	0.7605	0.4296	0.7950

n	x					
48	31	0.6458	0.4946	0.7784	0.4503	0.8117
	32	0.6667	0.5159	0.7960	0.4714	0.8281
	33	0.6875	0.5375	0.8134	0.4928	0.8441
	34	0.7083	0.5594	0.8305	0.5145	0.8597
	35	0.7292	0.5815	0.8472	0.5367	0.8749
	36	0.7500	0.6040	0.8636	0.5592	0.8897
	37	0.7708	0.6269	0.8797	0.5822	0.9041
	38	0.7917	0.6501	0.8953	0.6057	0.9179
	39	0.8125	0.6737	0.9105	0.6297	0.9311
	40	0.8333	0.6978	0.9252	0.6542	0.9438
	41	0.8542	0.7224	0.9393	0.6794	0.9557
	42	0.8750	0.7475	0.9527	0.7054	0.9668
	43	0.8958	0.7734	0.9653	0.7322	0.9768
	44	0.9167	0.8002	0.9768	0.7602	0.9856
	45	0.9375	0.8280	0.9869	0.7895	0.9928
	46	0.9583	0.8575	0.9949	0.8209	0.9978
	47	0.9792	0.8893	0.9995	0.8552	0.9999
	48	1.0000	0.9260	1.0000	0.8955	1.0000
49	0	0.0000	0.0000	0.0725	0.0000	0.1025
	1	0.0204	0.0005	0.1085	0.0001	0.1421
	2	0.0408	0.0050	0.1398	0.0021	0.1758
	3	0.0612	0.0128	0.1687	0.0070	0.2065
	4	0.0816	0.0227	0.1960	0.0141	0.2353
	5	0.1020	0.0340	0.2223	0.0227	0.2628
	6	0.1224	0.0463	0.2477	0.0325	0.2892
	7	0.1429	0.0594	0.2724	0.0434	0.3147
	8	0.1633	0.0732	0.2966	0.0550	0.3395
	9	0.1837	0.0876	0.3202	0.0674	0.3637
	10	0.2041	0.1024	0.3434	0.0803	0.3873
	11	0.2245	0.1177	0.3662	0.0939	0.4104
	12	0.2449	0.1334	0.3887	0.1079	0.4330
	13	0.2653	0.1495	0.4108	0.1223	0.4552
	14	0.2857	0.1658	0.4326	0.1372	0.4770
	15	0.3061	0.1825	0.4542	0.1524	0.4985
	16	0.3265	0.1995	0.4754	0.1681	0.5196
	17	0.3469	0.2167	0.4964	0.1840	0.5403
	18	0.3673	0.2342	0.5171	0.2003	0.5607
	19	0.3878	0.2520	0.5376	0.2169	0.5809
	20	0.4082	0.2700	0.5579	0.2339	0.6007
	21	0.4286	0.2882	0.5779	0.2511	0.6202
	22	0.4490	0.3067	0.5977	0.2686	0.6395
	23	0.4694	0.3253	0.6173	0.2864	0.6584
	24	0.4898	0.3442	0.6366	0.3045	0.6771
	25	0.5102	0.3634	0.6558	0.3229	0.6955

n	x					
46	45	0.9783	0.8847	0.9994	0.8493	0.9999
	46	1.0000	0.9229	1.0000	0.8912	1.0000
47	0	0.0000	0.0000	0.0755	0.0000	0.1066
	1	0.0213	0.0005	0.1129	0.0001	0.1477
	2	0.0426	0.0052	0.1454	0.0022	0.1827
	3	0.0638	0.0134	0.1754	0.0073	0.2145
	4	0.0851	0.0237	0.2038	0.0147	0.2444
	5	0.1064	0.0355	0.2310	0.0237	0.2729
	6	0.1277	0.0483	0.2574	0.0340	0.3002
	7	0.1489	0.0620	0.2831	0.0453	0.3266
	8	0.1702	0.0765	0.3081	0.0575	0.3523
	9	0.1915	0.0915	0.3326	0.0704	0.3773
	10	0.2128	0.1070	0.3566	0.0840	0.4016
	11	0.2340	0.1230	0.3803	0.0981	0.4255
	12	0.2553	0.1394	0.4035	0.1128	0.4488
	13	0.2766	0.1562	0.4264	0.1279	0.4717
	14	0.2979	0.1734	0.4489	0.1435	0.4942
	15	0.3191	0.1909	0.4712	0.1595	0.5163
	16	0.3404	0.2086	0.4931	0.1759	0.5380
	17	0.3617	0.2267	0.5148	0.1927	0.5594
	18	0.3830	0.2451	0.5362	0.2098	0.5804
	19	0.4043	0.2637	0.5573	0.2273	0.6011
	20	0.4255	0.2826	0.5782	0.2451	0.6214
	21	0.4468	0.3017	0.5988	0.2632	0.6414
	22	0.4681	0.3211	0.6192	0.2816	0.6611
	23	0.4894	0.3408	0.6394	0.3004	0.6805
	24	0.5106	0.3606	0.6592	0.3195	0.6996
	25	0.5319	0.3808	0.6789	0.3389	0.7184
	26	0.5532	0.4012	0.6983	0.3586	0.7368
	27	0.5745	0.4218	0.7174	0.3786	0.7549
	28	0.5957	0.4427	0.7363	0.3989	0.7727
	29	0.6170	0.4638	0.7549	0.4196	0.7902
	30	0.6383	0.4852	0.7733	0.4406	0.8073
	31	0.6596	0.5069	0.7914	0.4620	0.8241
	32	0.6809	0.5288	0.8091	0.4837	0.8405
	33	0.7021	0.5511	0.8266	0.5058	0.8565
	34	0.7234	0.5736	0.8438	0.5283	0.8721
	35	0.7447	0.5965	0.8606	0.5512	0.8872
	36	0.7660	0.6197	0.8770	0.5745	0.9019
	37	0.7872	0.6434	0.8930	0.5984	0.9160
	38	0.8085	0.6674	0.9085	0.6227	0.9296
	39	0.8298	0.6919	0.9235	0.6477	0.9425
	40	0.8511	0.7169	0.9380	0.6734	0.9547
	41	0.8723	0.7426	0.9517	0.6998	0.9660

Continued

Table B.11. Exact confidence limits for a binomial proportion: x events are observed in a sample sized n. $p = x/n$ is the observed proportion. p_l and p_u are the lower and upper confidence limits for the population proportion

Confidence level

n	x	p	95% p_l	95% p_u	99% p_l	99% p_u
49	26	0.5306	0.3827	0.6747	0.3416	0.7136
	27	0.5510	0.4023	0.6933	0.3605	0.7314
	28	0.5714	0.4221	0.7118	0.3798	0.7489
	29	0.5918	0.4421	0.7300	0.3993	0.7661
	30	0.6122	0.4624	0.7480	0.4191	0.7831
	31	0.6327	0.4829	0.7658	0.4393	0.7997
	32	0.6531	0.5036	0.7833	0.4597	0.8160
	33	0.6735	0.5246	0.8005	0.4804	0.8319
	34	0.6939	0.5458	0.8175	0.5015	0.8476
	35	0.7143	0.5674	0.8342	0.5230	0.8628
	36	0.7347	0.5892	0.8505	0.5448	0.8777
	37	0.7551	0.6113	0.8666	0.5670	0.8921
	38	0.7755	0.6338	0.8823	0.5896	0.9061
	39	0.7959	0.6566	0.8976	0.6127	0.9197
	40	0.8163	0.6798	0.9124	0.6363	0.9326
	41	0.8367	0.7034	0.9268	0.6605	0.9450
	42	0.8571	0.7276	0.9406	0.6853	0.9566
	43	0.8776	0.7523	0.9537	0.7108	0.9675
	44	0.8980	0.7777	0.9660	0.7372	0.9773
	45	0.9184	0.8040	0.9773	0.7647	0.9859
	46	0.9388	0.8313	0.9872	0.7935	0.9930
	47	0.9592	0.8602	0.9950	0.8242	0.9979
	48	0.9796	0.8915	0.9995	0.8579	0.9999
	49	1.0000	0.9275	1.0000	0.8975	1.0000
50	0	0.0000	0.0000	0.0711	0.0000	0.1005
	1	0.0200	0.0005	0.1065	0.0001	0.1394
	2	0.0400	0.0049	0.1371	0.0021	0.1725
	3	0.0600	0.0125	0.1655	0.0069	0.2027
	4	0.0800	0.0222	0.1923	0.0138	0.2311
	5	0.1000	0.0333	0.2181	0.0222	0.2580
	6	0.1200	0.0453	0.2431	0.0319	0.2840
	7	0.1400	0.0582	0.2674	0.0425	0.3091
	8	0.1600	0.0717	0.2911	0.0539	0.3335
	9	0.1800	0.0858	0.3144	0.0660	0.3573
	10	0.2000	0.1003	0.3372	0.0786	0.3805
	11	0.2200	0.1153	0.3596	0.0919	0.4032
	12	0.2400	0.1306	0.3817	0.1056	0.4255

Confidence level

n	x	p	95% p_l	95% p_u	99% p_l	99% p_u
51	6	0.1176	0.0444	0.2387	0.0312	0.2790
	7	0.1373	0.0570	0.2626	0.0416	0.3037
	8	0.1569	0.0702	0.2859	0.0528	0.3277
	9	0.1765	0.0840	0.3087	0.0646	0.3511
	10	0.1961	0.0982	0.3312	0.0770	0.3739
	11	0.2157	0.1129	0.3532	0.0899	0.3963
	12	0.2353	0.1279	0.3749	0.1033	0.4182
	13	0.2549	0.1433	0.3963	0.1172	0.4398
	14	0.2745	0.1589	0.4174	0.1314	0.4610
	15	0.2941	0.1749	0.4383	0.1459	0.4818
	16	0.3137	0.1911	0.4589	0.1609	0.5023
	17	0.3333	0.2076	0.4792	0.1761	0.5225
	18	0.3529	0.2243	0.4993	0.1917	0.5423
	19	0.3725	0.2413	0.5192	0.2075	0.5619
	20	0.3922	0.2584	0.5389	0.2237	0.5813
	21	0.4118	0.2758	0.5583	0.2401	0.6003
	22	0.4314	0.2935	0.5775	0.2568	0.6191
	23	0.4510	0.3113	0.5966	0.2737	0.6376
	24	0.4706	0.3293	0.6154	0.2910	0.6558
	25	0.4902	0.3475	0.6340	0.3084	0.6738
	26	0.5098	0.3660	0.6525	0.3262	0.6916
	27	0.5294	0.3846	0.6707	0.3442	0.7090
	28	0.5490	0.4034	0.6887	0.3624	0.7263
	29	0.5686	0.4225	0.7065	0.3809	0.7432
	30	0.5882	0.4417	0.7242	0.3997	0.7599
	31	0.6078	0.4611	0.7416	0.4187	0.7763
	32	0.6275	0.4808	0.7587	0.4381	0.7925
	33	0.6471	0.5007	0.7757	0.4577	0.8083
	34	0.6667	0.5208	0.7924	0.4775	0.8239
	35	0.6863	0.5411	0.8089	0.4977	0.8391
	36	0.7059	0.5617	0.8251	0.5182	0.8541
	37	0.7255	0.5826	0.8411	0.5390	0.8686
	38	0.7451	0.6037	0.8567	0.5602	0.8828
	39	0.7647	0.6251	0.8721	0.5818	0.8967
	40	0.7843	0.6468	0.8871	0.6037	0.9101
	41	0.8039	0.6688	0.9018	0.6261	0.9230
	42	0.8235	0.6913	0.9160	0.6489	0.9354
	43	0.8431	0.7141	0.9298	0.6723	0.9472

n	i					
50	13	0.2600	0.1463	0.4034	0.1197	0.4474
	14	0.2800	0.1623	0.4249	0.1342	0.4689
	15	0.3000	0.1786	0.4461	0.1491	0.4900
	16	0.3200	0.1952	0.4670	0.1644	0.5108
	17	0.3400	0.2121	0.4877	0.1800	0.5312
	18	0.3600	0.2292	0.5081	0.1959	0.5514
	19	0.3800	0.2465	0.5283	0.2121	0.5713
	20	0.4000	0.2641	0.5482	0.2287	0.5908
	21	0.4200	0.2819	0.5679	0.2455	0.6101
	22	0.4400	0.2999	0.5875	0.2626	0.6291
	23	0.4600	0.3181	0.6068	0.2799	0.6478
	24	0.4800	0.3366	0.6258	0.2976	0.6663
	25	0.5000	0.3553	0.6447	0.3155	0.6845
	26	0.5200	0.3742	0.6634	0.3337	0.7024
	27	0.5400	0.3932	0.6819	0.3522	0.7201
	28	0.5600	0.4125	0.7001	0.3709	0.7374
	29	0.5800	0.4321	0.7181	0.3899	0.7545
	30	0.6000	0.4518	0.7359	0.4092	0.7713
	31	0.6200	0.4717	0.7535	0.4287	0.7879
	32	0.6400	0.4919	0.7708	0.4486	0.8041
	33	0.6600	0.5123	0.7879	0.4688	0.8200
	34	0.6800	0.5330	0.8048	0.4892	0.8356
	35	0.7000	0.5539	0.8214	0.5100	0.8509
	36	0.7200	0.5751	0.8377	0.5311	0.8658
	37	0.7400	0.5966	0.8537	0.5526	0.8803
	38	0.7600	0.6183	0.8694	0.5745	0.8944
	39	0.7800	0.6404	0.8847	0.5968	0.9081
	40	0.8000	0.6628	0.8997	0.6195	0.9214
	41	0.8200	0.6856	0.9142	0.6427	0.9340
	42	0.8400	0.7089	0.9283	0.6665	0.9461
	43	0.8600	0.7326	0.9418	0.6909	0.9575
	44	0.8800	0.7569	0.9547	0.7160	0.9681
	45	0.9000	0.7819	0.9667	0.7420	0.9778
	46	0.9200	0.8077	0.9778	0.7689	0.9862
	47	0.9400	0.8345	0.9875	0.7973	0.9931
	48	0.9600	0.8629	0.9951	0.8275	0.9979
	49	0.9800	0.8935	0.9995	0.8606	0.9999
	50	1.0000	0.9289	1.0000	0.8995	1.0000
51	0	0.0000	0.0000	0.0698	0.0000	0.0987
	1	0.0196	0.0005	0.1045	0.0001	0.1368
	2	0.0392	0.0048	0.1346	0.0020	0.1694
	3	0.0588	0.0123	0.1624	0.0067	0.1990
	4	0.0784	0.0218	0.1888	0.0135	0.2269
	5	0.0980	0.0326	0.2141	0.0218	0.2535

n	i					
51	44	0.8627	0.7374	0.9430	0.6963	0.9584
	45	0.8824	0.7613	0.9556	0.7210	0.9688
	46	0.9020	0.7859	0.9674	0.7465	0.9782
	47	0.9216	0.8112	0.9782	0.7731	0.9865
	48	0.9412	0.8376	0.9877	0.8010	0.9933
	49	0.9608	0.8654	0.9952	0.8306	0.9980
	50	0.9804	0.8955	0.9995	0.8632	0.9999
	51	1.0000	0.9302	1.0000	0.9013	1.0000
52	0	0.0000	0.0000	0.0685	0.0001	0.0969
	1	0.0192	0.0005	0.1026	0.0001	0.1344
	2	0.0385	0.0047	0.1321	0.0020	0.1663
	3	0.0577	0.0121	0.1595	0.0066	0.1955
	4	0.0769	0.0214	0.1854	0.0132	0.2229
	5	0.0962	0.0320	0.2103	0.0213	0.2490
	6	0.1154	0.0435	0.2344	0.0306	0.2741
	7	0.1346	0.0559	0.2579	0.0408	0.2984
	8	0.1538	0.0688	0.2808	0.0517	0.3220
	9	0.1731	0.0823	0.3033	0.0633	0.3451
	10	0.1923	0.0963	0.3253	0.0754	0.3676
	11	0.2115	0.1106	0.3470	0.0881	0.3896
	12	0.2308	0.1253	0.3684	0.1012	0.4112
	13	0.2500	0.1403	0.3895	0.1147	0.4324
	14	0.2692	0.1557	0.4102	0.1286	0.4533
	15	0.2885	0.1713	0.4308	0.1429	0.4738
	16	0.3077	0.1872	0.4510	0.1575	0.4940
	17	0.3269	0.2033	0.4711	0.1724	0.5139
	18	0.3462	0.2197	0.4909	0.1876	0.5336
	19	0.3654	0.2362	0.5104	0.2031	0.5529
	20	0.3846	0.2530	0.5298	0.2189	0.5720
	21	0.4038	0.2701	0.5490	0.2349	0.5908
	22	0.4231	0.2873	0.5680	0.2512	0.6093
	23	0.4423	0.3047	0.5867	0.2678	0.6276
	24	0.4615	0.3223	0.6053	0.2846	0.6457
	25	0.4808	0.3401	0.6237	0.3017	0.6635
	26	0.5000	0.3581	0.6419	0.3190	0.6810
	27	0.5192	0.3763	0.6599	0.3365	0.6983
	28	0.5385	0.3947	0.6777	0.3543	0.7154
	29	0.5577	0.4133	0.6953	0.3724	0.7322
	30	0.5769	0.4320	0.7127	0.3907	0.7488
	31	0.5962	0.4510	0.7299	0.4092	0.7651
	32	0.6154	0.4702	0.7470	0.4280	0.7811
	33	0.6346	0.4896	0.7638	0.4471	0.7969
	34	0.6538	0.5091	0.7803	0.4664	0.8124
	35	0.6731	0.5289	0.7967	0.4861	0.8276

Continued

Table B.11. Exact confidence limits for a binomial proportion: x events are observed in a sample sized n. $p = x/n$ is the observed proportion. p_l and p_u are the lower and upper confidence limits for the population proportion

Confidence level

			95%		99%	
n	x	p	p_l	p_u	p_l	p_u
52	36	0.6923	0.5490	0.8128	0.5060	0.8425
	37	0.7115	0.5692	0.8287	0.5262	0.8571
	38	0.7308	0.5898	0.8443	0.5467	0.8714
	39	0.7500	0.6105	0.8597	0.5676	0.8853
	40	0.7692	0.6316	0.8747	0.5888	0.8988
	41	0.7885	0.6530	0.8894	0.6104	0.9119
	42	0.8077	0.6747	0.9037	0.6324	0.9246
	43	0.8269	0.6967	0.9177	0.6549	0.9367
	44	0.8462	0.7192	0.9312	0.6780	0.9483
	45	0.8654	0.7421	0.9441	0.7016	0.9592
	46	0.8846	0.7656	0.9565	0.7259	0.9694
	47	0.9038	0.7897	0.9680	0.7510	0.9787
	48	0.9231	0.8146	0.9786	0.7771	0.9868
	49	0.9423	0.8405	0.9879	0.8045	0.9934
	50	0.9615	0.8679	0.9953	0.8337	0.9980
	51	0.9808	0.8974	0.9995	0.8656	0.9999
	52	1.0000	0.9315	1.0000	0.9031	1.0000
53	0	0.0000	0.0000	0.0672	0.0000	0.0951
	1	0.0189	0.0005	0.1007	0.0001	0.1320
	2	0.0377	0.0046	0.1298	0.0020	0.1634
	3	0.0566	0.0118	0.1566	0.0065	0.1921
	4	0.0755	0.0209	0.1821	0.0130	0.2190
	5	0.0943	0.0313	0.2066	0.0209	0.2447
	6	0.1132	0.0427	0.2303	0.0300	0.2694
	7	0.1321	0.0548	0.2534	0.0400	0.2933
	8	0.1509	0.0675	0.2759	0.0507	0.3166
	9	0.1698	0.0807	0.2980	0.0620	0.3393
	10	0.1887	0.0944	0.3197	0.0739	0.3614
	11	0.2075	0.1084	0.3411	0.0863	0.3831
	12	0.2264	0.1228	0.3621	0.0992	0.4044
	13	0.2453	0.1376	0.3828	0.1124	0.4253
	14	0.2642	0.1526	0.4033	0.1260	0.4459
	15	0.2830	0.1679	0.4235	0.1400	0.4661
	16	0.3019	0.1834	0.4434	0.1543	0.4861
	17	0.3208	0.1992	0.4632	0.1689	0.5057
	18	0.3396	0.2152	0.4827	0.1837	0.5251
	19	0.3585	0.2314	0.5020	0.1989	0.5441

Confidence level

			95%		99%	
n	x	p	p_l	p_u	p_l	p_u
54	10	0.1852	0.0925	0.3143	0.0725	0.3555
	11	0.2037	0.1063	0.3353	0.0846	0.3769
	12	0.2222	0.1204	0.3560	0.0972	0.3978
	13	0.2407	0.1349	0.3764	0.1102	0.4185
	14	0.2593	0.1496	0.3965	0.1235	0.4387
	15	0.2778	0.1646	0.4164	0.1372	0.4587
	16	0.2963	0.1798	0.4361	0.1512	0.4783
	17	0.3148	0.1952	0.4555	0.1655	0.4977
	18	0.3333	0.2109	0.4747	0.1800	0.5168
	19	0.3519	0.2268	0.4938	0.1948	0.5356
	20	0.3704	0.2429	0.5126	0.2099	0.5542
	21	0.3889	0.2592	0.5312	0.2253	0.5726
	22	0.4074	0.2757	0.5497	0.2409	0.5907
	23	0.4259	0.2923	0.5679	0.2567	0.6085
	24	0.4444	0.3092	0.5860	0.2727	0.6262
	25	0.4630	0.3262	0.6039	0.2890	0.6436
	26	0.4815	0.3434	0.6216	0.3055	0.6608
	27	0.5000	0.3608	0.6392	0.3223	0.6777
	28	0.5185	0.3784	0.6566	0.3392	0.6945
	29	0.5370	0.3961	0.6738	0.3564	0.7110
	30	0.5556	0.4140	0.6908	0.3738	0.7273
	31	0.5741	0.4321	0.7077	0.3915	0.7433
	32	0.5926	0.4503	0.7243	0.4093	0.7591
	33	0.6111	0.4688	0.7408	0.4274	0.7747
	34	0.6296	0.4874	0.7571	0.4458	0.7901
	35	0.6481	0.5062	0.7732	0.4644	0.8052
	36	0.6667	0.5253	0.7891	0.4832	0.8200
	37	0.6852	0.5445	0.8048	0.5023	0.8345
	38	0.7037	0.5639	0.8202	0.5217	0.8488
	39	0.7222	0.5836	0.8354	0.5413	0.8628
	40	0.7407	0.6035	0.8504	0.5613	0.8765
	41	0.7593	0.6236	0.8651	0.5815	0.8898
	42	0.7778	0.6440	0.8796	0.6022	0.9028
	43	0.7963	0.6647	0.8937	0.6231	0.9154
	44	0.8148	0.6857	0.9075	0.6445	0.9275
	45	0.8333	0.7071	0.9208	0.6664	0.9392
	46	0.8519	0.7288	0.9338	0.6887	0.9503
	47	0.8704	0.7510	0.9463	0.7116	0.9608

n	r					
53	20	0.3774	0.2479	0.5211	0.2143	0.5630
	21	0.3962	0.2645	0.5400	0.2300	0.5815
	22	0.4151	0.2814	0.5587	0.2459	0.5999
	23	0.4340	0.2984	0.5772	0.2621	0.6179
	24	0.4528	0.3156	0.5955	0.2786	0.6358
	25	0.4717	0.3330	0.6136	0.2952	0.6534
	26	0.4906	0.3506	0.6316	0.3121	0.6707
	27	0.5094	0.3684	0.6494	0.3293	0.6879
	28	0.5283	0.3864	0.6670	0.3466	0.7048
	29	0.5472	0.4045	0.6844	0.3642	0.7214
	30	0.5660	0.4228	0.7016	0.3821	0.7379
	31	0.5849	0.4413	0.7186	0.4001	0.7541
	32	0.6038	0.4600	0.7355	0.4185	0.7700
	33	0.6226	0.4789	0.7521	0.4370	0.7857
	34	0.6415	0.4980	0.7686	0.4559	0.8011
	35	0.6604	0.5173	0.7848	0.4749	0.8163
	36	0.6792	0.5368	0.8008	0.4943	0.8311
	37	0.6981	0.5566	0.8166	0.5139	0.8457
	38	0.7170	0.5765	0.8321	0.5339	0.8600
	39	0.7358	0.5967	0.8474	0.5541	0.8740
	40	0.7547	0.6172	0.8624	0.5747	0.8876
	41	0.7736	0.6379	0.8772	0.5956	0.9008
	42	0.7925	0.6589	0.8916	0.6169	0.9137
	43	0.8113	0.6803	0.9056	0.6386	0.9261
	44	0.8302	0.7020	0.9193	0.6607	0.9380
	45	0.8491	0.7241	0.9325	0.6834	0.9493
	46	0.8679	0.7466	0.9452	0.7067	0.9600
	47	0.8868	0.7697	0.9573	0.7306	0.9700
	48	0.9057	0.7934	0.9687	0.7553	0.9791
	49	0.9245	0.8179	0.9791	0.7810	0.9870
	50	0.9434	0.8434	0.9882	0.8079	0.9935
	51	0.9623	0.8702	0.9954	0.8366	0.9980
	52	0.9811	0.8993	0.9995	0.8680	0.9999
	53	1.0000	0.9328	1.0000	0.9049	1.0000
54	0	0.0000	0.0000	0.0660	0.0000	0.0935
	1	0.0185	0.0005	0.0989	0.0001	0.1297
	2	0.0370	0.0045	0.1275	0.0019	0.1606
	3	0.0556	0.0116	0.1539	0.0064	0.1888
	4	0.0741	0.0206	0.1789	0.0127	0.2153
	5	0.0926	0.0308	0.2030	0.0205	0.2406
	6	0.1111	0.0419	0.2263	0.0294	0.2649
	7	0.1296	0.0537	0.2490	0.0392	0.2884
	8	0.1481	0.0662	0.2712	0.0497	0.3113
	9	0.1667	0.0792	0.2929	0.0608	0.3336

n	r					
54	48	0.8889	0.7737	0.9581	0.7351	0.9706
	49	0.9074	0.7970	0.9692	0.7594	0.9795
	50	0.9259	0.8211	0.9794	0.7847	0.9873
	51	0.9444	0.8461	0.9884	0.8112	0.9936
	52	0.9630	0.8725	0.9955	0.8394	0.9981
	53	0.9815	0.9011	0.9995	0.8703	0.9999
	54	1.0000	0.9340	1.0000	0.9065	1.0000
55	0	0.0000	0.0000	0.0649	0.0000	0.0918
	1	0.0182	0.0005	0.0972	0.0001	0.1275
	2	0.0364	0.0044	0.1253	0.0019	0.1579
	3	0.0545	0.0114	0.1512	0.0062	0.1856
	4	0.0727	0.0202	0.1759	0.0125	0.2117
	5	0.0909	0.0302	0.1995	0.0201	0.2366
	6	0.1091	0.0411	0.2225	0.0289	0.2605
	7	0.1273	0.0527	0.2448	0.0385	0.2837
	8	0.1455	0.0650	0.2666	0.0488	0.3062
	9	0.1636	0.0777	0.2880	0.0597	0.3282
	10	0.1818	0.0908	0.3090	0.0711	0.3497
	11	0.2000	0.1043	0.3297	0.0830	0.3708
	12	0.2182	0.1181	0.3501	0.0953	0.3915
	13	0.2364	0.1323	0.3702	0.1081	0.4118
	14	0.2545	0.1467	0.3900	0.1211	0.4318
	15	0.2727	0.1614	0.4096	0.1345	0.4515
	16	0.2909	0.1763	0.4290	0.1482	0.4708
	17	0.3091	0.1914	0.4481	0.1622	0.4900
	18	0.3273	0.2068	0.4671	0.1764	0.5088
	19	0.3455	0.2224	0.4858	0.1910	0.5274
	20	0.3636	0.2381	0.5044	0.2057	0.5457
	21	0.3818	0.2541	0.5227	0.2207	0.5639
	22	0.4000	0.2702	0.5409	0.2360	0.5817
	23	0.4182	0.2865	0.5589	0.2515	0.5994
	24	0.4364	0.3030	0.5768	0.2672	0.6168
	25	0.4545	0.3197	0.5945	0.2831	0.6340
	26	0.4727	0.3365	0.6120	0.2992	0.6510
	27	0.4909	0.3535	0.6293	0.3156	0.6678
	28	0.5091	0.3707	0.6465	0.3322	0.6844
	29	0.5273	0.3880	0.6635	0.3490	0.7008
	30	0.5455	0.4055	0.6803	0.3660	0.7169
	31	0.5636	0.4232	0.6970	0.3832	0.7328
	32	0.5818	0.4411	0.7135	0.4006	0.7485
	33	0.6000	0.4591	0.7298	0.4183	0.7640
	34	0.6182	0.4773	0.7459	0.4361	0.7793
	35	0.6364	0.4956	0.7619	0.4543	0.7943
	36	0.6545	0.5142	0.7776	0.4726	0.8090

Continued

Table B.11. Exact confidence limits for a binomial proportion: x events are observed in a sample sized n. $p = x/n$ is the observed proportion. p_l and p_u are the lower and upper confidence limits for the population proportion

			Confidence level			
			95%		99%	
n	x	p	p_l	p_u	p_l	p_u
55	37	0.6727	0.5329	0.7932	0.4912	0.8236
	38	0.6909	0.5519	0.8086	0.5100	0.8378
	39	0.7091	0.5710	0.8237	0.5292	0.8518
	40	0.7273	0.5904	0.8386	0.5485	0.8655
	41	0.7455	0.6100	0.8533	0.5682	0.8789
	42	0.7636	0.6298	0.8677	0.5882	0.8919
	43	0.7818	0.6499	0.8819	0.6085	0.9047
	44	0.8000	0.6703	0.8957	0.6292	0.9170
	45	0.8182	0.6910	0.9092	0.6503	0.9289
	46	0.8364	0.7120	0.9223	0.6718	0.9403
	47	0.8545	0.7334	0.9350	0.6938	0.9512
	48	0.8727	0.7552	0.9473	0.7163	0.9615
	49	0.8909	0.7775	0.9589	0.7395	0.9711
	50	0.9091	0.8005	0.9698	0.7634	0.9799
	51	0.9273	0.8241	0.9798	0.7883	0.9875
	52	0.9455	0.8488	0.9886	0.8144	0.9938
	53	0.9636	0.8747	0.9956	0.8421	0.9981
	54	0.9818	0.9028	0.9995	0.8725	0.9999
	55	1.0000	0.9351	1.0000	0.9082	1.0000
56	0	0.0000	0.0000	0.0638	0.0000	0.0903
	1	0.0179	0.0005	0.0955	0.0001	0.1253
	2	0.0357	0.0044	0.1231	0.0019	0.1552
	3	0.0536	0.0112	0.1487	0.0061	0.1825
	4	0.0714	0.0198	0.1729	0.0123	0.2082
	5	0.0893	0.0296	0.1962	0.0198	0.2327
	6	0.1071	0.0403	0.2188	0.0283	0.2563
	7	0.1250	0.0518	0.2407	0.0377	0.2791
	8	0.1429	0.0638	0.2622	0.0479	0.3013
	9	0.1607	0.0762	0.2833	0.0586	0.3230
	10	0.1786	0.0891	0.3040	0.0698	0.3442
	11	0.1964	0.1023	0.3243	0.0814	0.3649
	12	0.2143	0.1159	0.3444	0.0935	0.3853
	13	0.2321	0.1298	0.3642	0.1060	0.4053
	14	0.2500	0.1439	0.3837	0.1188	0.4250
	15	0.2679	0.1583	0.4030	0.1319	0.4445
	16	0.2857	0.1730	0.4221	0.1453	0.4636
	17	0.3036	0.1878	0.4410	0.1590	0.4824

			Confidence level			
			95%		99%	
n	x	p	p_l	p_u	p_l	p_u
57	5	0.0877	0.0291	0.1930	0.0194	0.2290
	6	0.1053	0.0396	0.2152	0.0278	0.2522
	7	0.1228	0.0508	0.2368	0.0371	0.2747
	8	0.1404	0.0626	0.2579	0.0470	0.2965
	9	0.1579	0.0748	0.2787	0.0575	0.3179
	10	0.1754	0.0875	0.2991	0.0685	0.3388
	11	0.1930	0.1005	0.3191	0.0799	0.3592
	12	0.2105	0.1138	0.3389	0.0918	0.3793
	13	0.2281	0.1274	0.3584	0.1040	0.3991
	14	0.2456	0.1413	0.3776	0.1166	0.4185
	15	0.2632	0.1554	0.3966	0.1294	0.4377
	16	0.2807	0.1697	0.4154	0.1426	0.4565
	17	0.2982	0.1843	0.4340	0.1560	0.4751
	18	0.3158	0.1991	0.4524	0.1697	0.4935
	19	0.3333	0.2140	0.4706	0.1836	0.5116
	20	0.3509	0.2291	0.4887	0.1978	0.5295
	21	0.3684	0.2445	0.5066	0.2122	0.5472
	22	0.3860	0.2600	0.5243	0.2268	0.5646
	23	0.4035	0.2756	0.5418	0.2417	0.5819
	24	0.4211	0.2914	0.5592	0.2567	0.5989
	25	0.4386	0.3074	0.5764	0.2720	0.6157
	26	0.4561	0.3236	0.5934	0.2874	0.6324
	27	0.4737	0.3398	0.6103	0.3031	0.6488
	28	0.4912	0.3563	0.6271	0.3189	0.6651
	29	0.5088	0.3729	0.6437	0.3349	0.6811
	30	0.5263	0.3897	0.6602	0.3512	0.6969
	31	0.5439	0.4066	0.6764	0.3676	0.7126
	32	0.5614	0.4236	0.6926	0.3843	0.7280
	33	0.5789	0.4408	0.7086	0.4011	0.7433
	34	0.5965	0.4582	0.7244	0.4181	0.7583
	35	0.6140	0.4757	0.7400	0.4354	0.7732
	36	0.6316	0.4934	0.7555	0.4528	0.7878
	37	0.6491	0.5113	0.7709	0.4705	0.8022
	38	0.6667	0.5294	0.7860	0.4884	0.8164
	39	0.6842	0.5476	0.8009	0.5065	0.8303
	40	0.7018	0.5660	0.8157	0.5249	0.8440
	41	0.7193	0.5846	0.8303	0.5435	0.8574
	42	0.7368	0.6034	0.8446	0.5623	0.8706

n						
56	18	0.3214	0.2029	0.4596	0.1730	0.5010
	19	0.3393	0.2181	0.4781	0.1872	0.5194
	20	0.3571	0.2336	0.4964	0.2017	0.5375
	21	0.3750	0.2492	0.5145	0.2164	0.5554
	22	0.3929	0.2650	0.5325	0.2313	0.5731
	23	0.4107	0.2810	0.5502	0.2465	0.5905
	24	0.4286	0.2971	0.5678	0.2618	0.6077
	25	0.4464	0.3134	0.5853	0.2774	0.6248
	26	0.4643	0.3299	0.6026	0.2932	0.6416
	27	0.4821	0.3466	0.6197	0.3092	0.6582
	28	0.5000	0.3634	0.6366	0.3254	0.6746
	29	0.5179	0.3803	0.6534	0.3418	0.6908
	30	0.5357	0.3974	0.6701	0.3584	0.7068
	31	0.5536	0.4147	0.6866	0.3752	0.7226
	32	0.5714	0.4322	0.7029	0.3923	0.7382
	33	0.5893	0.4498	0.7190	0.4095	0.7535
	34	0.6071	0.4675	0.7350	0.4269	0.7687
	35	0.6250	0.4855	0.7508	0.4446	0.7836
	36	0.6429	0.5036	0.7664	0.4625	0.7983
	37	0.6607	0.5219	0.7819	0.4806	0.8128
	38	0.6786	0.5404	0.7971	0.4990	0.8270
	39	0.6964	0.5590	0.8122	0.5176	0.8410
	40	0.7143	0.5779	0.8270	0.5364	0.8547
	41	0.7321	0.5970	0.8417	0.5555	0.8681
	42	0.7500	0.6163	0.8561	0.5750	0.8812
	43	0.7679	0.6358	0.8702	0.5947	0.8940
	44	0.7857	0.6556	0.8841	0.6147	0.9065
	45	0.8036	0.6757	0.8977	0.6351	0.9186
	46	0.8214	0.6960	0.9109	0.6558	0.9302
	47	0.8393	0.7167	0.9238	0.6770	0.9414
	48	0.8571	0.7378	0.9362	0.6987	0.9521
	49	0.8750	0.7593	0.9482	0.7209	0.9623
	50	0.8929	0.7812	0.9597	0.7437	0.9717
	51	0.9107	0.8038	0.9704	0.7673	0.9802
	52	0.9286	0.8271	0.9802	0.7918	0.9877
	53	0.9464	0.8513	0.9888	0.8175	0.9939
	54	0.9643	0.8769	0.9956	0.8448	0.9981
	55	0.9821	0.9045	0.9995	0.8747	0.9999
	56	1.0000	0.9362	1.0000	0.9097	1.0000
57	0	0.0000	0.0000	0.0627	0.0000	0.0888
	1	0.0175	0.0004	0.0939	0.0001	0.1232
	2	0.0351	0.0043	0.1211	0.0018	0.1527
	3	0.0526	0.0110	0.1462	0.0060	0.1796
	4	0.0702	0.0195	0.1700	0.0120	0.2048

n						
57	43	0.7544	0.6224	0.8587	0.5815	0.8834
	44	0.7719	0.6416	0.8726	0.6009	0.8960
	45	0.7895	0.6611	0.8862	0.6207	0.9082
	46	0.8070	0.6809	0.8995	0.6408	0.9201
	47	0.8246	0.7009	0.9125	0.6612	0.9315
	48	0.8421	0.7213	0.9252	0.6821	0.9425
	49	0.8596	0.7421	0.9374	0.7035	0.9530
	50	0.8772	0.7632	0.9492	0.7253	0.9629
	51	0.8947	0.7848	0.9604	0.7478	0.9722
	52	0.9123	0.8070	0.9709	0.7710	0.9806
	53	0.9298	0.8300	0.9805	0.7952	0.9880
	54	0.9474	0.8538	0.9890	0.8204	0.9940
	55	0.9649	0.8789	0.9957	0.8473	0.9982
	56	0.9825	0.9061	0.9996	0.8768	0.9999
	57	1.0000	0.9373	1.0000	0.9112	1.0000
58	0	0.0000	0.0000	0.0616	0.0000	0.0873
	1	0.0172	0.0004	0.0924	0.0001	0.1212
	2	0.0345	0.0042	0.1191	0.0018	0.1502
	3	0.0517	0.0108	0.1438	0.0059	0.1767
	4	0.0690	0.0191	0.1673	0.0118	0.2016
	5	0.0862	0.0286	0.1898	0.0191	0.2253
	6	0.1034	0.0389	0.2117	0.0273	0.2482
	7	0.1207	0.0499	0.2330	0.0364	0.2703
	8	0.1379	0.0615	0.2538	0.0461	0.2919
	9	0.1552	0.0735	0.2742	0.0564	0.3129
	10	0.1724	0.0859	0.2943	0.0672	0.3335
	11	0.1897	0.0987	0.3141	0.0785	0.3537
	12	0.2069	0.1117	0.3335	0.0901	0.3735
	13	0.2241	0.1251	0.3527	0.1021	0.3930
	14	0.2414	0.1387	0.3717	0.1144	0.4122
	15	0.2586	0.1526	0.3904	0.1270	0.4311
	16	0.2759	0.1666	0.4090	0.1399	0.4497
	17	0.2931	0.1809	0.4273	0.1531	0.4680
	18	0.3103	0.1954	0.4454	0.1665	0.4862
	19	0.3276	0.2101	0.4634	0.1802	0.5041
	20	0.3448	0.2249	0.4812	0.1941	0.5217
	21	0.3621	0.2399	0.4988	0.2082	0.5392
	22	0.3793	0.2551	0.5163	0.2225	0.5564
	23	0.3966	0.2705	0.5336	0.2370	0.5735
	24	0.4138	0.2860	0.5507	0.2518	0.5903
	25	0.4310	0.3016	0.5677	0.2667	0.6070
	26	0.4483	0.3174	0.5846	0.2818	0.6234
	27	0.4655	0.3334	0.6013	0.2972	0.6397
	28	0.4828	0.3495	0.6178	0.3127	0.6557

Continued

Table B.11. Exact confidence limits for a binomial proportion: x events are observed in a sample sized n. $p = x/n$ is the observed proportion. p_l and p_u are the lower and upper confidence limits for the population proportion

Confidence level

n	x	p	95% p_l	95% p_u	99% p_l	99% p_u
58	29	0.5000	0.3658	0.6342	0.3284	0.6716
	30	0.5172	0.3822	0.6505	0.3443	0.6873
	31	0.5345	0.3987	0.6666	0.3603	0.7028
	32	0.5517	0.4154	0.6826	0.3766	0.7182
	33	0.5690	0.4323	0.6984	0.3930	0.7333
	34	0.5862	0.4493	0.7140	0.4097	0.7482
	35	0.6034	0.4664	0.7295	0.4265	0.7630
	36	0.6207	0.4837	0.7449	0.4436	0.7775
	37	0.6379	0.5012	0.7601	0.4608	0.7918
	38	0.6552	0.5188	0.7751	0.4783	0.8059
	39	0.6724	0.5366	0.7899	0.4959	0.8198
	40	0.6897	0.5546	0.8046	0.5138	0.8335
	41	0.7069	0.5727	0.8191	0.5320	0.8469
	42	0.7241	0.5910	0.8334	0.5503	0.8601
	43	0.7414	0.6096	0.8474	0.5689	0.8730
	44	0.7586	0.6283	0.8613	0.5878	0.8856
	45	0.7759	0.6473	0.8749	0.6070	0.8979
	46	0.7931	0.6665	0.8883	0.6265	0.9099
	47	0.8103	0.6859	0.9013	0.6463	0.9215
	48	0.8276	0.7057	0.9141	0.6665	0.9328
	49	0.8448	0.7258	0.9265	0.6871	0.9436
	50	0.8621	0.7462	0.9385	0.7081	0.9539
	51	0.8793	0.7670	0.9501	0.7297	0.9636
	52	0.8966	0.7883	0.9611	0.7518	0.9727
	53	0.9138	0.8102	0.9714	0.7747	0.9809
	54	0.9310	0.8327	0.9809	0.7984	0.9882
	55	0.9483	0.8562	0.9892	0.8233	0.9941
	56	0.9655	0.8809	0.9958	0.8498	0.9982
	57	0.9828	0.9076	0.9996	0.8788	0.9999
	58	1.0000	0.9384	1.0000	0.9127	1.0000
59	**0**	0.0000	0.0000	0.0606	0.0000	0.0859
	1	0.0169	0.0004	0.0909	0.0001	0.1193
	2	0.0339	0.0041	0.1171	0.0018	0.1478
	3	0.0508	0.0106	0.1415	0.0058	0.1739
	4	0.0678	0.0188	0.1646	0.0116	0.1984
	5	0.0847	0.0281	0.1868	0.0187	0.2218
	6	0.1017	0.0382	0.2083	0.0269	0.2443

Confidence level

n	x	p	95% p_l	95% p_u	99% p_l	99% p_u
59	52	0.8814	0.7707	0.9509	0.7338	0.9642
	53	0.8983	0.7917	0.9618	0.7557	0.9731
	54	0.9153	0.8132	0.9719	0.7782	0.9813
	55	0.9322	0.8354	0.9812	0.8016	0.9884
	56	0.9492	0.8585	0.9894	0.8261	0.9942
	57	0.9661	0.8829	0.9959	0.8522	0.9982
	58	0.9831	0.9091	0.9996	0.8807	0.9999
	59	1.0000	0.9394	1.0000	0.9141	1.0000
60	**0**	0.0000	0.0000	0.0596	0.0000	0.0845
	1	0.0167	0.0004	0.0894	0.0001	0.1174
	2	0.0333	0.0041	0.1153	0.0017	0.1455
	3	0.0500	0.0104	0.1392	0.0057	0.1712
	4	0.0667	0.0185	0.1620	0.0114	0.1953
	5	0.0833	0.0276	0.1839	0.0184	0.2184
	6	0.1000	0.0376	0.2051	0.0264	0.2406
	7	0.1167	0.0482	0.2257	0.0351	0.2621
	8	0.1333	0.0594	0.2459	0.0445	0.2831
	9	0.1500	0.0710	0.2657	0.0545	0.3035
	10	0.1667	0.0829	0.2852	0.0649	0.3235
	11	0.1833	0.0952	0.3044	0.0757	0.3431
	12	0.2000	0.1078	0.3233	0.0869	0.3624
	13	0.2167	0.1207	0.3420	0.0985	0.3814
	14	0.2333	0.1338	0.3604	0.1104	0.4001
	15	0.2500	0.1472	0.3786	0.1225	0.4184
	16	0.2667	0.1607	0.3966	0.1349	0.4366
	17	0.2833	0.1745	0.4144	0.1476	0.4545
	18	0.3000	0.1885	0.4321	0.1605	0.4721
	19	0.3167	0.2026	0.4496	0.1737	0.4896
	20	0.3333	0.2169	0.4669	0.1870	0.5068
	21	0.3500	0.2313	0.4840	0.2006	0.5239
	22	0.3667	0.2459	0.5010	0.2144	0.5407
	23	0.3833	0.2607	0.5179	0.2283	0.5573
	24	0.4000	0.2756	0.5346	0.2425	0.5738
	25	0.4167	0.2907	0.5512	0.2568	0.5901
	26	0.4333	0.3059	0.5676	0.2713	0.6062
	27	0.4500	0.3212	0.5839	0.2860	0.6221
	28	0.4667	0.3367	0.6000	0.3009	0.6378

59

7	0.1186	0.0491	0.2293	0.0358	0.2662
8	0.1356	0.0604	0.2498	0.0453	0.2874
9	0.1525	0.0722	0.2699	0.0554	0.3082
10	0.1695	0.0844	0.2897	0.0660	0.3284
11	0.1864	0.0969	0.3091	0.0771	0.3483
12	0.2034	0.1098	0.3283	0.0885	0.3679
13	0.2203	0.1229	0.3473	0.1003	0.3871
14	0.2373	0.1362	0.3659	0.1124	0.4060
15	0.2542	0.1498	0.3844	0.1247	0.4247
16	0.2712	0.1636	0.4027	0.1374	0.4430
17	0.2881	0.1776	0.4208	0.1503	0.4612
18	0.3051	0.1919	0.4387	0.1635	0.4791
19	0.3220	0.2062	0.4564	0.1769	0.4967
20	0.3390	0.2208	0.4739	0.1905	0.5142
21	0.3559	0.2355	0.4913	0.2043	0.5314
22	0.3729	0.2504	0.5085	0.2184	0.5484
23	0.3898	0.2655	0.5256	0.2326	0.5653
24	0.4068	0.2807	0.5425	0.2470	0.5819
25	0.4237	0.2961	0.5593	0.2617	0.5984
26	0.4407	0.3116	0.5760	0.2765	0.6147
27	0.4576	0.3272	0.5925	0.2915	0.6308
28	0.4746	0.3430	0.6088	0.3067	0.6467
29	0.4915	0.3589	0.6250	0.3220	0.6624
30	0.5085	0.3750	0.6411	0.3376	0.6780
31	0.5254	0.3912	0.6570	0.3533	0.6933
32	0.5424	0.4075	0.6728	0.3692	0.7085
33	0.5593	0.4240	0.6884	0.3853	0.7235
34	0.5763	0.4407	0.7039	0.4016	0.7383
35	0.5932	0.4575	0.7193	0.4181	0.7530
36	0.6102	0.4744	0.7345	0.4347	0.7674
37	0.6271	0.4915	0.7496	0.4516	0.7816
38	0.6441	0.5087	0.7645	0.4686	0.7957
39	0.6610	0.5261	0.7792	0.4858	0.8095
40	0.6780	0.5436	0.7938	0.5033	0.8231
41	0.6949	0.5613	0.8081	0.5209	0.8365
42	0.7119	0.5792	0.8224	0.5388	0.8497
43	0.7288	0.5973	0.8364	0.5570	0.8626
44	0.7458	0.6156	0.8502	0.5753	0.8753
45	0.7627	0.6341	0.8638	0.5940	0.8876
46	0.7797	0.6527	0.8771	0.6129	0.8997
47	0.7966	0.6717	0.8902	0.6321	0.9115
48	0.8136	0.6909	0.9031	0.6517	0.9229
49	0.8305	0.7103	0.9156	0.6716	0.9340
50	0.8475	0.7301	0.9278	0.6918	0.9446
51	0.8644	0.7502	0.9396	0.7126	0.9547

60

60

29	0.4833	0.3523	0.6161	0.3160	0.6534
30	0.5000	0.3681	0.6319	0.3312	0.6688
31	0.5167	0.3839	0.6477	0.3466	0.6840
32	0.5333	0.4000	0.6633	0.3622	0.6991
33	0.5500	0.4161	0.6788	0.3779	0.7140
34	0.5667	0.4324	0.6941	0.3938	0.7287
35	0.5833	0.4488	0.7093	0.4099	0.7432
36	0.6000	0.4654	0.7244	0.4262	0.7575
37	0.6167	0.4821	0.7393	0.4427	0.7717
38	0.6333	0.4990	0.7541	0.4593	0.7856
39	0.6500	0.5160	0.7687	0.4761	0.7994
40	0.6667	0.5331	0.7831	0.4932	0.8130
41	0.6833	0.5504	0.7974	0.5104	0.8263
42	0.7000	0.5679	0.8115	0.5279	0.8395
43	0.7167	0.5856	0.8255	0.5455	0.8524
44	0.7333	0.6034	0.8393	0.5634	0.8651
45	0.7500	0.6214	0.8528	0.5816	0.8775
46	0.7667	0.6396	0.8662	0.5999	0.8896
47	0.7833	0.6580	0.8793	0.6186	0.9015
48	0.8000	0.6767	0.8922	0.6376	0.9131
49	0.8167	0.6956	0.9048	0.6569	0.9243
50	0.8333	0.7148	0.9171	0.6765	0.9351
51	0.8500	0.7343	0.9290	0.6965	0.9455
52	0.8667	0.7541	0.9406	0.7169	0.9555
53	0.8833	0.7743	0.9518	0.7379	0.9649
54	0.9000	0.7949	0.9624	0.7594	0.9736
55	0.9167	0.8161	0.9724	0.7816	0.9816
56	0.9333	0.8380	0.9815	0.8047	0.9886
57	0.9500	0.8608	0.9896	0.8288	0.9943
58	0.9667	0.8847	0.9959	0.8545	0.9983
59	0.9833	0.9106	0.9996	0.8826	0.9999
60	1.0000	0.9404	1.0000	0.9155	1.0000

61

0	0.0000	0.0000	0.0587	0.0000	0.0832
1	0.0164	0.0004	0.0880	0.0001	0.1156
2	0.0328	0.0040	0.1135	0.0017	0.1433
3	0.0492	0.0103	0.1371	0.0056	0.1686
4	0.0656	0.0182	0.1595	0.0112	0.1924
5	0.0820	0.0272	0.1810	0.0181	0.2151
6	0.0984	0.0370	0.2019	0.0259	0.2370
7	0.1148	0.0474	0.2222	0.0345	0.2582
8	0.1311	0.0584	0.2422	0.0438	0.2788
9	0.1475	0.0698	0.2617	0.0535	0.2990
10	0.1639	0.0815	0.2809	0.0638	0.3187
11	0.1803	0.0936	0.2998	0.0744	0.3381

Continued

Table B.11. Exact confidence limits for a binomial proportion: x events are observed in a sample sized n. $p = x/n$ is the observed proportion. p_l and p_u are the lower and upper confidence limits for the population proportion

Confidence level

n	x	p	95% p_l	95% p_u	99% p_l	99% p_u
61	12	0.1967	0.1060	0.3184	0.0854	0.3571
	13	0.2131	0.1186	0.3368	0.0968	0.3758
	14	0.2295	0.1315	0.3550	0.1084	0.3942
	15	0.2459	0.1446	0.3729	0.1204	0.4124
	16	0.2623	0.1580	0.3907	0.1326	0.4303
	17	0.2787	0.1715	0.4083	0.1450	0.4480
	18	0.2951	0.1852	0.4257	0.1577	0.4654
	19	0.3115	0.1990	0.4429	0.1706	0.4826
	20	0.3279	0.2131	0.4600	0.1837	0.4997
	21	0.3443	0.2273	0.4769	0.1970	0.5165
	22	0.3607	0.2416	0.4937	0.2105	0.5331
	23	0.3770	0.2561	0.5104	0.2242	0.5496
	24	0.3934	0.2707	0.5269	0.2381	0.5659
	25	0.4098	0.2855	0.5432	0.2521	0.5820
	26	0.4262	0.3004	0.5594	0.2664	0.5979
	27	0.4426	0.3155	0.5755	0.2808	0.6136
	28	0.4590	0.3306	0.5915	0.2954	0.6292
	29	0.4754	0.3460	0.6073	0.3101	0.6446
	30	0.4918	0.3614	0.6230	0.3250	0.6599
	31	0.5082	0.3770	0.6386	0.3401	0.6750
	32	0.5246	0.3927	0.6540	0.3554	0.6899
	33	0.5410	0.4085	0.6694	0.3708	0.7046
	34	0.5574	0.4245	0.6845	0.3864	0.7192
	35	0.5738	0.4406	0.6996	0.4021	0.7336
	36	0.5902	0.4568	0.7145	0.4180	0.7479
	37	0.6066	0.4731	0.7293	0.4341	0.7619
	38	0.6230	0.4896	0.7439	0.4504	0.7758
	39	0.6393	0.5063	0.7584	0.4669	0.7895
	40	0.6557	0.5231	0.7727	0.4835	0.8030
	41	0.6721	0.5400	0.7869	0.5003	0.8163
	42	0.6885	0.5571	0.8010	0.5174	0.8294
	43	0.7049	0.5743	0.8148	0.5346	0.8423
	44	0.7213	0.5917	0.8285	0.5520	0.8550
	45	0.7377	0.6093	0.8420	0.5697	0.8674
	46	0.7541	0.6271	0.8554	0.5876	0.8796
	47	0.7705	0.6450	0.8685	0.6058	0.8916
	48	0.7869	0.6632	0.8814	0.6242	0.9032
	49	0.8033	0.6816	0.8940	0.6429	0.9146

Confidence level

n	x	p	95% p_l	95% p_u	99% p_l	99% p_u
62	32	0.5161	0.3856	0.6450	0.3488	0.6809
	33	0.5323	0.4012	0.6602	0.3639	0.6955
	34	0.5484	0.4168	0.6752	0.3792	0.7100
	35	0.5645	0.4326	0.6901	0.3946	0.7243
	36	0.5806	0.4485	0.7049	0.4102	0.7384
	37	0.5968	0.4645	0.7195	0.4259	0.7524
	38	0.6129	0.4807	0.7340	0.4419	0.7662
	39	0.6290	0.4969	0.7484	0.4579	0.7798
	40	0.6452	0.5134	0.7626	0.4742	0.7932
	41	0.6613	0.5299	0.7767	0.4907	0.8065
	42	0.6774	0.5466	0.7906	0.5073	0.8195
	43	0.6935	0.5635	0.8044	0.5241	0.8324
	44	0.7097	0.5805	0.8180	0.5411	0.8451
	45	0.7258	0.5977	0.8315	0.5584	0.8575
	46	0.7419	0.6150	0.8447	0.5758	0.8697
	47	0.7581	0.6326	0.8578	0.5935	0.8817
	48	0.7742	0.6503	0.8707	0.6114	0.8934
	49	0.7903	0.6682	0.8834	0.6296	0.9049
	50	0.8065	0.6863	0.8958	0.6480	0.9160
	51	0.8226	0.7047	0.9080	0.6668	0.9268
	52	0.8387	0.7233	0.9198	0.6859	0.9373
	53	0.8548	0.7422	0.9314	0.7054	0.9474
	54	0.8710	0.7615	0.9426	0.7253	0.9570
	55	0.8871	0.7811	0.9534	0.7456	0.9660
	56	0.9032	0.8012	0.9637	0.7665	0.9745
	57	0.9194	0.8217	0.9733	0.7881	0.9822
	58	0.9355	0.8430	0.9821	0.8105	0.9889
	59	0.9516	0.8650	0.9899	0.8340	0.9945
	60	0.9677	0.8883	0.9961	0.8589	0.9983
	61	0.9839	0.9134	0.9996	0.8862	0.9999
	62	1.0000	0.9422	1.0000	0.9181	1.0000
63	0	0.0000	0.0000	0.0569	0.0000	0.0807
	1	0.0159	0.0004	0.0853	0.0001	0.1121
	2	0.0317	0.0039	0.1100	0.0017	0.1390
	3	0.0476	0.0099	0.1329	0.0054	0.1636
	4	0.0635	0.0176	0.1547	0.0109	0.1867
	5	0.0794	0.0263	0.1756	0.0175	0.2088

n	k					
61	50	0.8197	0.7002	0.9064	0.6619	0.9256
	51	0.8361	0.7191	0.9185	0.6813	0.9362
	52	0.8525	0.7383	0.9302	0.7010	0.9465
	53	0.8689	0.7578	0.9416	0.7212	0.9562
	54	0.8852	0.7778	0.9526	0.7418	0.9655
	55	0.9016	0.7981	0.9630	0.7630	0.9741
	56	0.9180	0.8190	0.9728	0.7849	0.9819
	57	0.9344	0.8405	0.9818	0.8076	0.9888
	58	0.9508	0.8629	0.9897	0.8314	0.9944
	59	0.9672	0.8865	0.9960	0.8567	0.9983
	60	0.9836	0.9120	0.9996	0.8844	0.9999
	61	1.0000	0.9413	1.0000	0.9168	1.0000
62	**0**	0.0000	0.0000	0.0578	0.0000	0.0819
	1	0.0161	0.0004	0.0866	0.0001	0.1138
	2	0.0323	0.0039	0.1117	0.0017	0.1411
	3	0.0484	0.0101	0.1350	0.0055	0.1660
	4	0.0645	0.0179	0.1570	0.0111	0.1895
	5	0.0806	0.0267	0.1783	0.0178	0.2119
	6	0.0968	0.0363	0.1988	0.0255	0.2335
	7	0.1129	0.0466	0.2189	0.0340	0.2544
	8	0.1290	0.0574	0.2385	0.0430	0.2747
	9	0.1452	0.0686	0.2578	0.0526	0.2946
	10	0.1613	0.0802	0.2767	0.0627	0.3141
	11	0.1774	0.0920	0.2953	0.0732	0.3332
	12	0.1935	0.1042	0.3137	0.0840	0.3520
	13	0.2097	0.1166	0.3318	0.0951	0.3704
	14	0.2258	0.1293	0.3497	0.1066	0.3886
	15	0.2419	0.1422	0.3674	0.1183	0.4065
	16	0.2581	0.1553	0.3850	0.1303	0.4242
	17	0.2742	0.1685	0.4023	0.1425	0.4416
	18	0.2903	0.1820	0.4195	0.1549	0.4589
	19	0.3065	0.1956	0.4365	0.1676	0.4759
	20	0.3226	0.2094	0.4534	0.1805	0.4927
	21	0.3387	0.2233	0.4701	0.1935	0.5093
	22	0.3548	0.2374	0.4866	0.2068	0.5258
	23	0.3710	0.2516	0.5031	0.2202	0.5421
	24	0.3871	0.2660	0.5193	0.2338	0.5581
	25	0.4032	0.2805	0.5355	0.2476	0.5741
	26	0.4194	0.2951	0.5515	0.2616	0.5898
	27	0.4355	0.3099	0.5674	0.2757	0.6054
	28	0.4516	0.3248	0.5832	0.2900	0.6208
	29	0.4677	0.3398	0.5988	0.3045	0.6361
	30	0.4839	0.3550	0.6144	0.3191	0.6512
	31	0.5000	0.3702	0.6298	0.3339	0.6661

n	k					
63	6	0.0952	0.0358	0.1959	0.0251	0.2300
	7	0.1111	0.0459	0.2156	0.0334	0.2507
	8	0.1270	0.0565	0.2350	0.0423	0.2708
	9	0.1429	0.0675	0.2539	0.0518	0.2904
	10	0.1587	0.0788	0.2726	0.0617	0.3096
	11	0.1746	0.0905	0.2910	0.0719	0.3284
	12	0.1905	0.1025	0.3091	0.0826	0.3470
	13	0.2063	0.1147	0.3270	0.0935	0.3652
	14	0.2222	0.1272	0.3446	0.1048	0.3831
	15	0.2381	0.1398	0.3621	0.1163	0.4008
	16	0.2540	0.1527	0.3794	0.1281	0.4183
	17	0.2698	0.1657	0.3965	0.1401	0.4355
	18	0.2857	0.1789	0.4135	0.1523	0.4525
	19	0.3016	0.1923	0.4302	0.1647	0.4693
	20	0.3175	0.2058	0.4469	0.1774	0.4859
	21	0.3333	0.2195	0.4634	0.1902	0.5024
	22	0.3492	0.2334	0.4797	0.2032	0.5186
	23	0.3651	0.2473	0.4960	0.2164	0.5347
	24	0.3810	0.2615	0.5120	0.2297	0.5506
	25	0.3968	0.2757	0.5280	0.2433	0.5664
	26	0.4127	0.2901	0.5438	0.2570	0.5819
	27	0.4286	0.3046	0.5595	0.2708	0.5974
	28	0.4444	0.3192	0.5751	0.2849	0.6126
	29	0.4603	0.3339	0.5906	0.2990	0.6277
	30	0.4762	0.3488	0.6059	0.3134	0.6427
	31	0.4921	0.3638	0.6211	0.3279	0.6575
	32	0.5079	0.3789	0.6362	0.3425	0.6721
	33	0.5238	0.3941	0.6512	0.3573	0.6866
	34	0.5397	0.4094	0.6661	0.3723	0.7010
	35	0.5556	0.4249	0.6808	0.3874	0.7151
	36	0.5714	0.4405	0.6954	0.4026	0.7292
	37	0.5873	0.4562	0.7099	0.4181	0.7430
	38	0.6032	0.4720	0.7243	0.4336	0.7567
	39	0.6190	0.4880	0.7385	0.4494	0.7703
	40	0.6349	0.5040	0.7527	0.4653	0.7836
	41	0.6508	0.5203	0.7666	0.4814	0.7968
	42	0.6667	0.5366	0.7805	0.4976	0.8098
	43	0.6825	0.5531	0.7942	0.5141	0.8226
	44	0.6984	0.5698	0.8077	0.5307	0.8353
	45	0.7143	0.5865	0.8211	0.5475	0.8477
	46	0.7302	0.6035	0.8343	0.5645	0.8599
	47	0.7460	0.6206	0.8473	0.5817	0.8719
	48	0.7619	0.6379	0.8602	0.5992	0.8837
	49	0.7778	0.6554	0.8728	0.6169	0.8952

Continued

Table B.11. Exact confidence limits for a binomial proportion: x events are observed in a sample sized n. $p = x/n$ is the observed proportion. p_l and p_u are the lower and upper confidence limits for the population proportion

n	x	p	95% p_l	95% p_u	99% p_l	99% p_u
63	50	0.7937	0.6730	0.8853	0.6348	0.9065
	51	0.8095	0.6909	0.8975	0.6530	0.9174
	52	0.8254	0.7090	0.9095	0.6716	0.9281
	53	0.8413	0.7274	0.9212	0.6904	0.9383
	54	0.8571	0.7461	0.9325	0.7096	0.9482
	55	0.8730	0.7650	0.9435	0.7292	0.9577
	56	0.8889	0.7844	0.9541	0.7493	0.9666
	57	0.9048	0.8041	0.9642	0.7700	0.9749
	58	0.9206	0.8244	0.9737	0.7912	0.9825
	59	0.9365	0.8453	0.9824	0.8133	0.9891
	60	0.9524	0.8671	0.9901	0.8364	0.9946
	61	0.9683	0.8900	0.9961	0.8610	0.9983
	62	0.9841	0.9147	0.9996	0.8879	0.9999
	63	1.0000	0.9431	1.0000	0.9193	1.0000
64	0	0.0000	0.0000	0.0560	0.0000	0.0795
	1	0.0156	0.0004	0.0840	0.0001	0.1104
	2	0.0313	0.0038	0.1084	0.0016	0.1369
	3	0.0469	0.0098	0.1309	0.0053	0.1612
	4	0.0625	0.0173	0.1524	0.0107	0.1840
	5	0.0781	0.0259	0.1730	0.0172	0.2057
	6	0.0938	0.0352	0.1930	0.0247	0.2267
	7	0.1094	0.0451	0.2125	0.0329	0.2471
	8	0.1250	0.0555	0.2315	0.0416	0.2669
	9	0.1406	0.0664	0.2502	0.0509	0.2862
	10	0.1563	0.0776	0.2686	0.0606	0.3052
	11	0.1719	0.0890	0.2868	0.0708	0.3238
	12	0.1875	0.1008	0.3046	0.0812	0.3421
	13	0.2031	0.1128	0.3223	0.0920	0.3601
	14	0.2188	0.1251	0.3397	0.1030	0.3778
	15	0.2344	0.1375	0.3569	0.1144	0.3953
	16	0.2500	0.1502	0.3740	0.1259	0.4125
	17	0.2656	0.1630	0.3909	0.1377	0.4295
	18	0.2813	0.1760	0.4076	0.1497	0.4463
	19	0.2969	0.1891	0.4242	0.1619	0.4629
	20	0.3125	0.2024	0.4406	0.1743	0.4794
	21	0.3281	0.2159	0.4569	0.1869	0.4956
	22	0.3438	0.2295	0.4730	0.1997	0.5117

n	x	p	95% p_l	95% p_u	99% p_l	99% p_u
65	2	0.0308	0.0037	0.1068	0.0016	0.1349
	3	0.0462	0.0096	0.1290	0.0053	0.1588
	4	0.0615	0.0170	0.1501	0.0105	0.1813
	5	0.0769	0.0254	0.1705	0.0170	0.2028
	6	0.0923	0.0346	0.1902	0.0243	0.2235
	7	0.1077	0.0444	0.2094	0.0323	0.2436
	8	0.1231	0.0547	0.2282	0.0410	0.2631
	9	0.1385	0.0653	0.2466	0.0501	0.2822
	10	0.1538	0.0763	0.2648	0.0597	0.3009
	11	0.1692	0.0876	0.2827	0.0696	0.3193
	12	0.1846	0.0992	0.3003	0.0799	0.3373
	13	0.2000	0.1110	0.3177	0.0905	0.3551
	14	0.2154	0.1231	0.3349	0.1014	0.3726
	15	0.2308	0.1353	0.3519	0.1125	0.3899
	16	0.2462	0.1477	0.3687	0.1238	0.4069
	17	0.2615	0.1603	0.3854	0.1354	0.4237
	18	0.2769	0.1731	0.4019	0.1472	0.4403
	19	0.2923	0.1860	0.4183	0.1592	0.4567
	20	0.3077	0.1991	0.4345	0.1714	0.4729
	21	0.3231	0.2123	0.4505	0.1838	0.4890
	22	0.3385	0.2257	0.4665	0.1964	0.5049
	23	0.3538	0.2392	0.4823	0.2091	0.5206
	24	0.3692	0.2528	0.4980	0.2220	0.5361
	25	0.3846	0.2665	0.5136	0.2350	0.5515
	26	0.4000	0.2804	0.5290	0.2482	0.5668
	27	0.4154	0.2944	0.5444	0.2616	0.5819
	28	0.4308	0.3085	0.5596	0.2751	0.5968
	29	0.4462	0.3227	0.5747	0.2888	0.6116
	30	0.4615	0.3370	0.5897	0.3026	0.6263
	31	0.4769	0.3515	0.6046	0.3165	0.6408
	32	0.4923	0.3660	0.6193	0.3306	0.6552
	33	0.5077	0.3807	0.6340	0.3448	0.6694
	34	0.5231	0.3954	0.6485	0.3592	0.6835
	35	0.5385	0.4103	0.6630	0.3737	0.6974
	36	0.5538	0.4253	0.6773	0.3884	0.7112
	37	0.5692	0.4404	0.6915	0.4032	0.7249
	38	0.5846	0.4556	0.7056	0.4181	0.7384
	39	0.6000	0.4710	0.7196	0.4332	0.7518

n	r					
64	23	0.3594	0.2432	0.4890	0.2127	0.5276
	24	0.3750	0.2570	0.5049	0.2258	0.5433
	25	0.3906	0.2710	0.5207	0.2391	0.5589
	26	0.4063	0.2851	0.5363	0.2525	0.5743
	27	0.4219	0.2994	0.5518	0.2661	0.5895
	28	0.4375	0.3137	0.5672	0.2799	0.6046
	29	0.4531	0.3282	0.5825	0.2938	0.6196
	30	0.4688	0.3428	0.5977	0.3079	0.6344
	31	0.4844	0.3575	0.6127	0.3221	0.6490
	32	0.5000	0.3723	0.6277	0.3364	0.6636
	33	0.5156	0.3873	0.6425	0.3510	0.6779
	34	0.5313	0.4023	0.6572	0.3656	0.6921
	35	0.5469	0.4175	0.6718	0.3804	0.7062
	36	0.5625	0.4328	0.6863	0.3954	0.7201
	37	0.5781	0.4482	0.7006	0.4105	0.7339
	38	0.5938	0.4637	0.7149	0.4257	0.7475
	39	0.6094	0.4793	0.7290	0.4411	0.7609
	40	0.6250	0.4951	0.7430	0.4567	0.7742
	41	0.6406	0.5110	0.7568	0.4724	0.7873
	42	0.6563	0.5270	0.7705	0.4883	0.8003
	43	0.6719	0.5431	0.7841	0.5044	0.8131
	44	0.6875	0.5594	0.7976	0.5206	0.8257
	45	0.7031	0.5758	0.8109	0.5371	0.8381
	46	0.7188	0.5924	0.8240	0.5537	0.8503
	47	0.7344	0.6091	0.8370	0.5705	0.8623
	48	0.7500	0.6260	0.8498	0.5875	0.8741
	49	0.7656	0.6431	0.8625	0.6047	0.8856
	50	0.7813	0.6603	0.8749	0.6222	0.8970
	51	0.7969	0.6777	0.8872	0.6399	0.9080
	52	0.8125	0.6954	0.8992	0.6579	0.9188
	53	0.8281	0.7132	0.9110	0.6762	0.9292
	54	0.8438	0.7314	0.9224	0.6948	0.9394
	55	0.8594	0.7498	0.9336	0.7138	0.9491
	56	0.8750	0.7685	0.9445	0.7331	0.9584
	57	0.8906	0.7875	0.9549	0.7529	0.9671
	58	0.9063	0.8070	0.9648	0.7733	0.9753
	59	0.9219	0.8270	0.9741	0.7943	0.9828
	60	0.9375	0.8476	0.9827	0.8160	0.9893
	61	0.9531	0.8691	0.9902	0.8388	0.9947
	62	0.9688	0.8916	0.9962	0.8631	0.9984
	63	0.9844	0.9160	0.9996	0.8896	0.9999
	64	1.0000	0.9440	1.0000	0.9205	1.0000
65	0	0.0000	0.0000	0.0552	0.0000	0.0783
	1	0.0154	0.0004	0.0828	0.0001	0.1088

n	r					
65	40	0.6154	0.4864	0.7335	0.4485	0.7650
	41	0.6308	0.5020	0.7472	0.4639	0.7780
	42	0.6462	0.5177	0.7608	0.4794	0.7909
	43	0.6615	0.5335	0.7743	0.4951	0.8036
	44	0.6769	0.5495	0.7877	0.5110	0.8162
	45	0.6923	0.5655	0.8009	0.5271	0.8286
	46	0.7077	0.5817	0.8140	0.5433	0.8408
	47	0.7231	0.5981	0.8269	0.5597	0.8528
	48	0.7385	0.6146	0.8397	0.5763	0.8646
	49	0.7538	0.6313	0.8523	0.5931	0.8762
	50	0.7692	0.6481	0.8647	0.6101	0.8875
	51	0.7846	0.6651	0.8769	0.6274	0.8986
	52	0.8000	0.6823	0.8890	0.6449	0.9095
	53	0.8154	0.6997	0.9008	0.6627	0.9201
	54	0.8308	0.7173	0.9124	0.6807	0.9304
	55	0.8462	0.7352	0.9237	0.6991	0.9403
	56	0.8615	0.7534	0.9347	0.7178	0.9499
	57	0.8769	0.7718	0.9453	0.7369	0.9590
	58	0.8923	0.7906	0.9556	0.7564	0.9677
	59	0.9077	0.8098	0.9654	0.7765	0.9757
	60	0.9231	0.8295	0.9746	0.7972	0.9830
	61	0.9385	0.8499	0.9830	0.8187	0.9895
	62	0.9538	0.8710	0.9904	0.8412	0.9947
	63	0.9692	0.8932	0.9963	0.8651	0.9984
	64	0.9846	0.9172	0.9996	0.8912	0.9999
	65	1.0000	0.9448	1.0000	0.9217	1.0000
66	0	0.0000	0.0000	0.0544	0.0000	0.0771
	1	0.0152	0.0004	0.0816	0.0001	0.1072
	2	0.0303	0.0037	0.1052	0.0016	0.1330
	3	0.0455	0.0095	0.1271	0.0052	0.1566
	4	0.0606	0.0168	0.1480	0.0104	0.1788
	5	0.0758	0.0251	0.1680	0.0167	0.1999
	6	0.0909	0.0341	0.1874	0.0239	0.2204
	7	0.1061	0.0437	0.2064	0.0318	0.2402
	8	0.1212	0.0538	0.2249	0.0403	0.2595
	9	0.1364	0.0643	0.2431	0.0493	0.2783
	10	0.1515	0.0751	0.2610	0.0587	0.2968
	11	0.1667	0.0862	0.2787	0.0685	0.3149
	12	0.1818	0.0976	0.2961	0.0786	0.3327
	13	0.1970	0.1093	0.3132	0.0890	0.3503
	14	0.2121	0.1211	0.3302	0.0997	0.3675
	15	0.2273	0.1331	0.3470	0.1107	0.3846
	16	0.2424	0.1454	0.3636	0.1218	0.4014
	17	0.2576	0.1578	0.3801	0.1332	0.4180

Continued

Table B.11. Exact confidence limits for a binomial proportion: x events are observed in a sample sized n. $p = x/n$ is the observed proportion. p_l and p_u are the lower and upper confidence limits for the population proportion

Confidence level

n	x	p	95% p_l	95% p_u	99% p_l	99% p_u
66	18	0.2727	0.1703	0.3964	0.1449	0.4344
	19	0.2879	0.1830	0.4125	0.1567	0.4506
	20	0.3030	0.1959	0.4285	0.1686	0.4667
	21	0.3182	0.2089	0.4444	0.1808	0.4825
	22	0.3333	0.2220	0.4601	0.1931	0.4982
	23	0.3485	0.2353	0.4758	0.2056	0.5138
	24	0.3636	0.2487	0.4913	0.2183	0.5292
	25	0.3788	0.2622	0.5066	0.2311	0.5444
	26	0.3939	0.2758	0.5219	0.2441	0.5595
	27	0.4091	0.2895	0.5371	0.2572	0.5744
	28	0.4242	0.3034	0.5521	0.2705	0.5892
	29	0.4394	0.3174	0.5670	0.2839	0.6039
	30	0.4545	0.3314	0.5819	0.2974	0.6184
	31	0.4697	0.3456	0.5966	0.3111	0.6328
	32	0.4848	0.3599	0.6112	0.3249	0.6470
	33	0.5000	0.3743	0.6257	0.3389	0.6611
	34	0.5152	0.3888	0.6401	0.3530	0.6751
	35	0.5303	0.4034	0.6544	0.3672	0.6889
	36	0.5455	0.4181	0.6686	0.3816	0.7026
	37	0.5606	0.4330	0.6826	0.3961	0.7161
	38	0.5758	0.4479	0.6966	0.4108	0.7295
	39	0.5909	0.4629	0.7105	0.4256	0.7428
	40	0.6061	0.4781	0.7242	0.4405	0.7559
	41	0.6212	0.4934	0.7378	0.4556	0.7689
	42	0.6364	0.5087	0.7513	0.4708	0.7817
	43	0.6515	0.5242	0.7647	0.4862	0.7944
	44	0.6667	0.5399	0.7780	0.5018	0.8069
	45	0.6818	0.5556	0.7911	0.5175	0.8192
	46	0.6970	0.5715	0.8041	0.5333	0.8314
	47	0.7121	0.5875	0.8170	0.5494	0.8433
	48	0.7273	0.6036	0.8297	0.5656	0.8551
	49	0.7424	0.6199	0.8422	0.5820	0.8668
	50	0.7576	0.6364	0.8546	0.5986	0.8782
	51	0.7727	0.6530	0.8669	0.6154	0.8893
	52	0.7879	0.6698	0.8789	0.6325	0.9003
	53	0.8030	0.6868	0.8907	0.6497	0.9110
	54	0.8182	0.7039	0.9024	0.6673	0.9214
	55	0.8333	0.7213	0.9138	0.6851	0.9315

Confidence level

n	x	p	95% p_l	95% p_u	99% p_l	99% p_u
67	34	0.5075	0.3824	0.6318	0.3470	0.6668
	35	0.5224	0.3967	0.6460	0.3610	0.6805
	36	0.5373	0.4112	0.6600	0.3751	0.6941
	37	0.5522	0.4258	0.6740	0.3893	0.7075
	38	0.5672	0.4404	0.6878	0.4037	0.7208
	39	0.5821	0.4552	0.7015	0.4182	0.7340
	40	0.5970	0.4700	0.7151	0.4328	0.7470
	41	0.6119	0.4850	0.7286	0.4476	0.7599
	42	0.6269	0.5001	0.7420	0.4626	0.7727
	43	0.6418	0.5153	0.7553	0.4776	0.7853
	44	0.6567	0.5306	0.7685	0.4928	0.7977
	45	0.6716	0.5460	0.7815	0.5082	0.8100
	46	0.6866	0.5616	0.7944	0.5237	0.8221
	47	0.7015	0.5773	0.8072	0.5394	0.8341
	48	0.7164	0.5931	0.8199	0.5553	0.8459
	49	0.7313	0.6090	0.8324	0.5713	0.8575
	50	0.7463	0.6251	0.8447	0.5875	0.8689
	51	0.7612	0.6414	0.8569	0.6039	0.8801
	52	0.7761	0.6578	0.8689	0.6205	0.8911
	53	0.7910	0.6743	0.8808	0.6374	0.9018
	54	0.8060	0.6911	0.8924	0.6544	0.9124
	55	0.8209	0.7080	0.9039	0.6718	0.9226
	56	0.8358	0.7252	0.9151	0.6893	0.9326
	57	0.8507	0.7426	0.9260	0.7072	0.9422
	58	0.8657	0.7603	0.9367	0.7255	0.9514
	59	0.8806	0.7782	0.9470	0.7441	0.9603
	60	0.8955	0.7965	0.9570	0.7631	0.9686
	61	0.9104	0.8152	0.9664	0.7827	0.9764
	62	0.9254	0.8344	0.9753	0.8028	0.9835
	63	0.9403	0.8541	0.9835	0.8237	0.9898
	64	0.9552	0.8747	0.9907	0.8456	0.9949
	65	0.9701	0.8963	0.9964	0.8689	0.9984
	66	0.9851	0.9196	0.9996	0.8943	0.9999
	67	1.0000	0.9464	1.0000	0.9240	1.0000
68	0	0.0000	0.0000	0.0528	0.0000	0.0750
	1	0.0147	0.0004	0.0792	0.0001	0.1042
	2	0.0294	0.0036	0.1022	0.0015	0.1293
	3	0.0441	0.0092	0.1236	0.0050	0.1522

66

	c1	c2	c3	c4	c5
56	0.8485	0.7390	0.9249	0.7032	0.9413
57	0.8636	0.7569	0.9357	0.7217	0.9507
58	0.8788	0.7751	0.9462	0.7405	0.9597
59	0.8939	0.7936	0.9563	0.7598	0.9682
60	0.9091	0.8126	0.9659	0.7796	0.9761
61	0.9242	0.8320	0.9749	0.8001	0.9833
62	0.9394	0.8520	0.9832	0.8212	0.9896
63	0.9545	0.8729	0.9905	0.8434	0.9948
64	0.9697	0.8948	0.9963	0.8670	0.9984
65	0.9848	0.9184	0.9996	0.8928	0.9999
66	1.0000	0.9456	1.0000	0.9229	1.0000

67

	c1	c2	c3	c4	c5
0	0.0000	0.0000	0.0536	0.0000	0.0760
1	0.0149	0.0004	0.0804	0.0001	0.1057
2	0.0299	0.0036	0.1037	0.0016	0.1311
3	0.0448	0.0093	0.1253	0.0051	0.1544
4	0.0597	0.0165	0.1459	0.0102	0.1763
5	0.0746	0.0247	0.1656	0.0165	0.1972
6	0.0896	0.0336	0.1848	0.0236	0.2173
7	0.1045	0.0430	0.2035	0.0314	0.2369
8	0.1194	0.0530	0.2218	0.0397	0.2559
9	0.1343	0.0633	0.2397	0.0486	0.2745
10	0.1493	0.0740	0.2574	0.0578	0.2928
11	0.1642	0.0849	0.2748	0.0674	0.3107
12	0.1791	0.0961	0.2920	0.0774	0.3282
13	0.1940	0.1076	0.3089	0.0876	0.3456
14	0.2090	0.1192	0.3257	0.0982	0.3626
15	0.2239	0.1311	0.3422	0.1089	0.3795
16	0.2388	0.1431	0.3586	0.1199	0.3961
17	0.2537	0.1553	0.3749	0.1311	0.4125
18	0.2687	0.1676	0.3910	0.1425	0.4287
19	0.2836	0.1801	0.4069	0.1541	0.4447
20	0.2985	0.1928	0.4227	0.1659	0.4606
21	0.3134	0.2056	0.4384	0.1779	0.4763
22	0.3284	0.2185	0.4540	0.1900	0.4918
23	0.3433	0.2315	0.4694	0.2023	0.5072
24	0.3582	0.2447	0.4847	0.2147	0.5224
25	0.3731	0.2580	0.4999	0.2273	0.5374
26	0.3881	0.2714	0.5150	0.2401	0.5524
27	0.4030	0.2849	0.5300	0.2530	0.5672
28	0.4179	0.2985	0.5448	0.2660	0.5818
29	0.4328	0.3122	0.5596	0.2792	0.5963
30	0.4478	0.3260	0.5742	0.2925	0.6107
31	0.4627	0.3400	0.5888	0.3059	0.6249
32	0.4776	0.3540	0.6033	0.3195	0.6390
33	0.4925	0.3682	0.6176	0.3332	0.6530

68

	c1	c2	c3	c4	c5
4	0.0588	0.0163	0.1438	0.0101	0.1738
5	0.0735	0.0243	0.1633	0.0162	0.1945
6	0.0882	0.0331	0.1822	0.0232	0.2144
7	0.1029	0.0424	0.2007	0.0309	0.2337
8	0.1176	0.0522	0.2187	0.0391	0.2525
9	0.1324	0.0623	0.2364	0.0478	0.2708
10	0.1471	0.0728	0.2539	0.0569	0.2888
11	0.1618	0.0836	0.2710	0.0664	0.3065
12	0.1765	0.0947	0.2880	0.0762	0.3239
13	0.1912	0.1059	0.3047	0.0863	0.3410
14	0.2059	0.1174	0.3212	0.0966	0.3578
15	0.2206	0.1290	0.3376	0.1072	0.3745
16	0.2353	0.1409	0.3538	0.1180	0.3909
17	0.2500	0.1529	0.3698	0.1291	0.4071
18	0.2647	0.1650	0.3857	0.1403	0.4231
19	0.2794	0.1773	0.4015	0.1517	0.4390
20	0.2941	0.1898	0.4171	0.1633	0.4546
21	0.3088	0.2024	0.4326	0.1751	0.4702
22	0.3235	0.2151	0.4479	0.1870	0.4855
23	0.3382	0.2279	0.4632	0.1991	0.5007
24	0.3529	0.2408	0.4783	0.2113	0.5158
25	0.3676	0.2539	0.4933	0.2237	0.5307
26	0.3824	0.2671	0.5082	0.2362	0.5454
27	0.3971	0.2803	0.5230	0.2489	0.5600
28	0.4118	0.2937	0.5377	0.2617	0.5745
29	0.4265	0.3072	0.5523	0.2746	0.5889
30	0.4412	0.3208	0.5668	0.2877	0.6031
31	0.4559	0.3345	0.5812	0.3009	0.6172
32	0.4706	0.3483	0.5955	0.3142	0.6312
33	0.4853	0.3622	0.6097	0.3277	0.6450
34	0.5000	0.3762	0.6238	0.3412	0.6588
35	0.5147	0.3903	0.6378	0.3550	0.6723
36	0.5294	0.4045	0.6517	0.3688	0.6858
37	0.5441	0.4188	0.6655	0.3828	0.6991
38	0.5588	0.4332	0.6792	0.3969	0.7123
39	0.5735	0.4477	0.6928	0.4111	0.7254
40	0.5882	0.4623	0.7063	0.4255	0.7383
41	0.6029	0.4770	0.7197	0.4400	0.7511
42	0.6176	0.4918	0.7329	0.4546	0.7638
43	0.6324	0.5067	0.7461	0.4693	0.7763
44	0.6471	0.5217	0.7592	0.4842	0.7887
45	0.6618	0.5368	0.7721	0.4993	0.8009
46	0.6765	0.5521	0.7849	0.5145	0.8130
47	0.6912	0.5674	0.7976	0.5298	0.8249
48	0.7059	0.5829	0.8102	0.5454	0.8367

Continued

Table B.11. Exact confidence limits for a binomial proportion: x events are observed in a sample sized n. $p = x/n$ is the observed proportion. p_l and p_u are the lower and upper confidence limits for the population proportion

n	x	p	95% p_l	95% p_u	99% p_l	99% p_u
68	49	0.7206	0.5985	0.8227	0.5610	0.8483
	50	0.7353	0.6143	0.8350	0.5769	0.8597
	51	0.7500	0.6302	0.8471	0.5929	0.8709
	52	0.7647	0.6462	0.8591	0.6091	0.8820
	53	0.7794	0.6624	0.8710	0.6255	0.8928
	54	0.7941	0.6788	0.8826	0.6422	0.9034
	55	0.8088	0.6953	0.8941	0.6590	0.9137
	56	0.8235	0.7120	0.9053	0.6761	0.9238
	57	0.8382	0.7290	0.9164	0.6935	0.9336
	58	0.8529	0.7461	0.9272	0.7112	0.9431
	59	0.8676	0.7636	0.9377	0.7292	0.9522
	60	0.8824	0.7813	0.9478	0.7475	0.9609
	61	0.8971	0.7993	0.9576	0.7663	0.9691
	62	0.9118	0.8178	0.9669	0.7856	0.9768
	63	0.9265	0.8367	0.9757	0.8055	0.9838
	64	0.9412	0.8562	0.9837	0.8262	0.9899
	65	0.9559	0.8764	0.9908	0.8478	0.9950
	66	0.9706	0.8978	0.9964	0.8707	0.9985
	67	0.9853	0.9208	0.9996	0.8958	0.9999
	68	1.0000	0.9472	1.0000	0.9250	1.0000
69	0	0.0000	0.0000	0.0521	0.0000	0.0739
	1	0.0145	0.0004	0.0781	0.0001	0.1028
	2	0.0290	0.0035	0.1008	0.0015	0.1275
	3	0.0435	0.0091	0.1218	0.0050	0.1502
	4	0.0580	0.0160	0.1418	0.0099	0.1715
	5	0.0725	0.0239	0.1611	0.0160	0.1918
	6	0.0870	0.0326	0.1797	0.0229	0.2115
	7	0.1014	0.0418	0.1979	0.0304	0.2305
	8	0.1159	0.0514	0.2157	0.0385	0.2491
	9	0.1304	0.0614	0.2332	0.0471	0.2672
	10	0.1449	0.0717	0.2504	0.0561	0.2850
	11	0.1594	0.0824	0.2674	0.0654	0.3025
	12	0.1739	0.0932	0.2841	0.0750	0.3196
	13	0.1884	0.1043	0.3006	0.0850	0.3365
	14	0.2029	0.1156	0.3169	0.0951	0.3532
	15	0.2174	0.1271	0.3331	0.1056	0.3696
	16	0.2319	0.1387	0.3491	0.1162	0.3858
	17	0.2464	0.1505	0.3649	0.1271	0.4019

n	x	p	95% p_l	95% p_u	99% p_l	99% p_u
69	64	0.9275	0.8389	0.9761	0.8082	0.9840
	65	0.9420	0.8582	0.9840	0.8285	0.9901
	66	0.9565	0.8782	0.9909	0.8498	0.9950
	67	0.9710	0.8992	0.9965	0.8725	0.9985
	68	0.9855	0.9219	0.9996	0.8972	0.9999
	69	1.0000	0.9479	1.0000	0.9261	1.0000
70	0	0.0000	0.0000	0.0513	0.0000	0.0729
	1	0.0143	0.0004	0.0770	0.0001	0.1014
	2	0.0286	0.0035	0.0994	0.0015	0.1258
	3	0.0429	0.0089	0.1202	0.0049	0.1481
	4	0.0571	0.0158	0.1399	0.0098	0.1692
	5	0.0714	0.0236	0.1589	0.0157	0.1893
	6	0.0857	0.0321	0.1773	0.0225	0.2087
	7	0.1000	0.0412	0.1952	0.0300	0.2275
	8	0.1143	0.0507	0.2128	0.0380	0.2458
	9	0.1286	0.0605	0.2301	0.0464	0.2637
	10	0.1429	0.0707	0.2471	0.0552	0.2813
	11	0.1571	0.0811	0.2638	0.0644	0.2985
	12	0.1714	0.0918	0.2803	0.0739	0.3155
	13	0.1857	0.1028	0.2966	0.0837	0.3322
	14	0.2000	0.1139	0.3127	0.0937	0.3486
	15	0.2143	0.1252	0.3287	0.1040	0.3649
	16	0.2286	0.1367	0.3445	0.1145	0.3809
	17	0.2429	0.1483	0.3601	0.1251	0.3967
	18	0.2571	0.1601	0.3756	0.1360	0.4124
	19	0.2714	0.1720	0.3910	0.1471	0.4279
	20	0.2857	0.1840	0.4062	0.1583	0.4432
	21	0.3000	0.1962	0.4213	0.1697	0.4584
	22	0.3143	0.2085	0.4363	0.1812	0.4734
	23	0.3286	0.2209	0.4512	0.1929	0.4882
	24	0.3429	0.2335	0.4660	0.2047	0.5030
	25	0.3571	0.2461	0.4807	0.2167	0.5176
	26	0.3714	0.2589	0.4952	0.2288	0.5320
	27	0.3857	0.2717	0.5097	0.2411	0.5463
	28	0.4000	0.2847	0.5241	0.2534	0.5605
	29	0.4143	0.2977	0.5383	0.2659	0.5746
	30	0.4286	0.3109	0.5525	0.2785	0.5886
	31	0.4429	0.3241	0.5666	0.2913	0.6024

70 / 71

Continued

S							
32	0.6161	0.3042	0.5806	0.3374	0.4571		0.4177
33	0.6297	0.3172	0.5945	0.3509	0.4714		0.4334
34	0.6432	0.3303	0.6083	0.3644	0.4857		0.4489
35	0.6565	0.3435	0.6220	0.3780	0.5000		0.4642
36	0.6697	0.3568	0.6356	0.3917	0.5143		0.4794
37	0.6828	0.3703	0.6491	0.4055	0.5286		0.4944
38	0.6958	0.3839	0.6626	0.4194	0.5429		0.5093
39	0.7087	0.3976	0.6759	0.4334	0.5571		0.5240
40	0.7215	0.4114	0.6891	0.4475	0.5714		0.5386
41	0.7341	0.4254	0.7023	0.4617	0.5857		0.5531
42	0.7466	0.4395	0.7153	0.4759	0.6000		0.5675
43	0.7589	0.4537	0.7283	0.4903	0.6143		0.5817
44	0.7712	0.4680	0.7411	0.5048	0.6286		0.5958
45	0.7833	0.4824	0.7539	0.5193	0.6429		0.6097
46	0.7953	0.4970	0.7665	0.5340	0.6571		0.6236
47	0.8071	0.5118	0.7791	0.5488	0.6714		0.6373
48	0.8188	0.5266	0.7915	0.5637	0.6857		0.6509
49	0.8303	0.5416	0.8038	0.5787	0.7000		0.6643
50	0.8417	0.5568	0.8160	0.5938	0.7143		0.6777
51	0.8529	0.5721	0.8280	0.6090	0.7286		0.6909
52	0.8640	0.5876	0.8399	0.6244	0.7429		0.7040
53	0.8749	0.6033	0.8517	0.6399	0.7571		0.7170
54	0.8855	0.6191	0.8633	0.6555	0.7714		0.7298
55	0.8960	0.6351	0.8748	0.6713	0.7857		0.7425
56	0.9063	0.6514	0.8861	0.6873	0.8000		0.7551
57	0.9163	0.6678	0.8972	0.7034	0.8143		0.7676
58	0.9261	0.6845	0.9082	0.7197	0.8286		0.7799
59	0.9356	0.7015	0.9189	0.7362	0.8429		0.7920
60	0.9448	0.7187	0.9293	0.7529	0.8571		0.8041
61	0.9536	0.7363	0.9395	0.7699	0.8714		0.8160
62	0.9620	0.7542	0.9493	0.7872	0.8857		0.8277
63	0.9700	0.7725	0.9588	0.8048	0.9000		0.8393
64	0.9775	0.7913	0.9679	0.8227	0.9143		0.8507
65	0.9843	0.8107	0.9764	0.8411	0.9286		0.8619
66	0.9902	0.8308	0.9842	0.8601	0.9429		0.8729
67	0.9951	0.8519	0.9911	0.8798	0.9571		0.8838
68	0.9985	0.8742	0.9965	0.9006	0.9714		0.8944
69	0.9999	0.8986	0.9996	0.9230	0.9857		0.9049
70	1.0000	0.9271	1.0000	0.9487	1.0000		0.9150

71

S						
0	0.0719	0.0000	0.0506	0.0000	0.0000	0.9250
1	0.1000	0.0001	0.0760	0.0004	0.0141	0.9346
2	0.1241	0.0015	0.0981	0.0034	0.0282	0.9439
3	0.1462	0.0048	0.1186	0.0088	0.0423	0.9529
4	0.1669	0.0096	0.1380	0.0156	0.0563	0.9615
5	0.1868	0.0155	0.1567	0.0233	0.0704	0.9696
						0.9771

69

S					
18	0.2609	0.1625	0.3806	0.1381	0.4177
19	0.2754	0.1746	0.3962	0.1493	0.4334
20	0.2899	0.1869	0.4116	0.1607	0.4489
21	0.3043	0.1992	0.4269	0.1723	0.4642
22	0.3188	0.2117	0.4421	0.1840	0.4794
23	0.3333	0.2244	0.4571	0.1959	0.4944
24	0.3478	0.2371	0.4721	0.2080	0.5093
25	0.3623	0.2499	0.4869	0.2201	0.5240
26	0.3768	0.2629	0.5017	0.2324	0.5386
27	0.3913	0.2760	0.5163	0.2449	0.5531
28	0.4058	0.2891	0.5308	0.2575	0.5675
29	0.4203	0.3024	0.5452	0.2702	0.5817
30	0.4348	0.3158	0.5596	0.2830	0.5958
31	0.4493	0.3292	0.5738	0.2960	0.6097
32	0.4638	0.3428	0.5880	0.3091	0.6236
33	0.4783	0.3565	0.6020	0.3223	0.6373
34	0.4928	0.3702	0.6159	0.3357	0.6509
35	0.5072	0.3841	0.6298	0.3491	0.6643
36	0.5217	0.3980	0.6435	0.3627	0.6777
37	0.5362	0.4120	0.6572	0.3764	0.6909
38	0.5507	0.4262	0.6708	0.3903	0.7040
39	0.5652	0.4404	0.6842	0.4042	0.7170
40	0.5797	0.4548	0.6976	0.4183	0.7298
41	0.5942	0.4692	0.7109	0.4325	0.7425
42	0.6087	0.4837	0.7240	0.4469	0.7551
43	0.6232	0.4983	0.7371	0.4614	0.7676
44	0.6377	0.5131	0.7501	0.4760	0.7799
45	0.6522	0.5279	0.7629	0.4907	0.7920
46	0.6667	0.5429	0.7756	0.5056	0.8041
47	0.6812	0.5579	0.7883	0.5206	0.8160
48	0.6957	0.5731	0.8008	0.5358	0.8277
49	0.7101	0.5884	0.8131	0.5511	0.8393
50	0.7246	0.6038	0.8254	0.5666	0.8507
51	0.7391	0.6194	0.8375	0.5823	0.8619
52	0.7536	0.6351	0.8495	0.5981	0.8729
53	0.7681	0.6509	0.8613	0.6142	0.8838
54	0.7826	0.6669	0.8729	0.6304	0.8944
55	0.7971	0.6831	0.8844	0.6468	0.9049
56	0.8116	0.6994	0.8957	0.6635	0.9150
57	0.8261	0.7159	0.9068	0.6804	0.9250
58	0.8406	0.7326	0.9176	0.6975	0.9346
59	0.8551	0.7496	0.9283	0.7150	0.9439
60	0.8696	0.7668	0.9386	0.7328	0.9529
61	0.8841	0.7843	0.9486	0.7509	0.9615
62	0.8986	0.8021	0.9582	0.7695	0.9696
63	0.9130	0.8203	0.9674	0.7885	0.9771

Table B.11. Exact confidence limits for a binomial proportion: x events are observed in a sample sized n. $p = x/n$ is the observed proportion. p_l and p_u are the lower and upper confidence limits for the population proportion

n	x	p	95% p_l	95% p_u	99% p_l	99% p_u
71	6	0.0845	0.0316	0.1749	0.0222	0.2059
	7	0.0986	0.0406	0.1926	0.0295	0.2245
	8	0.1127	0.0499	0.2100	0.0374	0.2426
	9	0.1268	0.0596	0.2270	0.0457	0.2603
	10	0.1408	0.0697	0.2438	0.0544	0.2777
	11	0.1549	0.0800	0.2603	0.0635	0.2947
	12	0.1690	0.0905	0.2766	0.0728	0.3114
	13	0.1831	0.1013	0.2927	0.0824	0.3279
	14	0.1972	0.1122	0.3086	0.0923	0.3442
	15	0.2113	0.1233	0.3244	0.1024	0.3602
	16	0.2254	0.1346	0.3400	0.1127	0.3761
	17	0.2394	0.1461	0.3554	0.1233	0.3917
	18	0.2535	0.1577	0.3708	0.1340	0.4072
	19	0.2676	0.1694	0.3859	0.1448	0.4225
	20	0.2817	0.1813	0.4010	0.1559	0.4377
	21	0.2958	0.1933	0.4159	0.1671	0.4527
	22	0.3099	0.2054	0.4308	0.1784	0.4675
	23	0.3239	0.2176	0.4455	0.1899	0.4822
	24	0.3380	0.2300	0.4601	0.2016	0.4968
	25	0.3521	0.2424	0.4746	0.2134	0.5112
	26	0.3662	0.2550	0.4890	0.2253	0.5256
	27	0.3803	0.2676	0.5033	0.2373	0.5397
	28	0.3944	0.2803	0.5175	0.2495	0.5538
	29	0.4085	0.2932	0.5316	0.2618	0.5677
	30	0.4225	0.3061	0.5456	0.2742	0.5815
	31	0.4366	0.3191	0.5595	0.2867	0.5952
	32	0.4507	0.3323	0.5734	0.2994	0.6088
	33	0.4648	0.3455	0.5871	0.3122	0.6223
	34	0.4789	0.3588	0.6008	0.3250	0.6356
	35	0.4930	0.3722	0.6144	0.3380	0.6488
	36	0.5070	0.3856	0.6278	0.3512	0.6620
	37	0.5211	0.3992	0.6412	0.3644	0.6750
	38	0.5352	0.4129	0.6545	0.3777	0.6878
	39	0.5493	0.4266	0.6677	0.3912	0.7006
	40	0.5634	0.4405	0.6809	0.4048	0.7133
	41	0.5775	0.4544	0.6939	0.4185	0.7258
	42	0.5915	0.4684	0.7068	0.4323	0.7382
	43	0.6056	0.4825	0.7197	0.4462	0.7505

n	x	p	95% p_l	95% p_u	99% p_l	99% p_u
72	16	0.2222	0.1327	0.3356	0.1111	0.3714
	17	0.2361	0.1440	0.3509	0.1214	0.3869
	18	0.2500	0.1554	0.3660	0.1320	0.4022
	19	0.2639	0.1670	0.3810	0.1427	0.4173
	20	0.2778	0.1786	0.3959	0.1536	0.4323
	21	0.2917	0.1905	0.4107	0.1646	0.4471
	22	0.3056	0.2024	0.4253	0.1758	0.4618
	23	0.3194	0.2144	0.4399	0.1871	0.4764
	24	0.3333	0.2266	0.4543	0.1986	0.4908
	25	0.3472	0.2388	0.4686	0.2101	0.5051
	26	0.3611	0.2512	0.4829	0.2219	0.5192
	27	0.3750	0.2636	0.4970	0.2337	0.5333
	28	0.3889	0.2762	0.5111	0.2457	0.5472
	29	0.4028	0.2888	0.5250	0.2578	0.5610
	30	0.4167	0.3015	0.5389	0.2700	0.5747
	31	0.4306	0.3143	0.5527	0.2823	0.5882
	32	0.4444	0.3272	0.5664	0.2948	0.6017
	33	0.4583	0.3402	0.5800	0.3073	0.6150
	34	0.4722	0.3533	0.5935	0.3200	0.6282
	35	0.4861	0.3665	0.6069	0.3328	0.6413
	36	0.5000	0.3798	0.6202	0.3457	0.6543
	37	0.5139	0.3931	0.6335	0.3587	0.6672
	38	0.5278	0.4065	0.6467	0.3718	0.6800
	39	0.5417	0.4200	0.6598	0.3850	0.6927
	40	0.5556	0.4336	0.6728	0.3983	0.7052
	41	0.5694	0.4473	0.6857	0.4118	0.7177
	42	0.5833	0.4611	0.6985	0.4253	0.7300
	43	0.5972	0.4750	0.7112	0.4390	0.7422
	44	0.6111	0.4889	0.7238	0.4528	0.7543
	45	0.6250	0.5030	0.7364	0.4667	0.7663
	46	0.6389	0.5171	0.7488	0.4808	0.7781
	47	0.6528	0.5314	0.7612	0.4949	0.7899
	48	0.6667	0.5457	0.7734	0.5092	0.8014
	49	0.6806	0.5601	0.7856	0.5236	0.8129
	50	0.6944	0.5747	0.7976	0.5382	0.8242
	51	0.7083	0.5893	0.8095	0.5529	0.8354
	52	0.7222	0.6041	0.8214	0.5677	0.8464
	53	0.7361	0.6190	0.8330	0.5827	0.8573

n	k					
71	44	0.6197	0.4967	0.7324	0.4603	0.7627
	45	0.6338	0.5110	0.7450	0.4744	0.7747
	46	0.6479	0.5254	0.7576	0.4888	0.7866
	47	0.6620	0.5399	0.7700	0.5032	0.7984
	48	0.6761	0.5545	0.7824	0.5178	0.8101
	49	0.6901	0.5692	0.7946	0.5325	0.8216
	50	0.7042	0.5841	0.8067	0.5473	0.8329
	51	0.7183	0.5990	0.8187	0.5623	0.8441
	52	0.7324	0.6141	0.8306	0.5775	0.8552
	53	0.7465	0.6292	0.8423	0.5928	0.8660
	54	0.7606	0.6446	0.8539	0.6083	0.8767
	55	0.7746	0.6600	0.8654	0.6239	0.8873
	56	0.7887	0.6756	0.8767	0.6398	0.8976
	57	0.8028	0.6914	0.8878	0.6558	0.9077
	58	0.8169	0.7073	0.8987	0.6721	0.9176
	59	0.8310	0.7234	0.9095	0.6886	0.9272
	60	0.8451	0.7397	0.9200	0.7053	0.9365
	61	0.8592	0.7562	0.9303	0.7223	0.9456
	62	0.8732	0.7730	0.9404	0.7397	0.9543
	63	0.8873	0.7900	0.9501	0.7574	0.9626
	64	0.9014	0.8074	0.9594	0.7755	0.9705
	65	0.9155	0.8251	0.9684	0.7941	0.9778
	66	0.9296	0.8433	0.9767	0.8132	0.9845
	67	0.9437	0.8620	0.9844	0.8331	0.9904
	68	0.9577	0.8814	0.9912	0.8538	0.9952
	69	0.9718	0.9019	0.9966	0.8759	0.9985
	70	0.9859	0.9240	0.9996	0.9000	0.9999
	71	1.0000	0.9494	1.0000	0.9281	1.0000
72	0	0.0000	0.0000	0.0499	0.0000	0.0709
	1	0.0139	0.0004	0.0750	0.0001	0.0987
	2	0.0278	0.0034	0.0968	0.0014	0.1225
	3	0.0417	0.0087	0.1170	0.0047	0.1442
	4	0.0556	0.0153	0.1362	0.0095	0.1648
	5	0.0694	0.0229	0.1547	0.0153	0.1844
	6	0.0833	0.0312	0.1726	0.0219	0.2033
	7	0.0972	0.0400	0.1901	0.0291	0.2216
	8	0.1111	0.0492	0.2072	0.0369	0.2395
	9	0.1250	0.0588	0.2241	0.0451	0.2570
	10	0.1389	0.0687	0.2406	0.0536	0.2741
	11	0.1528	0.0788	0.2569	0.0626	0.2909
	12	0.1667	0.0892	0.2730	0.0718	0.3075
	13	0.1806	0.0998	0.2889	0.0812	0.3238
	14	0.1944	0.1106	0.3047	0.0910	0.3399
	15	0.2083	0.1216	0.3202	0.1009	0.3557

n	k					
72	54	0.8680	0.5978	0.8446	0.6340	0.7500
	55	0.8786	0.6131	0.8560	0.6491	0.7639
	56	0.8889	0.6286	0.8673	0.6644	0.7778
	57	0.8991	0.6443	0.8784	0.6798	0.7917
	58	0.9090	0.6601	0.8894	0.6953	0.8056
	59	0.9188	0.6762	0.9002	0.7111	0.8194
	60	0.9282	0.6925	0.9108	0.7270	0.8333
	61	0.9374	0.7091	0.9212	0.7431	0.8472
	62	0.9464	0.7259	0.9313	0.7594	0.8611
	63	0.9549	0.7430	0.9412	0.7759	0.8750
	64	0.9631	0.7605	0.9508	0.7928	0.8889
	65	0.9709	0.7784	0.9600	0.8099	0.9028
	66	0.9781	0.7967	0.9688	0.8274	0.9167
	67	0.9847	0.8156	0.9771	0.8453	0.9306
	68	0.9905	0.8352	0.9847	0.8638	0.9444
	69	0.9953	0.8558	0.9913	0.8830	0.9583
	70	0.9986	0.8775	0.9966	0.9032	0.9722
	71	0.9999	0.9013	0.9996	0.9250	0.9861
	72	1.0000	0.9291	1.0000	0.9501	1.0000
73	0	0.0700	0.0000	0.0493	0.0000	0.0000
	1	0.0974	0.0001	0.0740	0.0003	0.0137
	2	0.1209	0.0014	0.0955	0.0033	0.0274
	3	0.1424	0.0047	0.1154	0.0086	0.0411
	4	0.1626	0.0094	0.1344	0.0151	0.0548
	5	0.1820	0.0151	0.1526	0.0226	0.0685
	6	0.2007	0.0216	0.1704	0.0308	0.0822
	7	0.2188	0.0287	0.1876	0.0394	0.0959
	8	0.2365	0.0363	0.2046	0.0485	0.1096
	9	0.2537	0.0444	0.2212	0.0580	0.1233
	10	0.2707	0.0529	0.2375	0.0677	0.1370
	11	0.2873	0.0617	0.2536	0.0777	0.1507
	12	0.3037	0.0707	0.2695	0.0879	0.1644
	13	0.3198	0.0801	0.2853	0.0984	0.1781
	14	0.3357	0.0897	0.3008	0.1090	0.1918
	15	0.3513	0.0995	0.3162	0.1198	0.2055
	16	0.3668	0.1095	0.3314	0.1308	0.2192
	17	0.3821	0.1197	0.3465	0.1419	0.2329
	18	0.3973	0.1301	0.3614	0.1532	0.2466
	19	0.4122	0.1406	0.3762	0.1645	0.2603
	20	0.4271	0.1513	0.3909	0.1761	0.2740
	21	0.4417	0.1622	0.4055	0.1877	0.2877
	22	0.4563	0.1732	0.4200	0.1994	0.3014
	23	0.4707	0.1843	0.4344	0.2113	0.3151
	24	0.4849	0.1956	0.4487	0.2233	0.3288

Continued

Table B.11. Exact confidence limits for a binomial proportion: x events are observed in a sample sized n. $p = x/n$ is the observed proportion. p_l and p_u are the lower and upper confidence limits for the population proportion

n	x	p	95% p_l	95% p_u	99% p_l	99% p_u
73	25	0.3425	0.2353	0.4628	0.2070	0.4991
	26	0.3562	0.2475	0.4769	0.2186	0.5131
	27	0.3699	0.2597	0.4909	0.2302	0.5270
	28	0.3836	0.2721	0.5048	0.2420	0.5407
	29	0.3973	0.2845	0.5186	0.2539	0.5544
	30	0.4110	0.2971	0.5323	0.2659	0.5679
	31	0.4247	0.3097	0.5459	0.2780	0.5814
	32	0.4384	0.3224	0.5595	0.2903	0.5947
	33	0.4521	0.3352	0.5730	0.3026	0.6079
	34	0.4658	0.3480	0.5863	0.3151	0.6210
	35	0.4795	0.3610	0.5996	0.3277	0.6340
	36	0.4932	0.3740	0.6128	0.3403	0.6469
	37	0.5068	0.3872	0.6260	0.3531	0.6597
	38	0.5205	0.4004	0.6390	0.3660	0.6723
	39	0.5342	0.4137	0.6520	0.3790	0.6849
	40	0.5479	0.4270	0.6648	0.3921	0.6974
	41	0.5616	0.4405	0.6776	0.4053	0.7097
	42	0.5753	0.4541	0.6903	0.4186	0.7220
	43	0.5890	0.4677	0.7029	0.4321	0.7341
	44	0.6027	0.4814	0.7155	0.4456	0.7461
	45	0.6164	0.4952	0.7279	0.4593	0.7580
	46	0.6301	0.5091	0.7403	0.4730	0.7698
	47	0.6438	0.5231	0.7525	0.4869	0.7814
	48	0.6575	0.5372	0.7647	0.5009	0.7930
	49	0.6712	0.5513	0.7767	0.5151	0.8044
	50	0.6849	0.5656	0.7887	0.5293	0.8157
	51	0.6986	0.5800	0.8006	0.5437	0.8268
	52	0.7123	0.5945	0.8123	0.5583	0.8378
	53	0.7260	0.6091	0.8239	0.5729	0.8487
	54	0.7397	0.6238	0.8355	0.5878	0.8594
	55	0.7534	0.6386	0.8468	0.6027	0.8699
	56	0.7671	0.6535	0.8581	0.6179	0.8803
	57	0.7808	0.6686	0.8692	0.6332	0.8905
	58	0.7945	0.6838	0.8802	0.6487	0.9005
	59	0.8082	0.6992	0.8910	0.6643	0.9103
	60	0.8219	0.7147	0.9016	0.6802	0.9199
	61	0.8356	0.7305	0.9121	0.6963	0.9293
	62	0.8493	0.7464	0.9223	0.7127	0.9383

n	x	p	95% p_l	95% p_u	99% p_l	99% p_u
74	33	0.4459	0.3302	0.5661	0.2981	0.6010
	34	0.4595	0.3429	0.5793	0.3103	0.6139
	35	0.4730	0.3557	0.5925	0.3227	0.6268
	36	0.4865	0.3685	0.6056	0.3352	0.6396
	37	0.5000	0.3814	0.6186	0.3477	0.6523
	38	0.5135	0.3944	0.6315	0.3604	0.6648
	39	0.5270	0.4075	0.6443	0.3732	0.6773
	40	0.5405	0.4207	0.6571	0.3861	0.6897
	41	0.5541	0.4339	0.6698	0.3990	0.7019
	42	0.5676	0.4472	0.6823	0.4121	0.7141
	43	0.5811	0.4606	0.6949	0.4253	0.7261
	44	0.5946	0.4741	0.7073	0.4386	0.7380
	45	0.6081	0.4877	0.7196	0.4521	0.7499
	46	0.6216	0.5013	0.7319	0.4656	0.7616
	47	0.6351	0.5151	0.7440	0.4792	0.7732
	48	0.6486	0.5289	0.7561	0.4930	0.7847
	49	0.6622	0.5428	0.7681	0.5068	0.7960
	50	0.6757	0.5568	0.7800	0.5208	0.8073
	51	0.6892	0.5710	0.7917	0.5349	0.8184
	52	0.7027	0.5852	0.8034	0.5492	0.8293
	53	0.7162	0.5995	0.8150	0.5636	0.8402
	54	0.7297	0.6139	0.8265	0.5781	0.8509
	55	0.7432	0.6284	0.8378	0.5927	0.8614
	56	0.7568	0.6431	0.8490	0.6075	0.8718
	57	0.7703	0.6579	0.8601	0.6225	0.8820
	58	0.7838	0.6728	0.8711	0.6376	0.8921
	59	0.7973	0.6878	0.8819	0.6530	0.9020
	60	0.8108	0.7030	0.8925	0.6685	0.9116
	61	0.8243	0.7183	0.9030	0.6842	0.9211
	62	0.8378	0.7339	0.9133	0.7001	0.9303
	63	0.8514	0.7496	0.9234	0.7163	0.9392
	64	0.8649	0.7655	0.9332	0.7327	0.9479
	65	0.8784	0.7816	0.9429	0.7494	0.9562
	66	0.8919	0.7980	0.9522	0.7665	0.9642
	67	0.9054	0.8148	0.9611	0.7840	0.9717
	68	0.9189	0.8318	0.9697	0.8019	0.9787
	69	0.9324	0.8493	0.9777	0.8203	0.9851
	70	0.9459	0.8673	0.9851	0.8394	0.9908

73 / 74

Index					
63	0.8630	0.7625	0.9323	0.7293	0.9471
64	0.8767	0.7788	0.9420	0.7463	0.9556
65	0.8904	0.7954	0.9515	0.7635	0.9637
66	0.9041	0.8124	0.9606	0.7812	0.9713
67	0.9178	0.8296	0.9692	0.7993	0.9784
68	0.9315	0.8474	0.9774	0.8180	0.9849
69	0.9452	0.8656	0.9849	0.8374	0.9906
70	0.9589	0.8846	0.9914	0.8576	0.9953
71	0.9726	0.9045	0.9967	0.8791	0.9986
72	0.9863	0.9260	0.9997	0.9026	0.9999
73	1.0000	0.9507	1.0000	0.9300	1.0000
0	0.0000	0.0000	0.0486	0.0000	0.0691
1	0.0135	0.0003	0.0730	0.0001	0.0962
2	0.0270	0.0033	0.0942	0.0014	0.1193
3	0.0405	0.0084	0.1139	0.0046	0.1406
4	0.0541	0.0149	0.1327	0.0092	0.1606
5	0.0676	0.0223	0.1507	0.0149	0.1797
6	0.0811	0.0303	0.1682	0.0213	0.1981
7	0.0946	0.0389	0.1852	0.0283	0.2160
8	0.1081	0.0478	0.2020	0.0358	0.2335
9	0.1216	0.0571	0.2184	0.0438	0.2506
10	0.1351	0.0668	0.2345	0.0521	0.2673
11	0.1486	0.0766	0.2504	0.0608	0.2837
12	0.1622	0.0867	0.2661	0.0697	0.2999
13	0.1757	0.0970	0.2817	0.0789	0.3158
14	0.1892	0.1075	0.2970	0.0884	0.3315
15	0.2027	0.1181	0.3122	0.0980	0.3470
16	0.2162	0.1289	0.3272	0.1079	0.3624
17	0.2297	0.1399	0.3421	0.1180	0.3775
18	0.2432	0.1510	0.3569	0.1282	0.3925
19	0.2568	0.1622	0.3716	0.1386	0.4073
20	0.2703	0.1735	0.3861	0.1491	0.4219
21	0.2838	0.1850	0.4005	0.1598	0.4364
22	0.2973	0.1966	0.4148	0.1707	0.4508
23	0.3108	0.2083	0.4290	0.1816	0.4651
24	0.3243	0.2200	0.4432	0.1927	0.4792
25	0.3378	0.2319	0.4572	0.2040	0.4932
26	0.3514	0.2439	0.4711	0.2153	0.5070
27	0.3649	0.2560	0.4849	0.2268	0.5208
28	0.3784	0.2681	0.4987	0.2384	0.5344
29	0.3919	0.2804	0.5123	0.2501	0.5479
30	0.4054	0.2927	0.5259	0.2620	0.5614
31	0.4189	0.3051	0.5394	0.2739	0.5747
32	0.4324	0.3177	0.5528	0.2859	0.5879

74 / 75

Index					
71	0.9595	0.8861	0.9916	0.8594	0.9954
72	0.9730	0.9058	0.9967	0.8807	0.9986
73	0.9865	0.9270	0.9997	0.9038	0.9999
74	1.0000	0.9514	1.0000	0.9309	1.0000
0	0.0000	0.0000	0.0480	0.0000	0.0682
1	0.0133	0.0003	0.0721	0.0001	0.0949
2	0.0267	0.0032	0.0930	0.0014	0.1178
3	0.0400	0.0083	0.1125	0.0046	0.1388
4	0.0533	0.0147	0.1310	0.0091	0.1585
5	0.0667	0.0220	0.1488	0.0147	0.1774
6	0.0800	0.0299	0.1660	0.0210	0.1957
7	0.0933	0.0384	0.1829	0.0279	0.2134
8	0.1067	0.0472	0.1994	0.0353	0.2306
9	0.1200	0.0564	0.2156	0.0432	0.2475
10	0.1333	0.0658	0.2316	0.0514	0.2640
11	0.1467	0.0756	0.2473	0.0599	0.2803
12	0.1600	0.0855	0.2628	0.0688	0.2963
13	0.1733	0.0957	0.2781	0.0778	0.3120
14	0.1867	0.1060	0.2933	0.0871	0.3275
15	0.2000	0.1165	0.3083	0.0967	0.3429
16	0.2133	0.1271	0.3232	0.1064	0.3580
17	0.2267	0.1379	0.3379	0.1163	0.3730
18	0.2400	0.1489	0.3525	0.1264	0.3878
19	0.2533	0.1599	0.3670	0.1366	0.4024
20	0.2667	0.1711	0.3814	0.1470	0.4169
21	0.2800	0.1824	0.3956	0.1575	0.4313
22	0.2933	0.1938	0.4098	0.1682	0.4455
23	0.3067	0.2053	0.4238	0.1790	0.4596
24	0.3200	0.2169	0.4378	0.1900	0.4736
25	0.3333	0.2286	0.4517	0.2010	0.4874
26	0.3467	0.2404	0.4654	0.2122	0.5011
27	0.3600	0.2523	0.4791	0.2235	0.5148
28	0.3733	0.2643	0.4927	0.2349	0.5283
29	0.3867	0.2764	0.5062	0.2465	0.5416
30	0.4000	0.2885	0.5196	0.2581	0.5549
31	0.4133	0.3008	0.5330	0.2699	0.5681
32	0.4267	0.3131	0.5462	0.2817	0.5812
33	0.4400	0.3255	0.5594	0.2937	0.5942
34	0.4533	0.3379	0.5725	0.3057	0.6070
35	0.4667	0.3505	0.5855	0.3179	0.6198
36	0.4800	0.3631	0.5985	0.3302	0.6325
37	0.4933	0.3758	0.6114	0.3425	0.6450
38	0.5067	0.3886	0.6242	0.3550	0.6575
39	0.5200	0.4015	0.6369	0.3675	0.6698

Continued

Table B.11. Exact confidence limits for a binomial proportion: x events are observed in a sample sized n. $p = x/n$ is the observed proportion. p_l and p_u are the lower and upper confidence limits for the population proportion

| | | | Confidence level | | | |
| | | | 95% | | 99% | |
n	x	p	p_l	p_u	p_l	p_u
75	**40**	0.5333	0.4145	0.6495	0.3802	0.6821
	41	0.5467	0.4275	0.6621	0.3930	0.6943
	42	0.5600	0.4406	0.6745	0.4058	0.7063
	43	0.5733	0.4538	0.6869	0.4188	0.7183
	44	0.5867	0.4670	0.6992	0.4319	0.7301
	45	0.6000	0.4804	0.7115	0.4451	0.7419
	46	0.6133	0.4938	0.7236	0.4584	0.7535
	47	0.6267	0.5073	0.7357	0.4717	0.7651
	48	0.6400	0.5209	0.7477	0.4852	0.7765
	49	0.6533	0.5346	0.7596	0.4989	0.7878
	50	0.6667	0.5483	0.7714	0.5126	0.7990
	51	0.6800	0.5622	0.7831	0.5264	0.8100
	52	0.6933	0.5762	0.7947	0.5404	0.8210
	53	0.7067	0.5902	0.8062	0.5545	0.8318
	54	0.7200	0.6044	0.8176	0.5687	0.8425
	55	0.7333	0.6186	0.8289	0.5831	0.8530
	56	0.7467	0.6330	0.8401	0.5976	0.8634
	57	0.7600	0.6475	0.8511	0.6122	0.8736

| | | | Confidence level | | | |
| | | | 95% | | 99% | |
n	x	p	p_l	p_u	p_l	p_u
75	58	0.7733	0.6621	0.8621	0.6270	0.8837
	59	0.7867	0.6768	0.8729	0.6420	0.8936
	60	0.8000	0.6917	0.8835	0.6571	0.9033
	61	0.8133	0.7067	0.8940	0.6725	0.9129
	62	0.8267	0.7219	0.9043	0.6880	0.9222
	63	0.8400	0.7372	0.9145	0.7037	0.9312
	64	0.8533	0.7527	0.9244	0.7197	0.9401
	65	0.8667	0.7684	0.9342	0.7360	0.9486
	66	0.8800	0.7844	0.9436	0.7525	0.9568
	67	0.8933	0.8006	0.9528	0.7694	0.9647
	68	0.9067	0.8171	0.9616	0.7866	0.9721
	69	0.9200	0.8340	0.9701	0.8043	0.9790
	70	0.9333	0.8512	0.9780	0.8226	0.9853
	71	0.9467	0.8690	0.9853	0.8415	0.9909
	72	0.9600	0.8875	0.9917	0.8612	0.9954
	73	0.9733	0.9070	0.9968	0.8822	0.9986
	74	0.9867	0.9279	0.9997	0.9051	0.9999
	75	1.0000	0.9520	1.0000	0.9318	1.0000

Table B.12. Exact confidence limits for a Poisson count: x is an observed Poisson count, x_l and x_u are the lower and upper limits for the population count

Confidence level	95%		99%	
x	x_l	x_u	x_l	x_u
0	0.000	3.689	0.000	5.298
1	0.025	5.572	0.005	7.430
2	0.242	7.225	0.103	9.274
3	0.619	8.767	0.338	10.977
4	1.090	10.242	0.672	12.594
5	1.623	11.668	1.078	14.150
6	2.202	13.059	1.537	15.660
7	2.814	14.423	2.037	17.134
8	3.454	15.763	2.571	18.578
9	4.115	17.085	3.132	19.998
10	4.795	18.390	3.717	21.398
11	5.491	19.682	4.321	22.779
12	6.201	20.962	4.943	24.145
13	6.922	22.230	5.580	25.497
14	7.654	23.490	6.231	26.836
15	8.395	24.740	6.893	28.164
16	9.145	25.983	7.567	29.482
17	9.903	27.219	8.251	30.791
18	10.668	28.448	8.943	32.091
19	11.439	29.671	9.644	33.383
20	12.217	30.888	10.353	34.668
21	12.999	32.101	11.069	35.946
22	13.787	33.308	11.792	37.218
23	14.580	34.511	12.521	38.484
24	15.377	35.710	13.255	39.745
25	16.179	36.905	13.995	41.000
26	16.984	38.096	14.741	42.251
27	17.793	39.284	15.491	43.497
28	18.606	40.468	16.245	44.738
29	19.422	41.649	17.004	45.976
30	20.241	42.827	17.767	47.209
31	21.063	44.002	18.534	48.439
32	21.888	45.174	19.305	49.665
33	22.716	46.344	20.079	50.888
34	23.546	47.512	20.857	52.107
35	24.379	48.677	21.638	53.324

Continued

Table B.12. *(Continued)* Exact confidence limits for a Poisson count: x is an observed Poisson count, x_l and x_u are the lower and upper limits for the population count

Confidence level	95%		99%	
x	x_l	x_u	x_l	x_u
36	25.214	49.839	22.422	54.537
37	26.051	51.000	23.208	55.748
38	26.891	52.158	23.998	56.955
39	27.733	53.314	24.791	58.161
40	28.577	54.469	25.586	59.363
41	29.422	55.621	26.384	60.563
42	30.270	56.772	27.184	61.761
43	31.119	57.921	27.986	62.956
44	31.970	59.068	28.791	64.149
45	32.823	60.214	29.598	65.341
46	33.678	61.358	30.407	66.530
47	34.534	62.500	31.218	67.717
48	35.391	63.641	32.032	68.902
49	36.250	64.781	32.847	70.085
50	37.111	65.919	33.664	71.266
51	37.973	67.056	34.483	72.446
52	38.836	68.191	35.303	73.624
53	39.701	69.325	36.125	74.800
54	40.566	70.458	36.949	75.974
55	41.434	71.590	37.775	77.147
56	42.302	72.721	38.602	78.319
57	43.171	73.850	39.431	79.489
58	44.042	74.978	40.261	80.657
59	44.914	76.106	41.093	81.824
60	45.786	77.232	41.926	82.990
61	46.660	78.357	42.760	84.154
62	47.535	79.481	43.596	85.317
63	48.411	80.604	44.433	86.479
64	49.288	81.727	45.272	87.639
65	50.166	82.848	46.111	88.798
66	51.044	83.968	46.952	89.956
67	51.924	85.088	47.794	91.113
68	52.805	86.206	48.637	92.269
69	53.686	87.324	49.482	93.423
70	54.568	88.441	50.327	94.577

Table B.12. *(Continued)*

Confidence level	95%		99%	
x	x_l	x_u	x_l	x_u
71	55.452	89.557	51.174	95.729
72	56.336	90.672	52.022	96.881
73	57.220	91.787	52.871	98.031
74	58.106	92.900	53.720	99.180
75	58.992	94.013	54.571	100.328
76	59.879	95.125	55.423	101.476
77	60.767	96.237	56.276	102.622
78	61.656	97.348	57.129	103.767
79	62.545	98.458	57.984	104.912
80	63.435	99.567	58.840	106.056
81	64.326	100.676	59.696	107.198
82	65.217	101.784	60.553	108.340
83	66.109	102.891	61.412	109.481
84	67.002	103.998	62.271	110.621
85	67.895	105.104	63.131	111.761
86	68.789	106.209	63.991	112.899
87	69.683	107.314	64.853	114.037
88	70.579	108.418	65.715	115.174
89	71.474	109.522	66.578	116.310
90	72.371	110.625	67.442	117.445
91	73.268	111.728	68.307	118.580
92	74.165	112.830	69.172	119.714
93	75.063	113.931	70.038	120.847
94	75.962	115.032	70.905	121.980
95	76.861	116.133	71.773	123.112
96	77.760	117.232	72.641	124.243
97	78.660	118.332	73.510	125.373
98	79.561	119.431	74.379	126.503
99	80.462	120.529	75.250	127.632
100	81.364	121.627	76.120	128.761

Table B.13(a). The F test: critical values for F distribution. For ANOVA $F = S_1^2/S_2^2$
d.f._1 = degrees of freedom for S_1^2. d.f._2 = degrees of freedom for S_2^2. $(S_1^2 > S_2^2)$

One-sided significance level: 0.05

d.f._1	1	2	3	4	5	6	7	8	9	10
d.f._2					Critical value F_c					
1	161	200	216	225	230	234	237	239	241	242
2	18.51	19.00	19.16	19.25	19.30	19.33	19.35	19.37	19.38	19.40
3	10.13	9.55	9.28	9.12	9.01	8.94	8.89	8.85	8.81	8.79
4	7.71	6.94	6.59	6.39	6.26	6.16	6.09	6.04	6.00	5.96
5	6.61	5.79	5.41	5.19	5.05	4.95	4.88	4.82	4.77	4.74
6	5.99	5.14	4.76	4.53	4.39	4.28	4.21	4.15	4.10	4.06
7	5.59	4.74	4.35	4.12	3.97	3.87	3.79	3.73	3.68	3.64
8	5.32	4.46	4.07	3.84	3.69	3.58	3.50	3.44	3.39	3.35
9	5.12	4.26	3.86	3.63	3.48	3.37	3.29	3.23	3.18	3.14
10	4.96	4.10	3.71	3.48	3.33	3.22	3.14	3.07	3.02	2.98
11	4.84	3.98	3.59	3.36	3.20	3.09	3.01	2.95	2.90	2.85
12	4.75	3.89	3.49	3.26	3.11	3.00	2.91	2.85	2.80	2.75
13	4.67	3.81	3.41	3.18	3.03	2.92	2.83	2.77	2.71	2.67
14	4.60	3.74	3.34	3.11	2.96	2.85	2.76	2.70	2.65	2.60
15	4.54	3.68	3.29	3.06	2.90	2.79	2.71	2.64	2.59	2.54
16	4.49	3.63	3.24	3.01	2.85	2.74	2.66	2.59	2.54	2.49
17	4.45	3.59	3.20	2.96	2.81	2.70	2.61	2.55	2.49	2.45
18	4.41	3.55	3.16	2.93	2.77	2.66	2.58	2.51	2.46	2.41
19	4.38	3.52	3.13	2.90	2.74	2.63	2.54	2.48	2.42	2.38
20	4.35	3.49	3.10	2.87	2.71	2.60	2.51	2.45	2.39	2.35
30	4.17	3.32	2.92	2.69	2.53	2.42	2.33	2.27	2.21	2.16
40	4.08	3.23	2.84	2.61	2.45	2.34	2.25	2.18	2.12	2.08
50	4.03	3.18	2.79	2.56	2.40	2.29	2.20	2.13	2.07	2.03
60	4.00	3.15	2.76	2.53	2.37	2.25	2.17	2.10	2.04	1.99
70	3.98	3.13	2.74	2.50	2.35	2.23	2.14	2.07	2.02	1.97
80	3.96	3.11	2.72	2.49	2.33	2.21	2.13	2.06	2.00	1.95
90	3.95	3.10	2.71	2.47	2.32	2.20	2.11	2.04	1.99	1.94
100	3.94	3.09	2.70	2.46	2.31	2.19	2.10	2.03	1.97	1.93
200	3.89	3.04	2.65	2.42	2.26	2.14	2.06	1.98	1.93	1.88
300	3.87	3.03	2.63	2.40	2.24	2.13	2.04	1.97	1.91	1.86
400	3.86	3.02	2.63	2.39	2.24	2.12	2.03	1.96	1.90	1.85
500	3.86	3.01	2.62	2.39	2.23	2.12	2.03	1.96	1.90	1.85

Significant result if $F \geqslant F_c$

Table B.13(b). The F test: critical values for F distribution. For ANOVA $F = S_1^2/S_2^2$
d.f.$_1$ = degrees of freedom for S_1^2. d.f.$_2$ = degrees of freedom for S_2^2. ($S_1^2 > S_2^2$)

One-sided significance level: 0.01

d.f.$_1$	1	2	3	4	5	6	7	8	9	10
d.f.$_2$					Critical value F_c					
1	4052	5000	5403	5625	5764	5859	5928	5981	6023	6056
2	98.50	99.00	99.17	99.25	99.30	99.33	99.36	99.37	99.39	99.40
3	34.12	30.82	29.46	28.71	28.24	27.91	27.67	27.49	27.35	27.23
4	21.20	18.00	16.69	15.98	15.52	15.21	14.98	14.80	14.66	14.55
5	16.26	13.27	12.06	11.39	10.97	10.67	10.46	10.29	10.16	10.05
6	13.75	10.92	9.78	9.15	8.75	8.47	8.26	8.10	7.98	7.87
7	12.25	9.55	8.45	7.85	7.46	7.19	6.99	6.84	6.72	6.62
8	11.26	8.65	7.59	7.01	6.63	6.37	6.18	6.03	5.91	5.81
9	10.56	8.02	6.99	6.42	6.06	5.80	5.61	5.47	5.35	5.26
10	10.04	7.56	6.55	5.99	5.64	5.39	5.20	5.06	4.94	4.85
11	9.65	7.21	6.22	5.67	5.32	5.07	4.89	4.74	4.63	4.54
12	9.33	6.93	5.95	5.41	5.06	4.82	4.64	4.50	4.39	4.30
13	9.07	6.70	5.74	5.21	4.86	4.62	4.44	4.30	4.19	4.10
14	8.86	6.51	5.56	5.04	4.69	4.46	4.28	4.14	4.03	3.94
15	8.68	6.36	5.42	4.89	4.56	4.32	4.14	4.00	3.89	3.80
16	8.53	6.23	5.29	4.77	4.44	4.20	4.03	3.89	3.78	3.69
17	8.40	6.11	5.18	4.67	4.34	4.10	3.93	3.79	3.68	3.59
18	8.29	6.01	5.09	4.58	4.25	4.01	3.84	3.71	3.60	3.51
19	8.18	5.93	5.01	4.50	4.17	3.94	3.77	3.63	3.52	3.43
20	8.10	5.85	4.94	4.43	4.10	3.87	3.70	3.56	3.46	3.37
30	7.56	5.39	4.51	4.02	3.70	3.47	3.30	3.17	3.07	2.98
40	7.31	5.18	4.31	3.83	3.51	3.29	3.12	2.99	2.89	2.80
50	7.17	5.06	4.20	3.72	3.41	3.19	3.02	2.89	2.78	2.70
60	7.08	4.98	4.13	3.65	3.34	3.12	2.95	2.82	2.72	2.63
70	7.01	4.92	4.07	3.60	3.29	3.07	2.91	2.78	2.67	2.59
80	6.96	4.88	4.04	3.56	3.26	3.04	2.87	2.74	2.64	2.55
90	6.93	4.85	4.01	3.53	3.23	3.01	2.84	2.72	2.61	2.52
100	6.90	4.82	3.98	3.51	3.21	2.99	2.82	2.69	2.59	2.50
200	6.76	4.71	3.88	3.41	3.11	2.89	2.73	2.60	2.50	2.41
300	6.72	4.68	3.85	3.38	3.08	2.86	2.70	2.57	2.47	2.38
400	6.70	4.66	3.83	3.37	3.06	2.85	2.68	2.56	2.45	2.37
500	6.69	4.65	3.82	3.36	3.05	2.84	2.68	2.55	2.44	2.36

Significant result if $F \geqslant F_c$

C

Statistical Analysis

C.1 Introduction

The purpose of this appendix is to summarize the statistical techniques discussed in the book by outlining their area of applicability and by providing step-by-step guides to their calculation.

Statistical analysis can be approached by using either confidence intervals to estimate relevant parameters or by hypothesis tests. A confidence interval gives, at a particular confidence level (usually 95% or 99%), a range of values within which the parameter being estimated is likely to lie.

Nearly all hypothesis tests follow the same general structure. A null hypothesis is postulated specifying a particular value for a relevant parameter. This null value is usually related to a lack of association between the variables being studied. A test statistic (e.g. t or χ^2), which is known to have a particular theoretical distribution if the null hypothesis is true, is calculated from the observed results. If, on the assumption of the null hypothesis, the probability of obtaining the value of this statistic, or one even more extreme, is less than a specified level — the significance level of the test — this is considered as evidence to reject the null hypothesis.

This probability is determined by referring the test statistic to a table which gives the critical values appropriate to the test and to the chosen one- or two-sided significance level (usually 5% or 1%). These critical values determine the acceptance and rejection regions for the test. If the test statistic lies in the acceptance region, the null hypothesis is not rejected and a non-significant result obtains. If, on the other hand, the test statistic lies in the rejection region — in the tail(s) of the particular distribution — the null hypothesis can be rejected and a significant result declared.

The simplest situation encountered is that of a single variable in one group or sample. In this case, simple population parameters can be estimated using confidence intervals, or one-sample hypothesis tests can be performed. Table C.1 lists the different techniques in this area and indicates where they are discussed in the body of the book and where they are to be found in this appendix.

Usually, however, analysis relates to a more complex situation than the one-group/one-variable case. Medical research in essence is concerned with examining

Table C.I. Statistical analysis in the one-group/one-variable situation (section and appendix numbers where the procedures are discussed are given in parentheses)

	Single-group analysis	
	Confidence intervals	Hypothesis tests
Means	(4.4; 4.7; C.2)	z test (6.6; C.2)
		t test (6.8; C.2)
Proportions	(4.8; C.3)	z test (6.9; C.3)
		χ^2 test (6.10; C.5)
Counts or rates	(4.9; C.4)	z test (6.11; C.4)

associations between variables, and as has been emphasised before, group membership can be considered a variable. Thus, one could examine the association or relationship of treatment to survival by comparing a treatment and control group. Such two-group comparisons are particularly common in medical research and much emphasis in this book has been on this situation. Table C.2 outlines the different techniques discussed. The significance tests for a null hypothesis of no group difference are given together with various comparative measures that can summarize that difference. These are either *difference* measures (such as the mean in one group minus the mean in the other group) or *ratio* measures (such as the relative risk).

When more than two groups are being compared somewhat different techniques are employed, and Table C.3 indicates the methods discussed. Gaps in the coverage are apparent but such situations do not arise that commonly in medical comparisons.

If an association between two quantitative variables is being analysed then regression or correlation are the appropriate techniques and these are considered in Chapter 9 and Sections C.19 and C.20 below. When more than two variables are involved in an analysis the statistical techniques become much more complex. Usually there is a single dependent variable, and there are two possible motives for the investigation. Interest may centre on the association between the dependent variable and a single explanatory variable, with the other variables being potential confounders of the association whose influence is to be adjusted for. Alternatively, the joint effects of the explanatory variables on the dependent variable may be of concern. These methods are all considered in Chapter 12, and Table C.4 (a repeat of Table 12.12) outlines the material covered. In this text the computations necessary to control confounding in 2×2 tables, using the Mantel–Haenzel methods, were described fully, while the other approaches, which really require

Table C.2. Hypothesis tests and summary measures of association (in italics) in the comparison of two groups (section and appendix numbers where the procedures are discussed are given in parentheses)

	Two-group comparisons		
	Independent	Frequency matched	Paired
Means	t test (7.4; C.6) *Difference* (7.4; C.6)	Two-way ANOVA *Difference* (12.3)*	Paired t test (7.6; C.8) *Difference* (7.6; C.8)
Medians	Wilcoxon rank sum test (7.5; C.7)	—	Sign test (7.7; C.9) Wilcoxon signed rank test (7.8; C.10)
Proportions	z test (7.9; C.11) χ^2 test (7.10; 7.12; C.12; C.14) Fisher's test (7.11; C.13) *Difference* (7.9; C.11) *Relative risk* (10.6; 10.10; C.12) *Odds ratio* (10.8; 10.10 C.12)	Mantel−Haenzel χ^2 (12.5) *Relative risk* (12.6) *Odds ratio* (12.6)	McNemar's χ^2 *Difference* (7.13; C.15) *Odds ratio* (10.8; 10.10; C.15)
Counts or rates	z test *Difference* (7.14; C.16) *Ratio* (10.11; C.16)	*SMR CMF* (13.3)	—
Lifetable survival (mortality)	z test Logrank test *Difference* (10.12) *O/E* (10.13)	Logrank test* *O/E* (10.13; 12.9)*	—

* Computational details not given in this text

Table C.3. Summary of techniques for multigroup comparisons (section and appendix numbers where the procedures are discussed are given in parentheses)

	Multigroup comparisons	
	Independent	Frequency matched
Means	One-way ANOVA (8.2−8.6; C.17)	Two-way ANOVA (12.3)*
Proportions	χ^2 test (8.7; C.14) χ^2 test for trend (8.8; C.18)	—

* Computational details not given in this text

Table C.4. Summary of multivariate techniques for the control of confounding and examination of the effects of explanatory variables

Explanatory or confounding variable(s)	Dependent variable			
	Mean	Binary proportion (risk)	Rate	Life table survival (mortality)
Qualitative only	ANOVA	Mantel–Haenzel techniques	Vital statistics methods (see Ch. 13)	Logrank methods
Quantitative and/or qualitative	Analysis of covariance Multiple regression	Logistic regression	–	Cox regression

computerized analysis, were discussed from the point of view of interpretation without computational detail.

The remaining sections of this appendix detail, in step-by-step form, the computations for the majority of the analytic techniques considered in this book. Life tables and the methods of Chapter 12 are not included, however, since these are best understood by following the text itself. It is hoped that this entire appendix will prove useful as a quick reference to the common techniques likely to be encountered by the medical researcher in analysing his or her own data.

C.2. The *z* and *t* tests for a single mean. Confidence intervals for a mean

These procedures are discussed in Sections 4.4, 4.7, 6.6 and 6.8.

Situation
Random sample size n from a population; quantitative variable of unknown mean μ.

Assumptions/requirements
That the distribution of the variable in the population is not markedly skewed.

Null hypothesis
That the mean μ of the population is equal to μ_0 (a numerical value).

Method
1 Calculate the mean, $\bar{x}$, and the standard deviation, S, in the sample.

2 If the standard deviation σ in the population is known, calculate the z statistic (equivalent to the t statistic on infinite degrees of freedom):

$$z = \frac{\bar{x} - \mu_0}{\sigma/\sqrt{n}}.$$

If the standard deviation in the population is not known, calculate the t statistic on $n - 1$ degrees of freedom:

$$t = \frac{\bar{x} - \mu_0}{S/\sqrt{n}}.$$

3 Look up the critical value t_c of the t distribution for degrees of freedom $n - 1$ or infinity at the required one- or two-sided significance level (Table B.3).

One-sided test
If $t \geqslant t_c$ $\qquad$ conclude $\mu > \mu_0$.
If $t \leqslant -t_c$ $\qquad$ conclude $\mu < \mu_0$.
If $-t_c < t < t_c$ $\qquad$ conclude $\mu = \mu_0$.

Two-sided test
If $t \geqslant t_c$ or $t \leqslant -t_c$ $\qquad$ conclude $\mu \neq \mu_0$.
If $-t_c < t < t_c$ $\qquad$ conclude $\mu = \mu_0$.

Confidence intervals
95% and 99% confidence intervals for μ are calculated as

$$\bar{x} \pm t_c\, \sigma/\sqrt{n} \quad (\sigma \text{ known})$$

or
$$\bar{x} \pm t_c\, S/\sqrt{n} \quad (\sigma \text{ unknown})$$

where t_c on $n - 1$ (σ unknown) or infinite (σ known) degrees of freedom is the two-sided 5% or 1% critical value for the t distribution.

C.3 The z test for a single proportion. Confidence intervals for a proportion

These procedures are discussed in Sections 4.8 and 6.9.

Situation
Random sample size n from a population; qualitative binary variable with unknown proportion π in one category.

Assumptions/requirements
That $n\pi$ and $n(1 - \pi)$ are both greater than 5.

Null hypothesis
That the proportion π in the population is equal to π_0 (a numerical value).

Method
1 Calculate the proportion p observed in the sample. ($p = x/n$)
2 Calculate the z statistic

$$z = \frac{p - \pi_0}{\sqrt{\dfrac{\pi_0 (1 - \pi_0)}{n}}}.$$

3 Look up the critical value z_c of the normal distribution at the required one- or two-sided significance level (Table B.2).

One-sided test
If $z \geqslant z_c$ conclude $\pi > \pi_0$.
If $z \leqslant -z_c$ conclude $\pi < \pi_0$.
If $-z_c < z < z_c$ conclude $\pi = \pi_0$.

Two-sided test
If $z \geqslant z_c$ or $z \leqslant -z_c$ conclude $\pi \neq \pi_0$.
If $-z_c < z < z_c$ conclude $\pi = \pi_0$.

Confidence intervals
Exact 95% and 99% confidence limits for a proportion are given in Table B.11 for sample sizes up to $n = 75$.
Look up n in the column on the left, and find x, the number of events in the next column. Succeeding columns give p and the lower (p_l) and upper (p_u) 95% and 99% limits for π.
Approximate 95% and 99% confidence intervals for π are calculated as

$$p \pm z_c \sqrt{p (1 - p)/n}$$

where z_c is the two-sided 5% or 1% critical value for the normal distribution. (See Section 4.8 on the accuracy of this approximation.)

C.4 The z test for a single count or rate. Confidence intervals for a count or rate

These procedures are discussed in Sections 4.9 and 6.11.

Situation
A single sample on which a count x has been determined, or a rate r calculated as a count divided by person-years at risk or person-years of follow-up ($r = x/\text{PYRS}$).

Assumptions/requirements
That the count be based on independent events, and that for the z test the count
be above 10.

Null hypothesis
1 That the underlying population count μ is μ_0 (a numerical value).
2 That the population rate θ is θ_0.

Method — null hypothesis (1)
1 Calculate the z statistic

$$z = \frac{x - \mu_0}{\sqrt{\mu_0}}.$$

2 Look up the critical value z_c of the normal distribution at the required one- or
two-sided significance level (Table B.2).

One-sided test
If $z \geqslant z_c$ conclude $\mu > \mu_0$.
If $z \leqslant -z_c$ conclude $\mu < \mu_0$.
If $-z_c < z < z_c$ conclude $\mu = \mu_0$.

Two-sided test
If $z \geqslant z_c$ or $z \leqslant -z_c$ conclude $\mu \neq \mu_0$.
If $-z_c < z < z_c$ conclude $\mu = \mu_0$.

Method — null hypothesis (2)
1 Calculate the z statistic

$$z = \frac{r - \theta_0}{\sqrt{\theta_0/\text{PYRS}}}.$$

2 Look up the critical value z_c of the normal distribution at the required one- or
two-sided significance level (Table B.2).

One sided test
If $z \geqslant z_c$ conclude $\theta > \theta_0$.
If $z \leqslant -z_c$ conclude $\theta < \theta_0$.
If $-z_c < z < z_c$ conclude $\theta = \theta_0$.

Two-sided test
If $z \geqslant z_c$ or $z \leqslant -z_c$ conclude $\theta \neq \theta_0$.
If $-z_c < z < z_c$ conclude $\theta = \theta_0$.

Confidence intervals for a count
Exact 95% and 99% confidence limits for a count are given in Table B.12 for

counts up to 100. Look up the observed count x in the left-hand column. Succeeding columns give the lower (x_l) and upper (x_u) 95% and 99% limits for μ.

Approximate 95% and 99% confidence intervals are calculated as

$$x \pm z_c \sqrt{x}$$

where z_c is the two-sided 5% or 1% critical value for the normal distribution. (This approximation should only be used for observed counts above 100.)

Confidence intervals for a rate
Confidence intervals for a rate ($r = x/\text{PYRS}$) can be obtained by calculating the limits for x as described above and dividing by PYRS. An alternative approximate formulae for the 95% and 99% limits directly is

$$r \pm z_c \sqrt{\frac{r}{\text{PYRS}}}$$

where z_c is the two-sided 5% or 1% critical value for the normal distribution. (This approximation should only be used for observed counts above 100.)

C.5 The χ^2 test for many proportions (in one group)

This procedure is discussed in Section 6.10.

Situation
Random sample size n from a population; qualitative variable with two or more categories.

Assumptions/requirements
That not more than 20% of the expected numbers (see below) in the categories are less than 5, and that no expected number is less than 1.

Null hypothesis
That the proportions in each category of the variable in the population have certain values defined independently of the data.

Method
1 Calculate the expected numbers (E) in each category of the variable by multiplying the sample size n by each of the hypothesized proportions.
2 Calculate the χ^2 statistic on degrees of freedom one less than the number of categories:

$$\chi^2 = \sum \frac{(O - E)^2}{E}$$

where O is the observed numbers in each category of the variable, and the summation is over all the categories.

3 Look up the critical value χ_c^2 of the chi-square distribution for the appropriate degrees of freedom at the required two-sided significance level (Table B.4).

If $\chi^2 \geqslant \chi_c^2$ reject the null hypothesis.
If $\chi^2 < \chi_c^2$ do not reject the null hypothesis.

C.6 The *t* test for two independent means. Confidence intervals for a mean difference

These procedures are discussed in Section 7.4.

Situation
Two independent random samples size n_1 and n_2 from two populations; quantitative variable with means μ_1 and μ_2 in the two populations.

Assumptions/requirements
That the distribution of the variable is not markedly skewed in either of the populations and either (a) that the population variances σ_1^2 and σ_2^2 are equal, or (b) that these variances are unequal and the sample size in both groups combined is greater than 60 with numbers in each group roughly the same.

Null hypothesis
That the means μ_1 and μ_2 of the two populations are equal, or that the mean difference is zero.

Method
1 Calculate the means $\bar{x}_1$ and $\bar{x}_2$ and the standard deviations S_1 and S_2 in the two samples.
2 Assumption a: calculate the pooled variance

$$S_p^2 = \frac{(n_1 - 1)\,S_1^2 + (n_2 - 1)\,S_2^2}{n_1 + n_2 - 2}$$

and the *t* statistic on $n_1 + n_2 - 2$ degrees of freedom

$$t = \frac{\bar{x}_1 - \bar{x}_2}{\sqrt{\dfrac{S_p^2}{n_1} + \dfrac{S_p^2}{n_2}}}.$$

3 Assumption b: calculate the z statistic (equivalent to the t statistic on infinite degrees of freedom)

$$z = \frac{\bar{x}_1 - \bar{x}_2}{\sqrt{\dfrac{S_1^2}{n_1} + \dfrac{S_2^2}{n_2}}}.$$

4 Look up the critical value t_c of the t distribution for degrees of freedom $n_1 + n_2 - 2$ (assumption a) or infinity (assumption b) at the required one- or two-sided significance level (Table B.3).

One-sided test

If $t \geqslant t_c$	conclude $\mu_1 > \mu_2$.
If $t \leqslant -t_c$	conclude $\mu_1 < \mu_2$.
If $-t_c < t < t_c$	conclude $\mu_1 = \mu_2$.

Two-sided test

If $t \geqslant t_c$ or $t \leqslant -t_c$	conclude $\mu_1 \neq \mu_2$.
If $-t_c < t < t_c$	conclude $\mu_1 = \mu_2$.

Confidence intervals for a mean difference (independent data)
95% and 99% confidence intervals for the mean difference $\mu_1 - \mu_2$ between the two populations are calculated from

$$(x_1 - x_2) \pm t_c \, SE \, (x_1 - x_2)$$

where SE $(x_1 - x_2)$ is the denominator of the test statistic above, and t_c on $n_1 + n_2 - 2$ (assumption a) or infinite (assumption b) degrees of freedom is the two-sided 5% or 1% critical value for the t distribution.

C.7 The Wilcoxon rank sum test for two independent medians

This procedure is discussed in Section 7.5.

Situation
Two independent random samples size n_1 and n_2 from two populations; quantitative or ordinal variable with medians m_1 and m_2 in the two populations.

Assumptions/requirements
That there is an underlying continuous distribution of the variable, even if it is only measured on an ordinal scale; that there are not too many tied observations.

Null hypothesis
That the medians m_1 and m_2 in the two populations are equal.

Method

1 Combine the observations from the two groups and order them from lowest to highest while still noting which observation came from which group. Assign a rank to each observation giving the smallest observation rank 1. If there are tied observations assign the mean of the ranks in the position concerned.

2 Calculate the sum of the ranks assigned to the observations in the group with sample size n_1. Call this T_1.

3 Locate the pages of the rank sum test table (Table B.5) corresponding to the sample size in group 1 (n_1). Choose the page that corresponds to the required one- or two-sided significance level, and look in the table for the entries corresponding to the sample sizes n_1 (in the row) and n_2 (in the column). These give the lower (T_l) and upper (T_u) critical values for the sum of ranks in group 1 (T_1). Relabel the groups if necessary to use the table.

One-sided test

If $T_1 \geq T_u$ conclude $m_1 > m_2$.

If $T_1 \leq T_l$ conclude $m_1 < m_2$.

If $T_l < T_1 < T_u$ conclude $m_1 = m_2$.

Two-sided test

If $T_1 \geq T_u$ or $T_1 \leq T_l$ conclude $m_1 \neq m_2$.

If $T_l < T_1 < T_u$ conclude $m_1 = m_2$.

C.8 The *t* test for paired means.
Confidence intervals for a mean difference

This procedure is discussed in Section 7.6.

Situation

Two individually matched samples each of sample size n (n pairs of observations); quantitative variable with population means μ_1 and μ_2.

Assumptions/requirements

That the distribution of the differences between pairs in the population is not too skewed.

Null hypothesis

That the population means μ_1 and μ_2 are equal, or that the mean difference is zero.

Method

1 Calculate the difference between each pair of values, $d = x_1 - x_2$, and compute the mean, $\bar{d}$, and standard deviation, S_d, of these n differences (include zero values of d).

2 Compute the t statistic on $n - 1$ degrees of freedom.

$$t = \frac{\bar{d}}{S_d/\sqrt{n}}.$$

3 Look up the critical value t_c of the t distribution for degrees of freedom $n - 1$ at the required one- or two-sided significance level (Table B.3).

One-sided test

If $t \geq t_c$	conclude $\mu_1 > \mu_2$.
If $t \leq -t_c$	conclude $\mu_1 < \mu_2$.
If $-t_c < t < t_c$	conclude $\mu_1 = \mu_2$.

Two-sided test

If $t \geq t_c$ or $t \leq -t_c$	conclude $\mu_1 \neq \mu_2$.
If $-t_c < t < t_c$	conclude $\mu_1 = \mu_2$.

Confidence intervals for a mean difference (paired data)
95% and 99% confidence intervals for the mean difference between the two populations are calculated from

$$\bar{d} \pm t_c \, S_d/\sqrt{n}$$

where t_c on $n - 1$ degrees of freedom is the two-sided 5% or 1% critical value for the t distribution.

C.9 The sign test for paired medians

This procedure is discussed in Section 7.7.

Situation
Two individually matched samples each of sample size N (N pairs of observations); quantitative or ordinal variable (in that one can determine which individual in each pair has a higher value than the other).

Assumptions/requirements
That there is an underlying continuous distribution of the variable even if it is only measured on an ordinal scale.

Null hypothesis
That the medians m_1 and m_2 in the two populations are equal.

Method

1 Calculate the sign (+ or −) of the differences $x_1 - x_2$ between each pair of values. If some pairs have the same value the difference is zero. Count the number of non-zero differences and call it n. If there are no ties $N = n$.

2 Count the number of positive (+) differences and call it n_+.

3 Look up the table for the sign test (Table B.6) corresponding to the chosen one- or two-sided significance level and the number of non-zero differences n. The entry gives the lower (S_l) and upper (S_u) critical values for the number of positive differences n_+.

One-sided test

If $n_+ \geqslant S_u$ conclude $m_1 > m_2$.

If $n_+ \leqslant S_l$ conclude $m_1 < m_2$.

If $S_l < n_+ < S_u$ conclude $m_1 = m_2$.

Two-sided test

If $n_+ \geqslant S_u$ or $n_+ \leqslant S_l$ conclude $m_1 \neq m_2$.

If $S_l < n_+ < S_u$ conclude $m_1 = m_2$.

C.10 The Wilcoxon signed rank test for paired medians

This procedure is discussed in Section 7.8.

Situation

Two individually matched samples each of sample size N (N pairs of observations); quantitative or ordinal variable in that the differences between each pair can be ordered.

Assumptions/requirements

That there is an underlying continuous distribution of the variable even if it is only measured on an ordinal scale; that there are not too many ties among the differences.

Null hypothesis

That the medians m_1 and m_2 in the two populations are equal.

Method

1 Calculate the differences between each pair of values, $d = x_1 - x_2$. Let n equal the number of non-zero differences.

2 Rank these non-zero differences from smallest to highest ignoring the sign of the difference. Assign a rank to each of these differences giving the smallest a rank of 1. If two differences have the same magnitude assign the mean of the ranks in the positions concerned. Now affix to each rank the sign (+ or −) of the difference it represents.

3 Add up the positive (+) ranks and call the sum T_+.

4 Look up the table for this test (Table B.7), and find the lower (T_l) and upper (T_u) critical values for T_+ corresponding to the number of non-zero differences n and the chosen one- or two-sided significance level.

One-sided test

If $T_+ \geqslant T_u$	conclude $m_1 > m_2$.
If $T_+ \leqslant T_l$	conclude $m_1 < m_2$.
If $T_l < T_+ < T_u$	conclude $m_1 = m_2$.

Two-sided test

If $T_+ \geqslant T_u$ or $T_+ \leqslant T_l$	conclude $m_1 \neq m_2$.
If $T_l < T_+ < T_u$	conclude $m_1 = m_2$.

C.11 The *z* test for two independent proportions. Confidence intervals for a difference between proportions

These procedures are discussed in Section 7.9.

Situation
Two independent random samples size n_1 and n_2 from two populations; qualitative binary variable with unknown population proportions, π_1 and π_2, in one category of the variable.

Assumptions/requirements
That for total sample size, $n_1 + n_2$, less than 40, the four quantities obtained by multiplying n_1 and n_2 by p and $1 - p$ are all greater than 5, where p is the pooled proportion in the two samples combined (see below). Thus, this test should not be used for total sample sizes less than 20.

Null hypothesis
That the proportions π_1 and π_2 in the populations are equal.

Method
1 Calculate the proportions p_1 and p_2 in each of the samples. Also calculate the overall sample proportion p in the two groups combined (the pooled value).

2 Calculate the z statistic

$$z = \frac{p_1 - p_2}{\sqrt{pq \left(\dfrac{1}{n_1} + \dfrac{1}{n_2}\right)}}$$

where $q = 1 - p$.

3 Look up the critical value z_c of the normal distribution at the required one- or two-sided significance level (Table B.2).

One-sided test

If $z \geqslant z_c$	conclude $\pi_1 > \pi_2$.
If $z \leqslant -z_c$	conclude $\pi_1 < \pi_2$.
If $-z_c < z < z_c$	conclude $\pi_1 = \pi_2$.

Two-sided test

If $z \geqslant z_c$ or $z \leqslant -z_c$	conclude $\pi_1 \neq \pi_2$.
If $-z_c < z < z_c$	conclude $\pi_1 = \pi_2$.

Confidence intervals for a difference between proportions
95% and 99% confidence intervals for the difference between the population proportions $\pi_1 - \pi_2$ are calculated from

$$(p_1 - p_2) \pm z_c \sqrt{\frac{p_1 q_1}{n_1} + \frac{p_2 q_2}{n_2}}$$

where $q_1 = 1 - p_1$, $q_2 = 1 - p_2$ and z_c is the two-sided 5% or 1% critical value for the normal distribution.

C.12 The χ^2 test for a 2 × 2 table. Confidence intervals for a relative risk (ratio of proportions) and for an odds ratio

These procedures are discussed in Sections 7.10, 10.6, 10.10 and A.3.

Situation
A 2 × 2 table with independent data laid out as below

a	b		r_1
c	d		r_2
c_1	c_2		n

where r_1, r_2, c_1 and c_2 are the row and column totals and n is the total sample size. Often the columns represent disease/non-disease and the rows represent exposed/non-exposed.

Assumptions
That none of the expected numbers (see below) be less than 5. (Recent work suggests that this may be too stringent a requirement.)

Null hypothesis
That the population proportions in the two groups are the same, or equivalently that the two variables defining group membership are independent.

Method
1 Calculate the expected numbers in each cell (E). These are obtained by multiplying the corresponding row and column totals and dividing by n.
2 Calculate the χ^2 statistic on 1 degree of freedom

$$\chi^2 = \sum \frac{(O - E)^2}{E}$$

where O are the observed numbers in the table and summation is over the four table cells. An equivalent formula is

$$\chi^2 = \frac{(ad - bc)^2 \, n}{r_1 \, r_2 \, c_1 \, c_2}.$$

3 Look up the critical value χ_c^2 of the chi-square distribution on 1 degree of freedom at the required two-sided significance level (one-sided tests are difficult to interpret).

$$\text{If } \chi^2 \geq \chi_c^2 \quad \text{reject the null hypothesis.}$$
$$\text{If } \chi^2 < \chi_c^2 \quad \text{do not reject the null hypothesis.}$$

Confidence intervals for a relative risk (ratio of independent proportions)
95% and 99% confidence intervals for the relative risk

$$RR = \frac{a/r_1}{c/r_2}$$

are calculated as

$$RR^{(1 \pm z_c/\chi)}$$

where χ is the square root of χ^2 and z_c is the critical two-sided 5% or 1% value of the normal distribution.

Confidence intervals for an odds ratio (independent data)
95% and 99% confidence intervals for the odds ratio

$$OR = \frac{a/b}{c/d}$$

are calculated as

$$OR^{(1 \pm z_c/\chi)}$$

where χ is the square root of χ^2 and z_c is the critical two-sided 5% or 1% value of the normal distribution.

C.13 Fisher's test for a 2 × 2 table

This procedure is discussed in Section 7.11.

Situation
Independent data laid out in a 2 × 2 table.

Assumptions/requirements
That the row and column totals are fixed.

Null hypothesis
That the row and column variables are not associated or, equivalently, that a binary variable is not associated with group membership in a two-sample situation.

Method
1   Rearrange the table so that the smallest cell frequency is in the top left-hand corner.
2   Create a new table by reducing the number in the top-left cell by 1 (unless it is zero to start with) and fill in the rest of the table so that it has the same row and column totals as the original.
3   Repeat step 2 until a table with a zero in the top left cell is obtained. There should now be a total of $V + 1$ tables, including the original, where V is the smallest cell frequency in the original. Label these tables from set 0 to set V according to the number in the top left cell. The table in set i has the form

$$
\begin{array}{cc|c}
a_i & b_i & r_1 \\
c_i & d_i & r_2 \\
\hline
s_1 & s_2 & n
\end{array}
$$

where, of course, r_1, r_2, s_1 and s_2 are the row and column totals which are the same for each table. $a_0 = 0$ and $a_i = i$.

4 Calculate the probability of the table in set 0, directly or using logs (Tables B.8 and B.9)

$$P_0 = \frac{r_2! \, s_2!}{d_0! \, n!}.$$

5 Calculate the probability of the table in the next set (if there is one) using

$$P_{i+1} = P_i \times \frac{b_i \times c_i}{a_{i+1} \times d_{i+1}}.$$

6 Repeat the last step until all the probabilities from P_0 to P_V have been calculated.

7 Sum these $V + 1$ probabilities. This is the one-sided p value for the test. Multiply this by 2 to obtain the two-sided value. If the (one- or two-sided) p value is less than 5% the null hypothesis can be rejected.

C.14 The χ^2 test for a general $I \times J$ table

This procedure is discussed in Sections 7.12 and 8.7.

Situation
Independent random samples from two or more populations; qualitative variable with two or more categories. The data are usually laid out in a $I \times J$ table where I is the number of rows and J is the number of columns. The number of observations in each cell of the table must be known. The situation also arises when two qualitative variables are being examined in a single sample.

Assumptions
That not more than 20% of the expected values in the cells (see below) should be less than 5 and no cell should have an expected value of less than 1.

Null hypothesis
That the distributions of the qualitative variable in the different populations are the same or, equivalently, that two qualitative variables in a single sample are not associated.

Method
1 Calculate the expected values (E) in each cell in the table. The expected value for the cell in the ith row and jth column is obtained by multiplying the totals of the corresponding row, r_i, and column, s_j, and dividing by the total sample size in all groups combined (n).

2 Calculate the χ^2 statistic on $(I - 1)(J - 1)$ degrees of freedom

$$\chi^2 = \Sigma \frac{(O - E)^2}{E}$$

where the O is the observed numbers in each cell and summation is over all cells in the table. (Eqn. 8.18 may be computationally simpler for a $2 \times k$ table.)
3 Look up the critical value χ_c^2 of the chi-square distribution for degrees of freedom $(I - 1)(J - 1)$ at the required two-sided significance level (Table B.4).

If $\chi^2 \geqslant \chi_c^2$ reject the null hypothesis.
If $\chi^2 < \chi_c^2$ do not reject the null hypothesis.

C.15 The McNemar and exact test for paired proportions. Confidence intervals for a difference between proportions and for an odds ratio

These procedures are discussed in Sections 7.13, 10.8 and 10.10.

Situation
Two individually matched groups each of size N (N pairs of observations); qualitative binary variable with unknown population proportions π_1 and π_2 in one category of the variable. This category is denoted by a plus sign below. Often the groups are cases and controls in a pair-matched case-control study, and the binary variable is exposure/non-exposure to a risk factor.

Assumptions/requirements
None.

Null hypothesis
That the proportions π_1 and π_2 in the two paired populations are equal.

Method
1 Lay out the data in a 2×2 table as

		Group 1	
		+	−
Group 2	+	a	b
	−	c	d

where the classification is based on the N pairs of observations, and the plus and minus refer to the categories of the binary variable.

2 For small sample sizes refer c (number of untied pairs in favour of group 1) to Table B.6, which gives the lower (S_l) and upper (S_u) critical values for the test, entered at $n = b + c$ which is the total number of untied pairs.

One-sided test

If $c \geqslant S_u$ conclude $\pi_1 > \pi_2$.

If $c \leqslant S_l$ conclude $\pi_1 < \pi_2$.

If $S_l < c < S_u$ conclude $\pi_1 = \pi_2$.

Two-sided test

If $c \geqslant S_u$ or $c \leqslant S_l$ conclude $\pi_1 \neq \pi_2$.

If $S_l < c < S_u$ conclude $\pi_1 = \pi_2$.

3 For large sample sizes calculate

$$\chi^2 = \frac{(c - b)^2}{b + c}$$

on 1 degree of freedom.

4 Look up the critical value χ_c^2 of the chi-square distribution on 1 degree of freedom at the required one- or two-sided significance level (Table B.4).

If $\chi^2 \geqslant \chi_c^2$ conclude $\pi_1 \neq \pi_2$.

If $\chi^2 < \chi_c^2$ conclude $\pi_1 = \pi_2$.

Confidence intervals for a difference between paired proportions
95% and 99% confidence intervals for the difference between the population proportions $\pi_1 - \pi_2$ are calculated from

$$(p_1 - p_2) \pm z_c \frac{1}{N} \sqrt{c + b - \frac{(c - b)^2}{N}}$$

where $p_1 = (a + c)/N$ and $p_2 = (a + b)/N$ are the observed proportions and z_c is the two-sided 5% or 1% critical value for the normal distribution.

Confidence interval for an odds ratio (paired data)
95% and 99% confidence intervals for the odds ratio from a pair matched study

$$OR = c/b$$

are given by

$$OR^{(1 \pm z_c/\chi)},$$

where χ is the square root of χ^2, and z_c is the critical two-sided 5% or 1% value of the normal distribution.

C.16 The z test for two independent counts or rates. Confidence intervals for a difference between counts or rates, and for a ratio of counts or rates

These procedures are discussed in Sections 7.14 and 10.11

Situation
Two independent samples, over the same time period or spatial area, on which two counts x_1 and x_2 are observed, or rates r_1 and r_2 based on counts per person-years at risk or person-years of follow-up in two groups ($r_1 = x_1/PYRS_1$, $r_2 = x_2/PYRS_2$).

Assumptions/requirements
That the counts are independent and greater than about 10 in each group.

Null hypothesis
1 That the underlying population counts μ_1 and μ_2 are equal.
2 That the underlying population rates θ_1 and θ_2 are equal.

Method — null hypothesis (1)
1 Calculate the z statistic

$$z = \frac{x_1 - x_2}{\sqrt{(x_1 + x_2)}}$$

where x_1 and x_2 are the two counts.
2 Look up the critical value z_c of the normal distribution at the required one- or two-sided significance level (Table B.2).

One-sided test

If $z \geqslant z_c$	conclude $\mu_1 > \mu_2$.
If $z \leqslant -z_c$	conclude $\mu_1 < \mu_2$.
If $-z_c < z < z_c$	conclude $\mu_1 = \mu_2$.

Two-sided test

If $z \geqslant z_c$ or $z \leqslant -z_c$	conclude $\mu_1 \neq \mu_2$.
If $-z_c < z < z_c$	conclude $\mu_1 = \mu_2$.

Method — null hypothesis (2)
1 Calculate the rates in the two populations $r_1 = x_1/PYRS_1$, $r_2 = x_2/PYRS_2$.
2 Calculate the overall (pooled) rate in the two populations combined

$$r = \frac{PYRS_1 \, (r_1) + PYRS_2 \, (r_2)}{PYRS_1 + PYRS_2}.$$

3 Calculate the z statistic

$$z = \frac{r_1 - r_2}{\sqrt{\dfrac{r}{\text{PYRS}_1} + \dfrac{r}{\text{PYRS}_2}}}.$$

4 Look up the critical value z_c of the normal distribution at the required one- or two-sided significance level (Table B.2).

One-sided test

If $z \geqslant z_c$	conclude $\theta_1 > \theta_2$.
If $z \leqslant -z_c$	conclude $\theta_1 < \theta_2$.
If $-z_c < z < z_c$	conclude $\theta_1 = \theta_2$.

Two-sided test

If $z \geqslant z_c$ or $z \leqslant -z_c$	conclude $\theta_1 \neq \theta_2$.
If $-z_c < z < z_c$	conclude $\theta_1 = \theta_2$.

Confidence interval for a difference in counts
95% and 99% confidence intervals for the difference between two population counts μ_1 and μ_2 (if based on the same time period or spatial area) are calculated from

$$(x_1 - x_2) \pm z_c \sqrt{(x_1 + x_2)}$$

where z_c is the two-sided 5% or 1% critical value of the normal distribution.

Confidence interval for a difference between rates
95% and 99% confidence intervals for the difference between the population rates θ_1 and θ_2 are calculated from

$$(r_1 - r_2) \pm z_c \sqrt{\frac{r_1}{\text{PYRS}_1} + \frac{r_2}{\text{PYRS}_2}}$$

where z_c is the two-sided 5% or 1% critical value of the normal distribution.

Confidence intervals for a ratio of counts
Exact 95% and 99% confidence intervals for the ratio of two population counts μ_1/μ_2 (not necessarily from the same time periods or spatial areas) can be obtained by considering $p = x_1/(x_1 + x_2)$ as a binomial proportion. The lower (p_l) and upper (p_u) limits for this proportion can be obtained using the method described in Section C.3 The lower and upper limits for the population ratio of the counts are then

$$\frac{p_l}{1 - p_l} \quad \text{and} \quad \frac{p_u}{1 - p_u}.$$

Confidence intervals for the ratio of rates
The ratio of rates is $RR = (x_1/x_2)(PYRS_2/PYRS_1)$ and lower (RR_l) and upper (RR_u) confidence limits are obtained by multiplying the confidence limits for the ratio of the counts x_1/x_2 by $PYRS_2/PYRS_1$ (see above):

$$RR_l = \frac{p_l}{1 - p_l} \frac{PYRS_2}{PYRS_1}$$

$$RR_u = \frac{p_u}{1 - p_u} \frac{PYRS_2}{PYRS_1}.$$

C.17 One way analysis of variance for means in more than two groups. Confidence intervals for means and mean differences

These procedures are discussed in Sections 8.2 to 8.6 and A.4.

Situation
Independent random samples from k groups. Sample size in group i is n_i and total sample size is N. Quantitative variable with population mean in group i of μ_i.

Assumptions/requirements
That the population variances in the k groups are equal and that the distribution of the variable is approximately normal in each group.

Null hypothesis
1 That the k population means μ_i are all equal.
2 That the population means μ_1 and μ_2 are equal (if a significant F value was obtained and the comparison was prespecified).

Method − null hypothesis (1)
1 Calculate the within- and between-group SSq using the methods of Section A.4. Also calculate the sample means $\bar{x}_i$ in each group.
2 Calculate

$$S_W^2 = \text{Within-group SSq}/N - k.$$
$$S_B^2 = \text{Between-group SSq}/k - 1.$$

3 Calculate the F statistic on $k - 1$ and $N - k$ degrees of freedom:

$$F = S_B^2/S_W^2.$$

4 Look up the critical value F_c of the F distribution on $k - 1$ and $N - k$ degrees of freedom at the required (one-sided) significance level (Table B.14).

If $F \geqslant F_c$ conclude that the μ_i are not all equal.
If $F < F_c$ conclude that the μ_i are all equal.

Method − null hypothesis (2)

1 Calculate the t statistic on $N - k$ degrees of freedom:

$$t = \frac{\bar{x}_1 - \bar{x}_2}{\sqrt{\dfrac{S_W^2}{n_1} + \dfrac{S_W^2}{n_2}}}.$$

2 Look up the critical value t_c of the t distribution for degrees of freedom $N - k$.

One-sided test

If $t \geqslant t_c$	conclude $\mu_1 > \mu_2$.
If $t \leqslant -t_c$	conclude $\mu_1 < \mu_2$.
If $-t_c < t < t_c$	conclude $\mu_1 = \mu_2$.

Two-sided test

If $t \geqslant t_c$ or $t \leqslant -t_c$	conclude $\mu_1 \neq \mu_2$.
If $-t_c < t < t_c$	conclude $\mu_1 = \mu_2$.

Confidence interval for a single mean

95% and 99% confidence for a particular population mean μ_i are calculated from

$$\bar{x}_i \pm t_c \frac{S_W}{\sqrt{n_i}}$$

where t_c on $N - k$ degrees of freedom is the two-sided 5% or 1% critical value for the t distribution.

Confidence intervals for a mean difference

95% and 99% confidence intervals for the mean difference $\mu_1 - \mu_2$ between the two corresponding populations are calculated from

$$(\bar{x}_1 - \bar{x}_2) \pm t_c \sqrt{\frac{S_W^2}{n_1} + \frac{S_W^2}{n_2}}$$

where t_c on $N - k$ degrees of freedom is the two-sided 5% or 1% critical value for the t distribution.

C.18 The χ^2 test for a trend in proportions in a 2 × k table

This procedure is discussed in Section 8.8

Situation

Independent random samples from k groups that have some intrinsic order. Sample size in group i is n_i and total sample size is N. Binary variable with a proportion d_i/n_i in each group and a total number of 'events' $D = \Sigma\, d_i$.

Assumptions/requirements
That not more than 20% of the expected numbers in the cells should fall below 5 or any fall below 1.

Null hypothesis
That there is no linear trend in the population proportions with group membership.

Method
1 Assign a score x_i to each group that reflects the relative ordering of the groups.
2 Calculate the following quantities from the data

$$\mathscr{B} = \Sigma\, n_i\, x_i$$
$$\mathscr{C} = \Sigma\, d_i\, x_i$$
$$\mathscr{D} = \Sigma\, n_i\, x_i^2.$$

3 Calculate the χ^2_{TR} statistic for trend on 1 degree of freedom:

$$\chi^2_{TR} = \frac{N\,(N\,\mathscr{C} - D\,\mathscr{B})^2}{D\,(N - D)\,(N\,\mathscr{D} - \mathscr{B}^2)}.$$

4 Calculate the usual χ^2 statistic for the $2 \times k$ table (see Section C.14), and obtain the χ^2_{DEP} for a departure from a linear trend on $k - 2$ degrees of freedom using

$$\chi^2_{DEP} = \chi^2 - \chi^2_{TR}.$$

5 Look up the critical value χ^2_c of the χ^2 distribution for 1 degree of freedom at the required one-sided significance level.

If $\chi^2_{TR} \geqslant \chi^2_c$ conclude there is a linear trend.
If $\chi^2_{TR} < \chi^2_c$ conclude there is no linear trend.

6 Look up the critical value χ^2_c of the χ^2 distribution for $k - 2$ degrees of freedom at the required one-sided significance level.

If $\chi^2_{DEP} \geqslant \chi^2_c$ conclude there is a departure from a linear trend.
If $\chi^2_{DEP} < \chi^2_c$ conclude there is no departure from a linear trend.

C.19 Tests for regression and correlation

These procedures are discussed in Section 9.5

Situation
Random samples of a y variable at different values of an x variable; both variables

quantitative; often assumed in random sampling from a single group; n pairs of values in all.

Assumptions / requirements
That the population distribution of y at each fixed x is normal and that the variances of these y distributions are all equal; that the means of the y distributions are linearly related to x.

Null hypotheses
1   That the population regression coefficient β is equal to a fixed value β_0 or
2   That the population correlation coefficient ρ is equal to zero.

Method — null hypothesis (1)
1   Calculate the regression coefficient b, the sum of squares $\Sigma\,(x - \bar{x})^2$ and the standard error of the estimate, $S_{y.x}$, using the methods outlined in Section A.4.
2   Calculate the t statistic on $n - 2$ degrees of freedom

$$t = \frac{b - \beta_0}{\text{SE}\,(b)}$$

where

$$\text{SE}\,(b) = \frac{S_{y.x}}{\sqrt{\Sigma(x - \bar{x})^2}}.$$

3   Look up the critical value t_c of the t distribution on $n - 2$ degrees of freedom at the required two-sided (usually) significance level (Table B.3).

$$\text{If } t \geq t_c \text{ or } t \leq -t_c \qquad \text{conclude } \beta \neq \beta_0.$$
$$\text{If } -t_c < t < t_c \qquad \text{conclude } \beta = \beta_0.$$

Confidence intervals
95% and 99% confidence intervals for β are calculated from

$$b \pm t_c\,\text{SE}\,(b)$$

where t_c is the appropriate critical value of the t distribution on $n - 1$ degrees of freedom.

Method — null hypothesis (2)
1   Calculate the correlation coefficient r (see Section A.4).
2   Calculate the t statistic on $n - 2$ degrees of freedom.

$$t = r\,\sqrt{\frac{n - 2}{1 - r^2}}.$$

3 Look up the critical value t_c of the t distribution on $n - 2$ degrees of freedom at the required two-sided (usually) significance level (Table B.3).

$$\text{If } t \geqslant t_c \text{ or } t \leqslant - t_c \qquad \text{conclude } \rho \neq 0.$$
$$\text{If } - t_c < t < t_c \qquad \text{conclude } \rho = 0.$$

C.20 Spearman's rank order correlation coefficient

This procedure is discussed in Section 9.7.

Situation
n pairs of observations on an x and y variable. Both variables quantitative or ordered.

Assumptions/requirements
That there are not too many ties in the ranks of the variables.

Null hypothesis
That the population correlation ρ_S between the two variables is zero.

Method
1 Assign ranks to the x and y variables separately, from lowest to highest, giving the average rank to tied observations.
2 For each pair subtract the rank of variable y from the rank of variable x and call the result d.
3 Square each d and add to obtain Σd^2.
4 Spearman's rank correlation coefficient is calculated as

$$r_S = 1 - \frac{6\Sigma d^2}{n\,(n^2 - 1)}.$$

5 Look up the critical value r_c for Spearman's rank correlation coefficient in Table B.10 for n equal to the number of pairs at the appropriate (usually) two-sided significance level.

$$\text{If } r_S \geqslant r_c \text{ or } r_S \leqslant - r_c \qquad \text{conclude } \rho_S \neq 0.$$
$$\text{If } - r_c < r_S < r_c \qquad \text{conclude } \rho_S = 0.$$

D

Sample-Size Calculations

D.I Introduction

As has been discussed, the sample size required for an investigation should be estimated at the planning stage. No study should be carried out unless it has a reasonable chance of detecting an important effect at a given level of statistical significance. If the sample size of a study is too small, important differences may be declared statistically non-significant. This appendix gives, without derivation, some sample-size formulae for use in two-group comparisons with equal numbers in each group. The sample sizes calculated assume that there are no losses from the study, and thus extra allowance should be made for patient withdrawals. The formulae also assume that (in prospective studies or clinical trials) a variable follow-up is not involved, so that the end-point of interest must be known to be either present or absent at a fixed time from study commencement in all patients.

Before a sample size can be estimated, some preliminary decisions must be made. Firstly, the investigators must decide on the minimum difference between the two groups they wish to detect. Thus, in a clinical trial, a standard treatment may be known to have a 5 year survival of 50%, and it is wished to see if a new therapy could increase this survival to 60%. The sample size for a two-group trial would then be estimated on the basis of a minimum survival difference between the groups of 10%. It would be accepted that a smaller effect than this might not be detected. Obviously, there will often be more than one variable of interest in a two-group comparison, and sample sizes may have to be calculated for comparisons of each of these variables, and the largest sample size chosen.

If a difference in a quantitative variable is to be tested, in addition to the minimum difference to be detected, the standard deviation of the variable is also required. If this is not available from previous studies, a pilot study would have to be performed to obtain a rough estimate.

Two other parameters must also be specified. These are the significance level (p value, probability of a type I error, α error) at which the group difference is to be detected, and the required probability of making a type II (β) error in detecting this difference. Often the β probability is set at four times the α probability. Thus, for a 5% level of significance, β might be set equal to 0·2. See Section 6.7 for a fuller discussion of type I and type II errors in significance testing.

In the next section, sample-size formulae are given for the comparison of means in independent samples, proportions in independent samples, and means in paired samples. The formulae are approximate and are not accurate for small sample sizes. Professional advice should usually be sought for sample-size estimation, although the formulae presented below will give some guide as to how large a particular study should be.

D.2 Sample-size formulae

For the comparison of mean values in two independent samples

$$n > \frac{2K \sigma^2}{\Delta^2} \tag{D.1}$$

where n is the sample size required in each of the groups. K is a constant (based on tables of the standard normal curve) which depends on the desired α and β probabilities for the comparison, and whether the significance test is to be one-sided or two-sided. Table D.1 gives these constants for varying levels of α and β. σ^2 is the variance in each of the groups being compared (equal variances are assumed). Usually, only a rough estimate of this will be available. Δ is the magnitude of the difference between the populations that it is required to detect at the stated α and β values.

Suppose a clinical trial is to be carried out to compare two different treatments for blood pressure reduction. The researchers want to have a fairly large chance of detecting, as statistically significant, a real (population) difference between the mean systolic blood pressures in the two groups of 10 mmHg or greater. A non-stratified randomization is to be employed, so that the two groups may be considered independent. The researchers decide on a two-sided significance test at a 5% level, and on a β probability of 0·2. This means that the resulting study should have an 80% $(1 - \beta$; the power of the test) chance of detecting this treatment effect. A preliminary estimate of the standard deviation of the systolic

Table D.I. Multiplying factor K for sample-size formulae. α = significance level (probability of a type I error). β = probability of a type II error

		One-sided test				Two-sided test	
		α				α	
		0·05	0·01			0·05	0·01
	0·05	10·8	15·8		0·05	13·0	17·8
β	0·10	8·6	13·0	β	0·10	10·5	14·9
	0·20	6·2	10·0		0·20	7·8	11·7

blood pressure is 20 mmHg. Thus from Table D.1, $K = 7.9$ while $\sigma^2 = 400$ and $\Delta^2 = 100$. Using Eqn. D.1, a sample size of over 63·2 is necessary in each group. This value is rounded up to the nearest integer so that a total of 128 patients will be required.

For the comparison of means in a paired situation

$$n > \frac{K \sigma_d^2}{\Delta^2}.$$ (D.2)

n in this case is the number of pairs required in the study, σ_d^2 is the variance of the differences between the values of the two populations, Δ is the minimum difference to be detected. K is determined as before from Table D.1 on the basis of the chosen α and β values.

Suppose that in the clinical trial discussed above, a cross-over design was to be used with each patient receiving each treatment, and that the same statistical requirements were chosen. If a preliminary estimate of the standard deviation of the paired differences was obtained as $\sigma_d = 25$ mmHg, n (the number of pairs required) turns out to be, from Eqn. D.2, 49·375 or 50 patients, since this is a self-paired experiment.

For the comparison of proportions in two independent groups

$$n > \frac{K (p_1 q_1 + p_2 q_2)}{\Delta^2}.$$ (D.3)

Again, n is the number of individuals required in each group, p_1 and p_2 are the presumed proportions in the two groups being compared, while, as usual, $q_1 = 1 - p_1$ and $q_2 = 1 - p_2$. Δ is the minimum difference to be detected which, of course, is nothing more than $p_1 - p_2$. Note that in this case no estimate of a standard deviation is required.

Again, taking a clinical trial example, the sample-size requirements for the situation discussed in Section D.1 will be examined. The usual 5-year survival for breast cancer patients is known to be around 50% (or, expressed as a proportion, 0·5) and it is hoped to study the effectiveness of a new therapy which might increase this to at least 60% (0·6). It is desired that this effect should be detected at a two-sided 1% significance level, with only a 0·05 chance of missing it if it does exist. A non-stratified randomization is to be employed, with follow-up of each patient for a full 5 years. Thus K from Table D.1 is 17·8. $p_1 = 0.5$, $q_1 = 0.5$, $p_2 = 0.6$, $q_2 = 0.4$, and $\Delta = 0.6 - 0.5 = 0.1$. Substituting these values into Eqn. D.3, the required sample size in each group is 872·2 or a total requirement of 1746 patients. Large sample sizes such as this are not uncommon in many situations.

Bibliography and References

The bibliography lists a number of books and articles for further reading. Some of these have already been referred to in the text and the selection, although by no means comprehensive, should guide the interested reader to a more advanced treatment of some of the topics covered. The reference section includes all works cited in the text from which illustrative examples were taken. Reproduction or adaptation of tables or figures from any of these works was by kind permission of the authors, editors and publishers concerned.

Bibliography

Abramson, J. H. (1984) *Survey Methods in Community Medicine*, 3rd edn. Churchill Livingstone, Edinburgh. A comprehensive text book on the planning and performance of medical surveys and clinical trials.

Armitage, P. (1975) *Sequential Medical Trials*. Blackwell Scientific Publications, Oxford. An excellent and detailed description of the sequential clinical trial. The mathematical level is considerably higher than that of this book.

Armitage, P. & Berry, G. (1987) *Statistical Methods in Medical Research*, 2nd edn. Blackwell Scientific Publications, Oxford. A standard reference work in medical statistics which includes details of many of the more complex techniques used in medical research. A good deal more advanced than this book.

Asbury, A. J. (1983) *ABC of Computing*. British Medical Association, London. Reprints of articles from the British Medical Journal which explain basic computer configurations and their application to medicine. A very useful introductory guide.

Benjamin, B. (1968) *Health and Vital Statistics*. Heinemann, London. Good introductory text covering demography, mortality, morbidity, fertility, hospital statistics and analysis of disease mortality.

Bennett, A. E. & Ritchie, K. (1975) *Questionnaires in Medicine*, Oxford University Press, Oxford. A useful book on the design and use of questionnaires in medical research.

Breslow, N. E. & Day, N. E. (1980, 1987) Statistical Methods in Cancer Research. Vols I and II. International Agency for Research on Cancer, Lyon. An excellent exposition of case-control and cohort studies, including a detailed discussion of design and implementation. Heavy emphasis is placed on the analytic techniques for the control of confounders. Appropriate multiple regression techniques are described in detail and computer programs are given in appendices. (More up-to-date programs may be available from the authors.)

Castle, W. M. (1972) *Statistics in Small Doses*, 2nd edn. Churchill Livingstone, Edinburgh. A programmed instruction text which leads the reader through some of the more simple aspects of data description and analysis.

Cohen, J. (1977) *Statistical Power Analysis for the Behavioral Sciences*. Academic Press, London. A very useful handbook for the calculation of sample sizes for many types of investigations. Extensive tables are given.

Colton, T. (1974) *Statistics in Medicine*. Little, Brown & Co., Boston. A textbook at about the same level as this work with extensive examples from the medical literature and a good introduction to study design. More recent methods are not covered.

Cox, D. R. (1972) Regression models and life-tables (with discussion). *Journal of the Royal Statistical Association* **B34**, 187−220. A difficult statistical paper which details the applications and theory of Cox's regression model for life-table analysis.

D'Agostino, R. B., Chase, W. & Belanger, A. (1988) The appropriateness of some common procedures for testing the equality of two independent binomial populations. *The American Statistician* **42**, 198−201. A paper that argues against Fisher's test for a 2 × 2 table and suggests that the usual χ^2 is more appropriate even for very small sample sizes.

Ederer, F. & Mantel, N. (1974) Confidence limits on the ratio of two Poisson variables. *American Journal of Epidemiology* **100**, 165−7. The paper which describes how the binomial confidence limits can be used to calculate limits for the ratio of two Poisson counts.

Emerson, J. D. & Colditz, G. A. (1983) Use of statistical analysis in the New England Journal of Medicine. *New England Journal of Medicine* **309**, 709−13. A survey of research articles in a general medical journal detailing the statistical techniques used.

Feinstein, A. R. (1977) *Clinical Biostatistics*. C. V. Mosby & Co., St Louis. A collection of articles on various topics in biostatistics, which originally appeared as essays in the *Journal of Clinical Pharmacology and Therapeutics*. This is a very readable book which discusses many of the problems and pitfalls to be encountered in epidemiological research.

Fleiss, J. L. (1981) *Statistical Methods for Rates and Proportions*, 2nd edn. John Wiley & Sons, New York. A standard reference work on the analysis of categorical or qualitative data.

Gardner, M. J. & Altman, D. G. (1989) *Statistics with Confidence*. British Medical Journal, London. Reprints and expansions of articles from the British Medical Journal on the use of confidence intervals in the analysis of data. A truly excellent book which details the calculations required in most situations. Much of the material in this text book is covered, but confidence interval calculations are described for many of the non-parametric tests also. A computer program implementing the techniques is available.

Geigy Scientific Tables (1982) Vol. 2, 8th edn. Ciba-Geigy, Basle. Edited by C. Lentner. A useful and comprehensive handbook of statistical tables with a summary section outlining a large body of statistical theory and significance tests.

Gore, S. M. & Altman, D. G. (1982) *Statistics in Practice*. British Medical Association, London. Reprints of articles from the *British Medical Journal* with emphasis on the methodology and execution of clinical trials. Most of the text is in a question and answer format but should be most useful for anyone involved in the design of a trial.

Gore, S. M., Jones, I. G. & Rytter, E. C. (1977) Misuse of statistical methods: critical assessment of articles in BMJ from January to March 1976. *British Medical Journal* **1**, 85−7. A survey of statistical errors in the medical literature.

Hill, A. B. (1963) Medical ethics and controlled trials. *British Medical Journal* **1**, 1043−9. An early but key paper on the ethics of the clinical trial.

Hill, A. B. (1971) *Principles of Medical Statistics*. Lancet, London. A classic textbook of medical statistics, at about the same level as this book.

Hills, M. & Armitage, P. (1979) The two-period cross-over clinical trial. *British Journal of Clinical Pharmacology* **8**, 7−20. A detailed description of the design and analysis of the cross-over clinical trial.

Kalbfleisch, J. D. & Prentice, R. L. (1980) *The Statistical Analysis of Failure Time Data*. John

Wiley & Sons, New York. A standard reference on the techniques for the analysis of censored data. A difficult and theoretical book.

Kleinbaum, D. G., Kupper, L. L. & Morgenstern, H. (1982) *Epidemiologic Research*, Lifetime Learning Publications, London. A detailed book on the analysis and design of epidemiological studies. Very good examples with detailed discussion of confounder controlling. Much more advanced than this book.

Last, J. M. (1988) *A Dictionary of Epidemiology*, 2nd edn., Oxford University, Press, Oxford. A dictionary of the terms used in epidemiology. Includes many statistical terms also. A useful reference work.

MacMahon, B. & Pugh, T. F. (1970) *Epidemiology: Principles and Methods*. Little, Brown & Co., Boston. A general textbook on epidemiology in which are described most of the measures used in summarizing epidemiological data.

Mantel, N. & Haenzel, W. (1959) Statistical aspects of the analysis of data from retrospective studies of disease. *Journal of the National Cancer Institute* **22**, 719–48. The paper that first described the Mantel–Haenzel test and summary measures.

Miettinen, O. S. (1976) Estimability and estimation in case-referent studies. *American Journal of Epidemiology* **103**, 226–35. The original description of 'test-based' confidence limits.

Peto, R., Pike, M. C., Armitage, P., Breslow, N. E., Cox, D. R., Howard, S. V., Mantel, N., McPherson, K., Peto J. & Smith, P. G. (1976) Design and analysis of randomized clinical trials requiring prolonged observation of each patient. I. Introduction and design. *British Journal of Cancer* **34**, 585–612.

Peto, R., Pike, M. C., Armitage, P., Breslow, N. E., Cox, D. R., Howard, S. V., Mantel, N., McPherson, K., Peto, J. & Smith, P. G. (1977) Design and analysis of randomized clinical trials requiring prolonged observation of each patient. II. Analysis and examples. *British Journal of Cancer* **35**, 1–39. Two articles on the design and analysis of clinical trials with particular emphasis on survival as an end-point. This article describes life tables and the logrank test in a readily understandable manner and is required reading for those interested in this area. A computer program to implement life table analysis is available from the authors.

Remington, R. D. & Schork, M. A. (1970) *Statistics with Applications to the Biological and Health Sciences*. Prentice-Hall Inc., New Jersey. A very readable textbook which goes into somewhat more mathematical detail than the present text, though with less coverage.

Sackett, D. L. (1979) Bias in analytic research. *Journal of Chronic Disease* **32**, 51–63. A catalogue of biases in medical research with references to their occurrence in the literature.

SAS User's Guide: Basics, 5th edn. (1985) Cary N. C. SAS Institute Inc. One of the manuals for a very powerful statistics/data management computer package.

Siegel, S. (1956) *Nonparametric Statistics for the Behavioural Sciences*. McGraw-Hill Kogakusha, Ltd., Tokyo. A textbook describing most of the non-parametric statistical tests in a readable comprehensible manner.

Smoking and Health (1964) A report of the advisory committee to the Surgeon General of the Public Health Service. U.S. Department of Health, Education and Welfare, Washington DC. A report including a description of the criteria for judging the causal significance of an association.

Sokal, R. R. & Rohlf, F. J. (1981) *Biometry*. W. H. Freeman & Co., San Francisco. A large and detailed text with emphasis on statistics in biological applications. Many complex techniques are covered but the application of each is explained in a simple step-by-step manner. Much more advanced than this book but a useful book to have available. Statistical tables are unfortunately published in a separate volume.

Swinscow, D. V. (1976) *Statistics at Square One*. British Medical Association, London. A short book which outlines the computations required for some of the simpler statistical tests.

Zelen, M. (1979) A new design for randomized clinical trials. *New England Journal of Medicine* **300**, 1242–6. A paper describing a particular design for a clinical trial which avoids some of the ethical problems caused by the demands of informed consent.

References

Barry, J. & Daly, L. (1988) *The Travellers' Health Status Study: Census of Travelling People, November 1986*. Health Research Board, Dublin.

Barry, J., Herity, B. & Solan, J. (1989) *The Travellers' Health Status Study: Vital Statistics of Travelling People, 1987*. Health Research Board, Dublin.

Daly, L. E. (1991) The first international Urokinase/Warfarin trial in colo-rectal carcinoma. *Clinical and Experimental Metastases* **9**, 3–12.

Daly, L. E., Mulcahy, R., Graham, I. & Hickey, N. (1983) Long term effect on mortality of stopping smoking after unstable angina and myocardial infarction. *British Medical Journal* **287**, 324–6.

Dawber, T. R. (1980) *The Framingham Study: The Epidemiology of Atherosclerotic Disease*. Harvard University Press, Cambridge, Mass.

Doll, R. & Peto, R. (1976) Mortality in relation to smoking: 20 years' observations on male British doctors. *British Medical Journal* **2**, 1525–36.

Green, T. P., Thompson, T. R., Johnson, D. E. & Lock, J. E. (1983) Furosemide promotes patent ductus arteriosus in premature infants with the respiratory-distress syndrome. *New England Journal of Medicine* **308**, 743–8.

Gregg, N. M. (1941) Congenital cataract following German measles in the mother. *Transactions of the Ophthalmological Society of Australia* **III**, 35–46.

Hayes, A., Daly, L., O'Brien, N. G. & MacDonald, D. (1983) Anthropometric standards for Irish newborn. *Irish Medical Journal* **76**, 60–70.

Herity, B., Moriarty, M., Bourke, G. J. & Daly, L. (1981) A case-control study of head and neck cancer in the Republic of Ireland. *British Journal of Cancer* **43**, 177–82.

Hickey, N., Mulchay, R., Daly, L., Bourke, G. & Moriarty, J. (1979) The relationship between blood glucose and prevalence of coronary heart disease: a study in the Republic of Ireland. *Journal of Chronic Diseases* **32**, 767–72.

Irish Statistical Bulletin (1985) *Irish Life Table No. 10 1980–82. Vol. LX, No. 4*. Stationery Office, Dublin.

Lagos, P., Lagona, E., Kattamis, C. & Matsaniotis, N. (1980) Serum ferritin in β-thalassaemia intermedia. *Lancet* **1**, 204–5.

Lowes, J. A., Williams, G., Tabaqchali, S., Hill, I. M., Hamer, J., Houang, E., Shaw, E. J., & Rees, G. M. (1980) 10 years of infective endocarditis at St. Bartholomew's Hospital: analysis of clinical features and treatment in relation to prognosis and mortality. *Lancet* **1**, 133–6.

Mitchell, J. R. A. (1981) Timolol after myocardial infarction: an answer or a new set of questions? *British Medical Journal* **282**, 1565–70.

O'Connor, J. & Daly, M. (1983) *Smoking and Drinking Behaviour. Vol. 1*. Health Education Bureau, Dublin.

Office of Population Censuses and Surveys (1986) *Occupational Mortality 1979–80 and 1982–83, Part 1*. HMSO, London.

Palmeri, S. T., Harrison, D. G., Cobb, F. R., Morris, K. G., Harrell, F. E., Ideker, R. E., Selvester, R. H. & Wagner, G. S. (1982) A QRS scoring system for assessing left ventricular function after myocardial infarction. *New England Journal of Medicine* **306**, 4–9.

Parks, J. H., Coe, F. L. & Strauss, A. L. (1982) Calcium nephrolithiasis and medullary sponge kidney in women. *New England Journal of Medicine* **306**, 1088–91.

Pollock, E., Wines, W. & Hall, D. (1981) A survey of blood pressure in 10-year-old children of a health district together with a consideration of screening policy for hypertension. *Community Medicine* **3**, 199–204.

Puska, P., Tuomilehto, J., Salonen, J., Nissinen, A., Virtamo, J., Björkqvist, S., Koskela, K., Neittaanmäki, L., Takalo, T., Kottke, T.E., Mäki, J., Sipilä, P. & Varvikko, P. (1981) *Community Control of Cardiovascular Diseases. The North Karelia Project*, World Health Organization, Copenhagen.

Salonen, J. T. & Vohlonen, I. (1982) Longitudinal cross-national analysis of coronary mortality. *International Journal of Epidemiology* **11**, 229–38.

The Norwegian Multicentre Study Group (1981). Timolol-induced reduction in mortality and reinfarction in patients surviving acute myocardial infarction. *New England Journal of Medicine* **304**, 801–7.

United Nations (1987) *Demographic Yearbook*. United Nations, New York.

Index